P9-CEC-075

The Horse from Conception to Maturity

PETER D. ROSSDALE
F.R.C.V.S
with Melanie Bailey

The Horse from Conception to Maturity

J A ALLEN
London

First published in Great Britain 2002

ISBN 0 85131 822 3

J. A. Allen
Clerkenwell House
Clerkenwell Green
London EC1R 0HT

J. A. Allen is an imprint of Robert Hale Ltd

British Library Catàloguing in Publication Data
A catalogue record for this book is available from the British Library

Copy preparation and proof reading: Brigitte Heard and Lindsey Abeyasekere
Design and book production: Bill Ireson
Jacket design: Paul Saunders
Colour separation by Tenon & Polert Colour Scanning Ltd, Hong Kong
Printed in Midas Printing International Ltd

Contents

Acknowledgements

The authors would like to express their thanks and appreciation to:

Jan Puzio, MRCVS, of Endell Veterinary Group, Salisbury, who advised on the technical detail with regard to the sections on artificial insemination and embryo transfer, as well as providing a number of the new photographic illustrations.

Kate Whetren, equine photographer, who provided an enormous number of new colour photographs for this book.

Cheveley Park, Shadwell, Side Hill and Littleton Studs.

Nick Wingfield Digby and colleagues at Beaufort Cottage Stables, for their advice and assistance.

Brigitte Heard and Lindsey Abeyasekere, for their assistance in the preparation and proofreading of this book.

CHAPTER ONE

The Horse in its Natural State

Introduction

Understanding is the core ingredient in our lives. To understand the cause and components of a problem is the first essential step to solving it, and to understand the way in which our bodies function opens the way to healthier living.

The aim of this book is to assist the reader in understanding the bodily functions of the horse as it develops from the time of conception to the fulfilment of maturity and performance potential. An understanding of these bodily functions is, indeed, crucial for good management and the avoidance of pitfalls in our approach to the breeding and rearing of horses.

The biological story recounted in the book starts at the beginning of the cycle of reproduction with the mating of stallion and mare. After conception the newly formed individual (fertilised egg) descends the fallopian tube and enters the uterus, where it is nurtured for some eleven months, growing tremendously in size to the being that we recognise as the newborn foal. This key moment in the transition from life within to life outside the womb is marked by the wonderful natural process of birth.

From the time of the birth, the story of the individual is one of a more gradual but nonetheless important and sustained growth pattern towards complete maturity, when the individual is ready to perform the challenging tasks imposed upon it by mankind, with both love and expectation.

In the first instance, before embarking on the story of the biological functions of the modern horse, it is prudent to consider the horse in its natural state and how it has evolved from the miniature form of the dawn horse (Eohippus) to the modern horse (*Equus caballus*), which already had been in existence for 50,000 years as an undomesticated species.

The evolutionary story explains why the form and function of the horse of today is such as it is, standing on four legs, each with four single digits (toes), and with an oestrous cycle confined naturally to spring and summer months. A knowledge of the evolution of the horse helps us to understand many of the quirks we encounter in equine nutrition, social behaviour, reproductive performance and its use for our own purposes of transport, work, pleasure and performance.

The horse on tiptoe

Those who work with horses should know something of the species' evolutionary history. This subject is by no means of academic interest alone; we cannot hope to tackle successfully the problems which beset us in the care and management of the horse unless we are aware of the fundamental properties of structure and function contained within its body.

In essence, the horse has a body which combines size and speed; other animals may be as fast or as large, but in *Equus caballus* (the modern horse) the dual combination has been brought near to perfection. It is, of course, the feature which has gripped the imagination of man and for centuries he has used the horse for transport as well as military ambitions. Nowadays its use is confined mainly to the pleasures of riding, racing, three-day eventing and similar pursuits.

To a certain extent, the horse's body has been modified by man through careful selection in breeding, to meet particular requirements, such as pulling heavy loads in agriculture or for racing, polo playing, and so on. The fundamental structures of its body have not, however, been affected; the modern horse is a creature whose bones, muscles and organs conform to a plan which is common to all breeds whether they be Shires, Thoroughbreds, Standardbreds or Shetland ponies.

Changes in Body Structure

Because of the horse's grazing habits and its tendency to live in large herds, it has been buried and fossilised in large numbers. The horse's evolutionary history is therefore the most well known of any species. The sequence from Eocene times to the present day is recorded in fossils discovered in North America. This story is well known and many books have appeared on the subject so it is not necessary to repeat it here in detail. Here we are more concerned with presenting changes in body structure which have occurred between the earliest-known horse called Hyracotherium (Eohippus, the dawn horse) and the horse we use today, in terms of their relevance to the problems of management in the present century.

The dawn horse was a small creature about the size of a fox, possessing four toes on its front limbs and three on the hind limbs. The limbs were slender and some authors claim that this horse, which lived 40 million years ago, may have been nearly as fast as the modern racehorse.

Limbs

The evolution of the horse has seen a remarkable lengthening of the legs and a reduction of the side (lateral) toes with increasing emphasis on the middle toe (Figure 1.1). Humans have retained the five-toed condition which was the original plan in the ancestors of both horse and man; when we run we raise ourselves onto our toes, but at rest we stand flat on our heels. The modern horse stands virtually on the tips of the

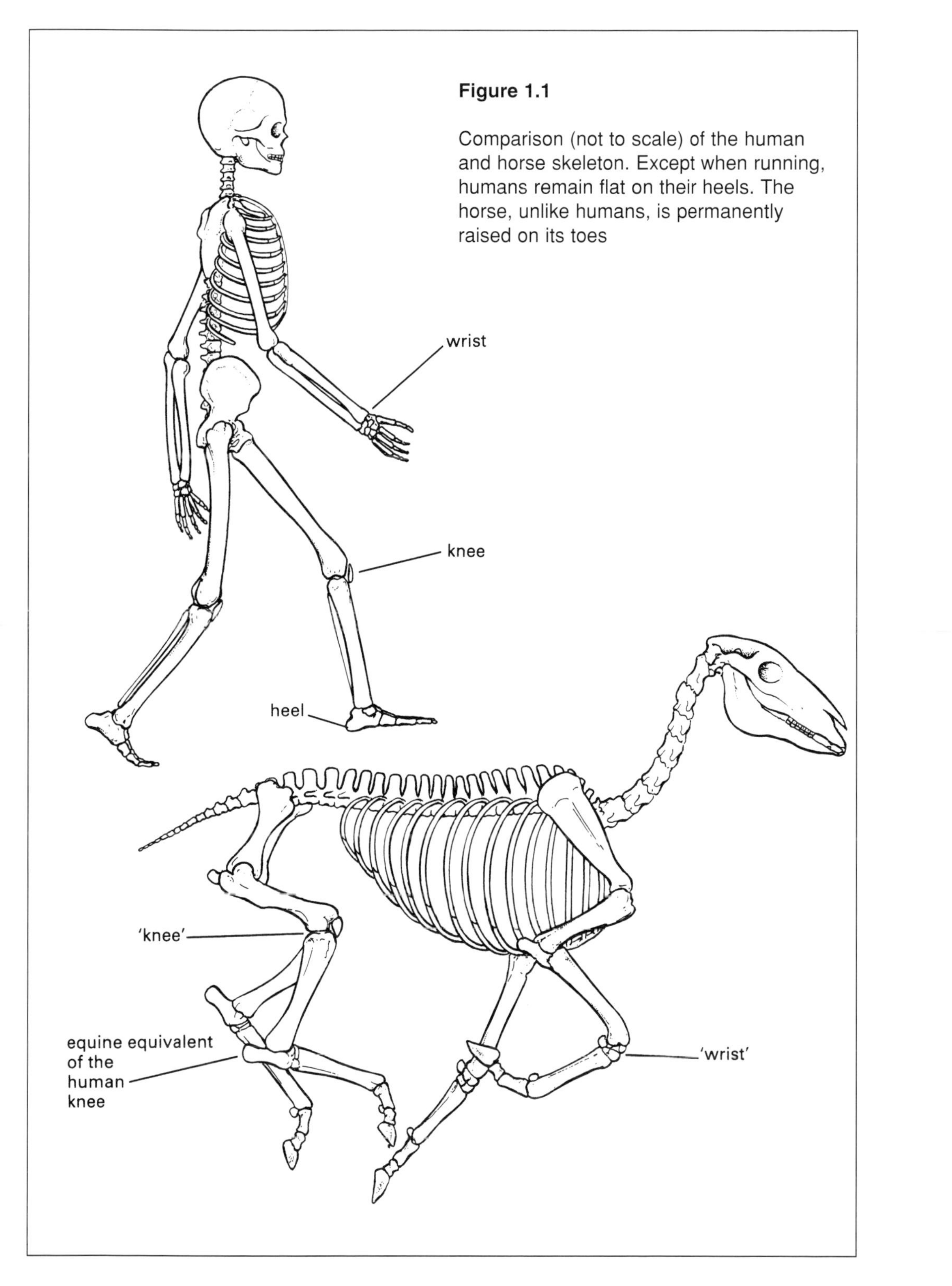

Figure 1.1

Comparison (not to scale) of the human and horse skeleton. Except when running, humans remain flat on their heels. The horse, unlike humans, is permanently raised on its toes

middle fingers and the toes of the fore and hind limbs, and thus its stride is lengthened and it is permanently raised into the position of running tiptoe.

The hoof is a specialist structure, developed at the tips of each limb for protection of the extremities. This may be likened to the nail of our own fingers or toes and serves not only to protect the deeper structures against injury, but also to absorb shock as the limb strikes the ground.

A number of bones in the horse's limbs have been reduced during evolution. The reduction has involved a simplification in the bones of the fore-arm and shin or gaskin (that is, those between the stifle and the hock). The dawn horse possessed two separate bones in the forearm (ulna and radius) and two in the gaskin (the tibia and fibula); this is the arrangement still retained in our own bodies. In the modern horse these bones have become fused, with the result that horses have lost the capacity to rotate their limbs in the same way that we can. They have, in addition, lost the power of grasping. In consequence, the muscles which carry out these processes have been discarded

Figure 1.2

In the horse, the muscles of locomotion are bunched above the carpus (knee) and tarsus (hock)

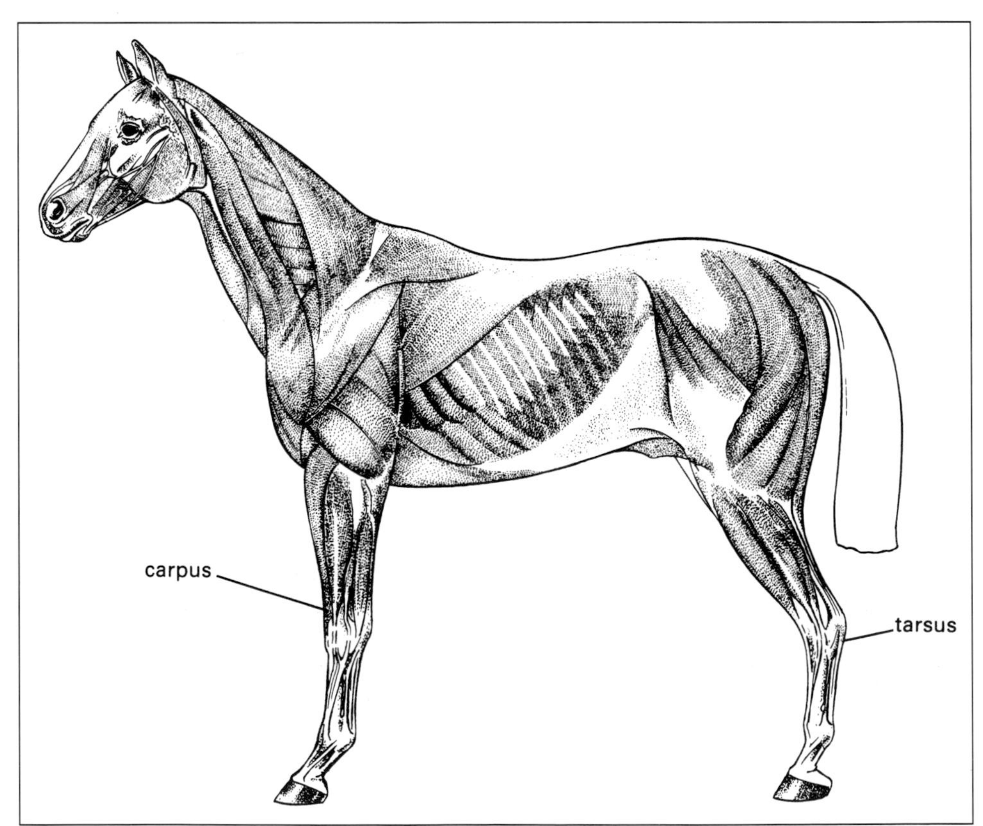

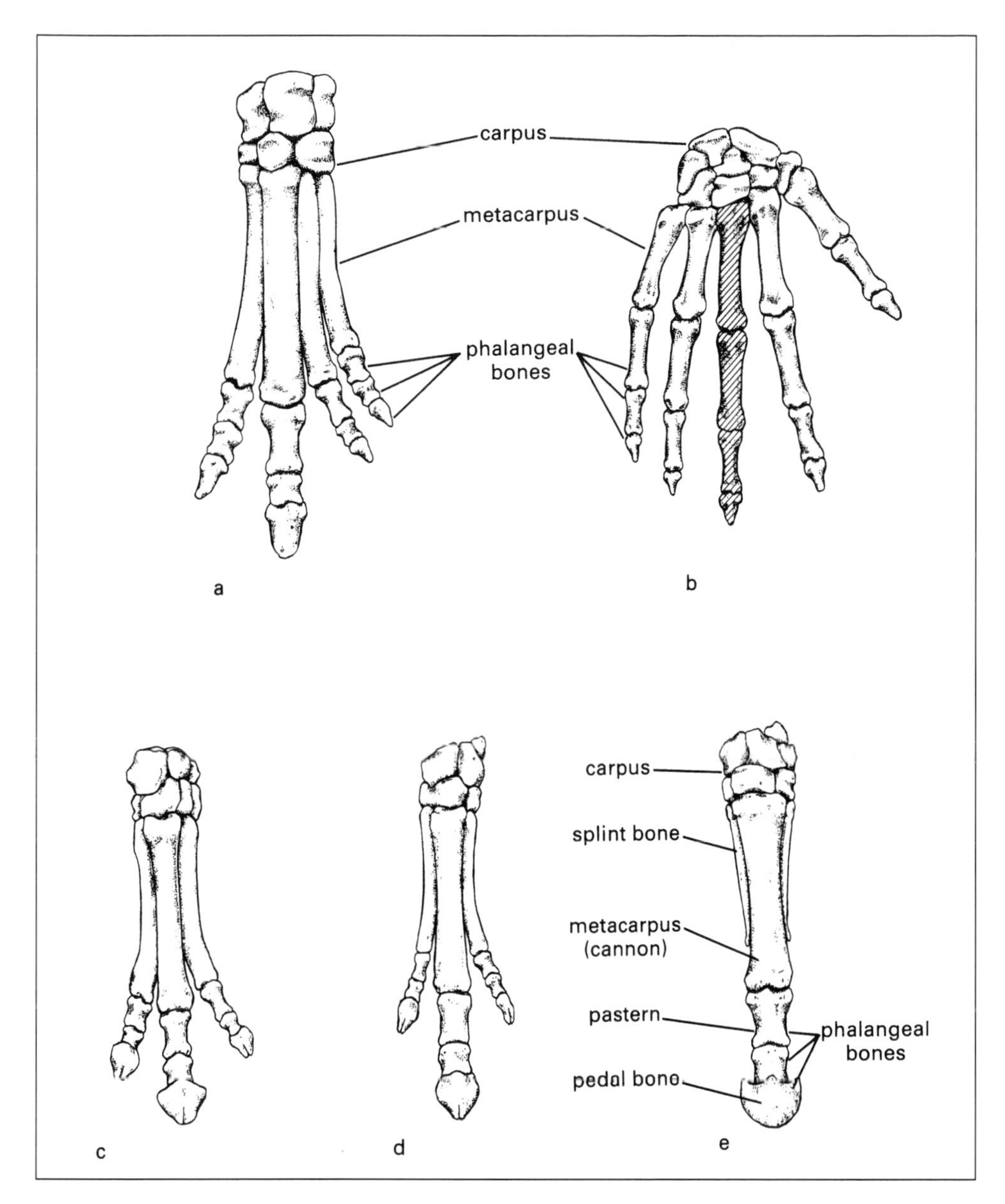

Figure 1.3

The forelimb (a) of the dawn horse showing carpal bones, called the knee and equivalent to the human wrist, and the four metacarpal bones, equivalent to those between the human wrist and knuckles, to each of which are attached first, second and third phalangeal bones; (b) the five-digital plan has been retained in the human hand, whereas only the middle one (shaded area) remains for the horse; and (c), (d) and (e) the intermediary forms between the dawn horse and the modern horse in favour of tendons to reduce the weight below the knee, and if we examine the body of the modern horse we find no muscles below the carpus (knee) or tarsus (hock) (Figure 1.2). The equivalent of these joints in the human body are the wrist and ankle (Figure 1.3).

It is obvious that the development of the limbs has achieved its evolutionary object – the horse has been able to use its speed to evade its enemies. The horse has also become useful to man, who would otherwise undoubtedly have become its most deadly predator. The associated modifications of body structure have meant, however, that we are presented with certain potential weaknesses which may lead to unsoundness.

For example, the practical implication of the enormous lengthening of the horse's limb below the hock and knee is that the tendons have become correspondingly elongated and susceptible to injuries. The residual third and fourth metacarpal and metatarsal bones, usually referred to as splint bones, are another source of trouble. Injuries to the first phalanx (pastern bone), the sesamoid bones behind the fetlock joint, and the pedal bone are frequent causes of unsoundness as are various inflammatory conditions of the bones and joints (osselets, ringbones, carpitis) from which horses suffer. The foot is particularly exposed to risks of injury and the old saying 'no foot, no horse' is a truism many a horse owner has learned to his cost.

Back

Significant changes have also occurred in other parts of the horse's body. For instance, the back has become straightened and stiffened, while a relatively heavy head is supported on the end of a long and flexible neck. The extension of the neck was, of course, necessary as the horse grew taller and at the same time adopted grazing habits. The condition of the vertebral column (spine) was an essential consideration for a species used to carry a rider but, in placing weight on its back, we have exposed the structures of the back to risks of trauma (especially as it does not finish growing until the horse is five years old); risks which are a direct result of the way horses are ridden. In particular, jumping a horse subjects the ligaments and bones of the spine to unnatural stresses. It is not surprising, therefore, that many unsoundnesses are associated with inflammatory reactions in the back which may be of a temporary or permanent nature.

Neck

Injuries to the neck are another common source of trouble and lead to damage to the nerves which pass down the spine (from the brain) to the body, including its extremities. The condition known as 'wobbler' disease, the signs of which include incoordination of the hind limbs, is such an example. This may have an inherited basis and if so it is interesting to speculate whether, in fact, horses suffered from the disease during their evolutionary history or whether it has been brought into the modern horse by untoward selection of breeding stock.

Head

As the horse grew in size, the weight of its head must have presented a problem (Figure 1.4).

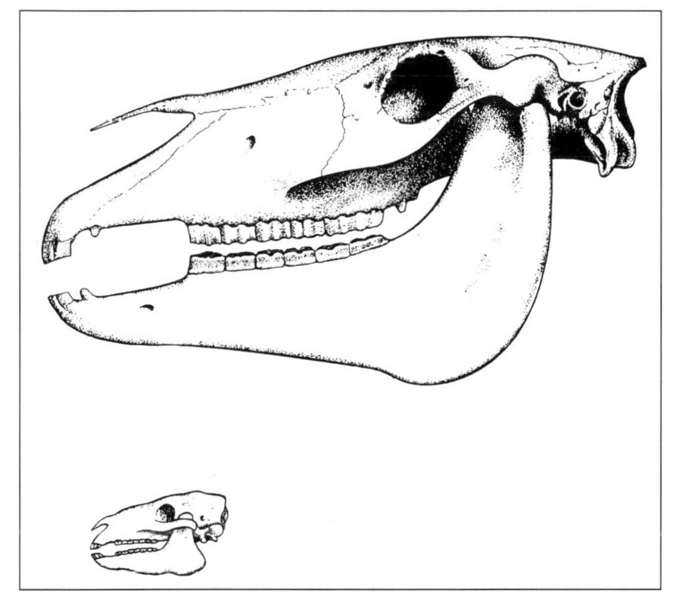

Figure 1.4

The skull of the modern horse (top) contrasted with that of the much smaller dawn horse (below). Apart from the size increase, the modern horse has the eye socket placed relatively far back and the jaws have become deeper to house more substantial teeth

To a large extent this was solved by the development of large cavities of air within the bones of the skull. These cavities are called sinuses and occasionally we find that they have become infected; because they communicate with the nasal passages the affected horse then suffers from a purulent discharge from the nose.

The enlargement of the skull has also caused the eye sockets to become raised so that they are well placed to observe the surroundings for the approach of danger while the horse is grazing. Natural selection would have also allowed those with better vision (that is, those with the eyes set in higher eye sockets) to see predators, and thus escape. These survivors would pass on their genes, unlike those with inferior vision, who succumbed more easily to their attackers.

As the head became larger so it was able to accommodate teeth that were adapted to meet the special requirements of the diet. The earliest horses browsed on the succulent foods which they found hanging on bushes, shrubs and trees; alterations in climate necessitated a change to grazing and the digestion of hard, fibrous grasses. To meet the demands of this diet, the cheek teeth became broader and their crowns were increased in height and complicated by patterns or ridges ideally suited to grinding food (Figure 1.5). As the teeth increased in size, so it was necessary for the skull to become deeper and the lower jaw broader to accommodate them.

In the modern horse the front teeth (incisors) are designed for cutting grass so that it can be pulled back through the mouth by a mobile tongue and then brought to molar teeth to be ground between their surfaces acting like a mill. It is perhaps fortunate that there is a gap between the incisors and the molars into which a bit can be conveniently placed! The grinding action of the jaws tends to produce sharp edges along the inside of the lower and the outside of the upper molar teeth. These sharp edges may be removed by rasping, a

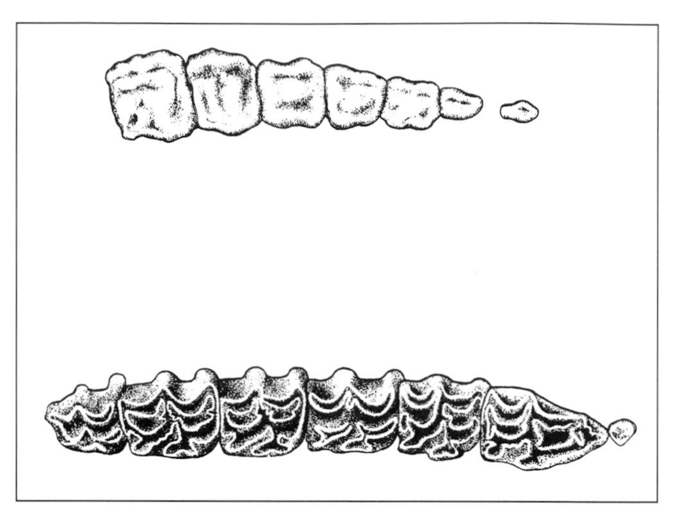

Figure 1.5

The dawn horse had teeth (top) with simple crowns adapted to eating soft food; the modern horse (below) has teeth suited for grinding hard fibrous foods, and crowns that are complicated by ridged patterns

procedure which should be carried out routinely about once a year or when there are indications that the horse is not chewing normally.

Alimentary tract (gut)

Evidence from fossils consists of parts of the body, such as teeth and bone, but we know less of the development of soft tissue such as the gut. However, we may infer that the present-day horse possesses the means of digestion that suited the harsh coarse fibrous food encountered in its more recent evolutionary past. The horse now digests its food mainly through the action of bacteria in the hind gut (colon and caecum) that break down the cellulose and fibrous material that passes, largely, through the small intestine in an undigested state. More soluble components of the diet are digested, as in ourselves, by the means of enzymes and digestive juices produced by the lining of the stomach and small intestines.

Both hind and fore gut are concerned with the conservation of body water which is absorbed through the gut wall in such a manner as to maintain moisture within the lumen of the gut while retaining water in the bloodstream and tissue spaces of the body.

In summary, food is taken in by the grasping motion of the lips and front teeth acting in unison to bite or tear vegetable matter, then ground by the molar teeth and mixed with saliva before being swallowed to pass down the gullet (oesophagus) into the stomach. From this part of the gut the food is propelled by muscular waves (peristalsis) which deliver the food material into the colon and caecum for the final stages of digestion, before finally exiting as faeces from the small colon and rectum (Figure 1.6).

The questions we must address in management include those that relate to the means of offering food and water to horses and composition and quantity of the diet against a background of the anatomical and functional status of the modern horse.

Many scientific investigations and trials of feeding and management have resulted in a great deal of advice and text being available on nutritional matters. Here it is sufficient to state the

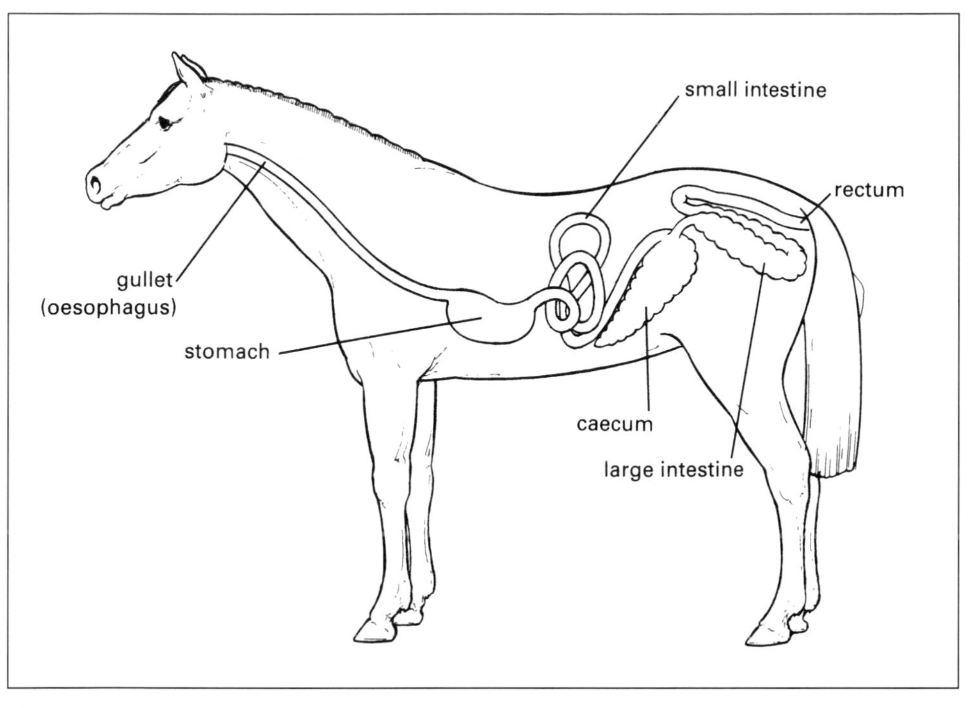

Figure 1.6

The gastrointestinal (alimentary) tract of the horse

simple corollary between the digestive requirements and the natural evolutionary needs of the individual, namely that of a relatively high-fibre diet consumed continuously over long periods in order to meet the peculiar form of a horse's digestive tract, particularly the relatively small capacity of the stomach and the voluminous, cavernous content of the hind gut. These features give rise to the potential risks of colic, disturbances due to diets which disturb the bacterial content of the hind gut (for example, antibiotics) and parasitic infestation. The latter is not a direct result of the peculiarity of the horse's digestive system but is dependent upon the continual grazing habits of the horse on pasture on which parasites, especially strongyle species, reside.

In evolutionary terms, it is probable that the shortage of grazing caused the horse to travel long distances in search of food, with the benefit not only of finding food, but of leaving worm egg contaminated pasture behind; a habit resembling modern-day pasture management.

Social Behaviour

Evolution has imbued horses with the herd instinct (that is, grouping), probably in order to give the horse an increased chance of survival with a safety in numbers principle.

Cohesion of mares around a stallion

also provided the means of conserving genes and of reproductive efficiency. Sexual behaviour became based upon the oestrous cycle, with its alternating periods of rejection and receptivity on the part of the mare coinciding with the production of an egg from the ovary (ovulation). In addition, oestrus (heat) and the cycle of sexual activity became strictly controlled to occur only in the months of late spring and summer, tailing off in autumn and not being present during winter. The logic of this control of sexual activity was to ensure that foals were delivered, eleven months later, when grass was relatively plentiful and climatic conditions were favourable to survival of the foal.

The cohesion of the herd and sexual behaviour evolved on the basis of instinctive reactions underwritten by hormonal control produced by the various glands of the body, including those that secrete pheromones externally; and the organs of smell (olfactory) having highly-developed sensitivity to identify the sexual status of each individual. Thus mares and foals come to recognise each other, as does each member of the herd; and the stallion has recognition of his harem.

The horse's behaviour is therefore based on the existence of groups of up to about twenty mares per stallion which last for many years, sometimes gaining an occasional outsider or losing one of their members to another group, but essentially remaining as a unit at least throughout their sexual life. The young male (or occasionally a more mature individual separated from its own group) becomes separated at weaning and after grouping with other young males matures as a sexual individual (stallion) and separates to attract a group of other weaned fillies.

The importance of herd behaviour and cohesion to modern-day management of horses cannot be over-stressed if we wish to understand some of the problems we encounter in the manner we put them to use.

In summary, we detach them from their natural herd relationship, placing strangers together and generally isolating individuals for long periods; often in looseboxes or stalls where they are subjected to an atmosphere which is laden with potentially harmful particles of fungus, bacteria and irritant non-vegetative matter that cause allergies, infection and physical damage to the airways. In addition, we mate them, especially Thoroughbreds, outside the natural breeding period of late spring to early autumn and provide them with food in meals, as if they were carnivores, not the continual herbivorous feeders that they are naturally.

Fortunately, most horses are very adaptable and come to cooperate in the dictates of man. In some respects, man has helped by selection and there has been something of a modern period of evolution based upon this artificial selection for characters that we ourselves require, from miniature ponies to Suffolk Punches and from Thoroughbred racehorses to jumping and other performance horses, all requiring their special size and type to meet man's specific requirements.

CHAPTER TWO

Breeding Organs of the Mare

Anatomy and Function

The genital organs (genitalia) (Figures 2.1 and 2.2) and glands which perform and control the breeding functions of the mare comprise two ovaries, from which eggs are shed, the fallopian tubes down which the egg travels and in which fertilisation occurs, the uterus with its two horns each of which communicate with the fallopian tubes and the uterine body which communicates through the cervix with the vagina that passes to the exterior through the vulval lips and perineum.

The associated endocrine glands which control the breeding organs are the hypothalamus (producing gonadotrophin releasing hormone: GnRH), the pituitary gland (producing follicle stimulating hormone: FSH and lutenising hormone: LH) and, because they release hormones into the bloodstream, the ovaries (oestrogen and progesterone) and the uterus (prostaglandins: PFG).

Ovaries

The ovaries (Figures 2.3 and 2.4) are roughly bean-shaped. Their size varies in different individuals and in the same mare at various times of the year. On average, they measure about 7 cm x 4 cm. Each ovary consists of a fibrous-like mass (stroma) containing numerous sacs of fluid (follicles) in which an egg (ovum) is to be found. Every individual is born with a complement of many thousands of eggs and does not produce more during her lifetime. In addition to the follicles and their eggs, the stroma may contain one or more structures, each known as a 'yellow body' (corpus luteum). Their formation and function is discussed below.

Fallopian tubes

The fallopian tubes (see Figure 2.1) or oviducts lie in the membrane which supports the ovaries and uterus. Each tube is coiled and measures about 25 cm in length. It is open at one end and enters directly into the uterus at the other.

Uterus

The uterus (see Figures 2.1, 2.2 and

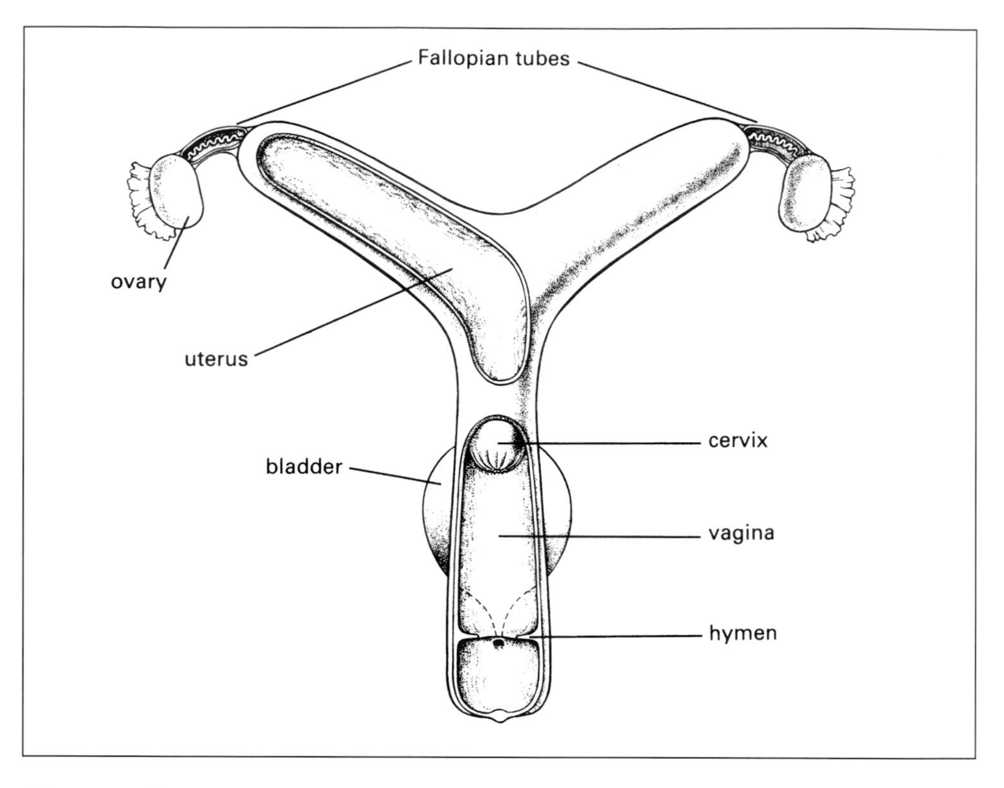

Figure 2.1 The mare's breeding organs (viewed from above), with sections exposing internal structures

Figure 2.2 The mare's breeding organs (viewed from the side)

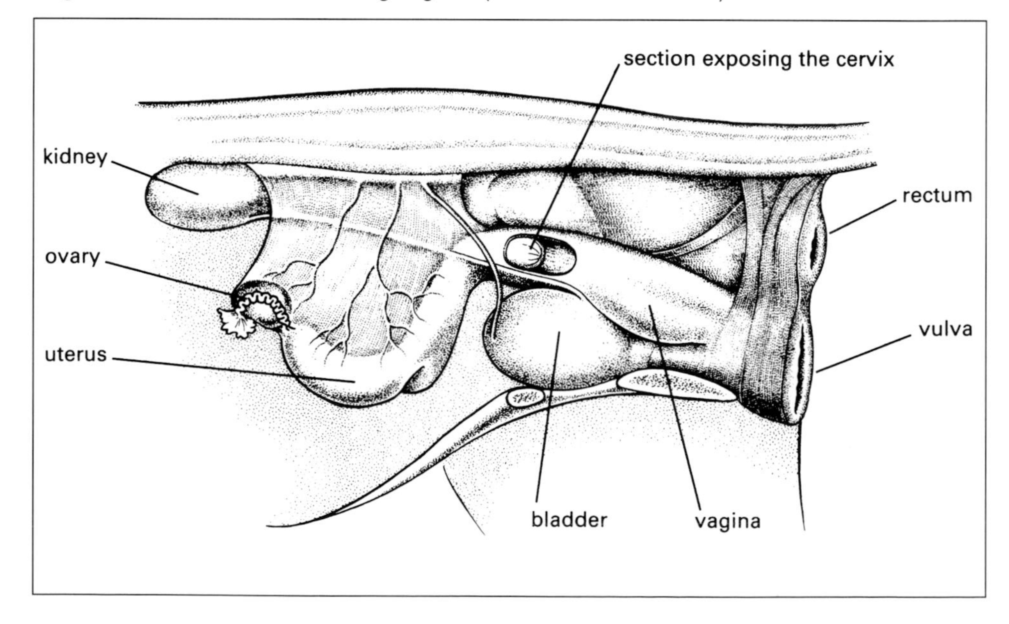

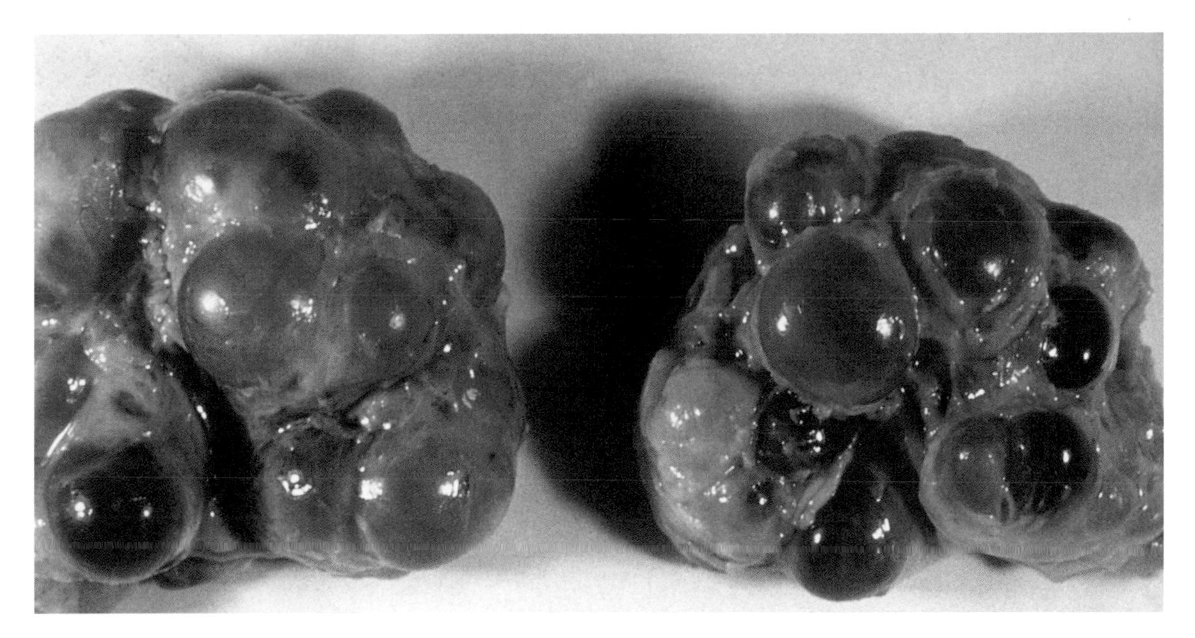

Figure 2.3

Ovaries showing follicle development. Only one follicle will reach maturity and ovulate on each oestrous period

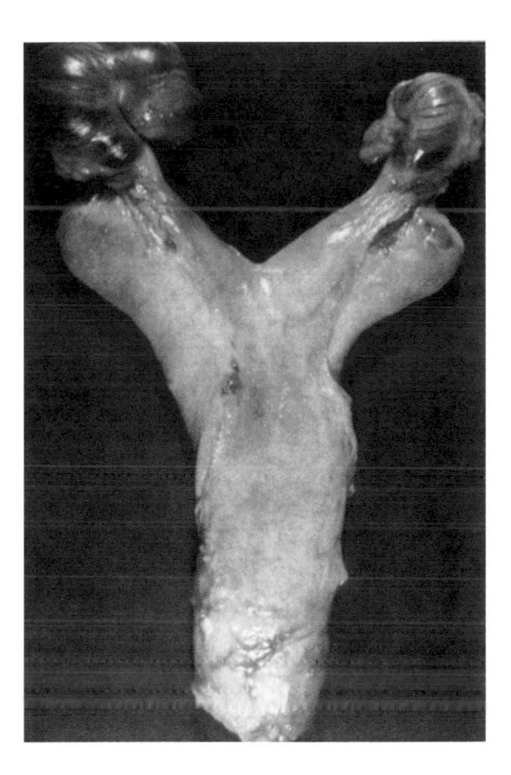

Figure 2.4

The uterus and ovaries; the left horn shows follicle development in the ovary

2.4) is a hollow organ with muscular walls lined on the inside with a layer of cells containing numerous small glands. It is roughly T-shaped and composed of a body and two horns; the horns are joined to the fallopian tubes and the body communicates with the exterior through the cervix and vagina.

The uterus is capable of undergoing profound changes during pregnancy when it accommodates the growing fetus, besides acting as a surface for attachment of the placenta. It also acts as a gland by secreting PFG. During pregnancy the uterine lining develops an intimate relationship with the placenta and acts to nourish and support the fetus during its eleven months' sojourn within the organ.

Cervix, vagina and vulva

The interior of the uterus is connected to the outside through the cervix. The cervix forms a highly muscular neck to the uterus and, like the uterus, is able to change under varying circumstances; these include a capacity to dilate to facilitate passage of the stallion's semen and at the termination of pregnancy to allow passage of the foal during birth.

The vagina is also capable of undergoing certain changes which will be described when we come to consider the reproductive cycle. Together with the vulva, the vagina acts as a vestibule of protection between the outside world and the interior of the uterus, the importance of which will be discussed later in relation to the problems of infection. The vulval lips are part of the perineum which includes the skin on either side bounded above by the anus and on either side by its attachment to the buttocks. At the lower end of the vulva, just inside the lips, is the clitoris.

The clitoris is the terminal part of the genital tract extending from the ovaries through the fallopian tubes, uterus, cervix and vagina. The clitoris is the equivalent of the penis in the male and actually possesses similar parts. The body is about 5 cm long and its diameter about 3 cm. The glans is the rounded and enlarged free end of the organ and occupies a depression in the lower part of the vulval lips. The organ is covered by a thin membrane equivalent to the prepuce in the male. The clitoris is composed of erectile tissue and is attached to the connective tissue overlying the rim of the pelvis.

Mammary glands

The mammary glands are modified skin glands closely associated in function with the genital organs. The mare has two mammary glands and each has the form of a very short flattened cone compressed to have a flat middle surface. The glands possess a body and a propeller or teat. At the apex of each teat there are two small openings placed close together through which the ducts leading to the glandular tissue discharge milk. These glands are divided into lobes and lobules with their tubules and alveoli which forms a mass analogous to the air sacs and ducts of the lungs but, of course, not containing air but secreting milk. The functions of the mammary glands are described later.

Pituitary gland

The pituitary gland is a very small body which is situated immediately beneath the brain in a small recess in the bony floor of the cranium. It is composed of anterior and posterior parts (lobes) each of which produces hormones.

The posterior part (lobe) produces oxytocin, the hormone involved in causing contraction of the uterine wall during foaling. It also produces prolactin which acts on the mammary glands causing the formation of milk and an antidiuretic hormone involved in regulating the flow of urine from the kidney.

The anterior part (lobe) produces the hormone FSH that acts on the ovaries to cause the development of follicles and the hormone LH which causes the follicles to ovulate (break) and develop the yellow body (corpus luteum). The anterior pituitary also produces non-reproductive hormones, namely adrenocorticotrophic hormone (ACTH), therotrophic hormone (TH) and, in the stallion, interstitial cell stimulating hormone (ICSH).

Uterine lining

The lining of the uterus produces a hormone known specifically as prostaglandin F2 alpha (PGF 2alpha). This hormone dissolves the yellow body and stops it producing progesterone.

Hypothalamus

The hypothalamus is a small area in the brain which controls the gonadotrophin-releasing hormone (GnRH). This acts on the pituitary, causing it to release the hormones FSH and LH.

Pineal gland

The pineal gland lies close to the hypothalamus and controls the release of the GnRH in response to light falling on the retina of the eyes.

Summary

The organs and glands that have been described above act in an intrarelated manner to stimulate or respond to stimulation in a way which can externally be recognised as the sexual signs. The pathways are shown in Figure 2.5. The central theme of activity is the oestrous cycle, an alternating sequence of oestrus (when the mare accepts the stallion for mating) and dioestrus (when she rejects the advances of the male). The cycle is controlled by hormones produced by the pituitary gland, the ovaries and the uterine lining.

Oestrous cycles operate during the breeding season (naturally in spring and summer); and this activity is controlled by the pineal gland and hypothalamus of the brain mediated by the length of daylight hours, interpreted through the light received by the retina of the eyes. In periods of the year when oestrous cyclic activity is absent (anoestrus) mares do not show the behaviour associated with the cycle. The cycles are also abolished during pregnancy. In the following section, the hormonal control and behavioural consequences of the oestrous cycle, anoestrus and pregnancy will be described.

Oestrous Cycle

The oestrous cycle is so named because of the two recurring periods of events which describe the mare as in oestrus (in heat, receptive, on) which alternates

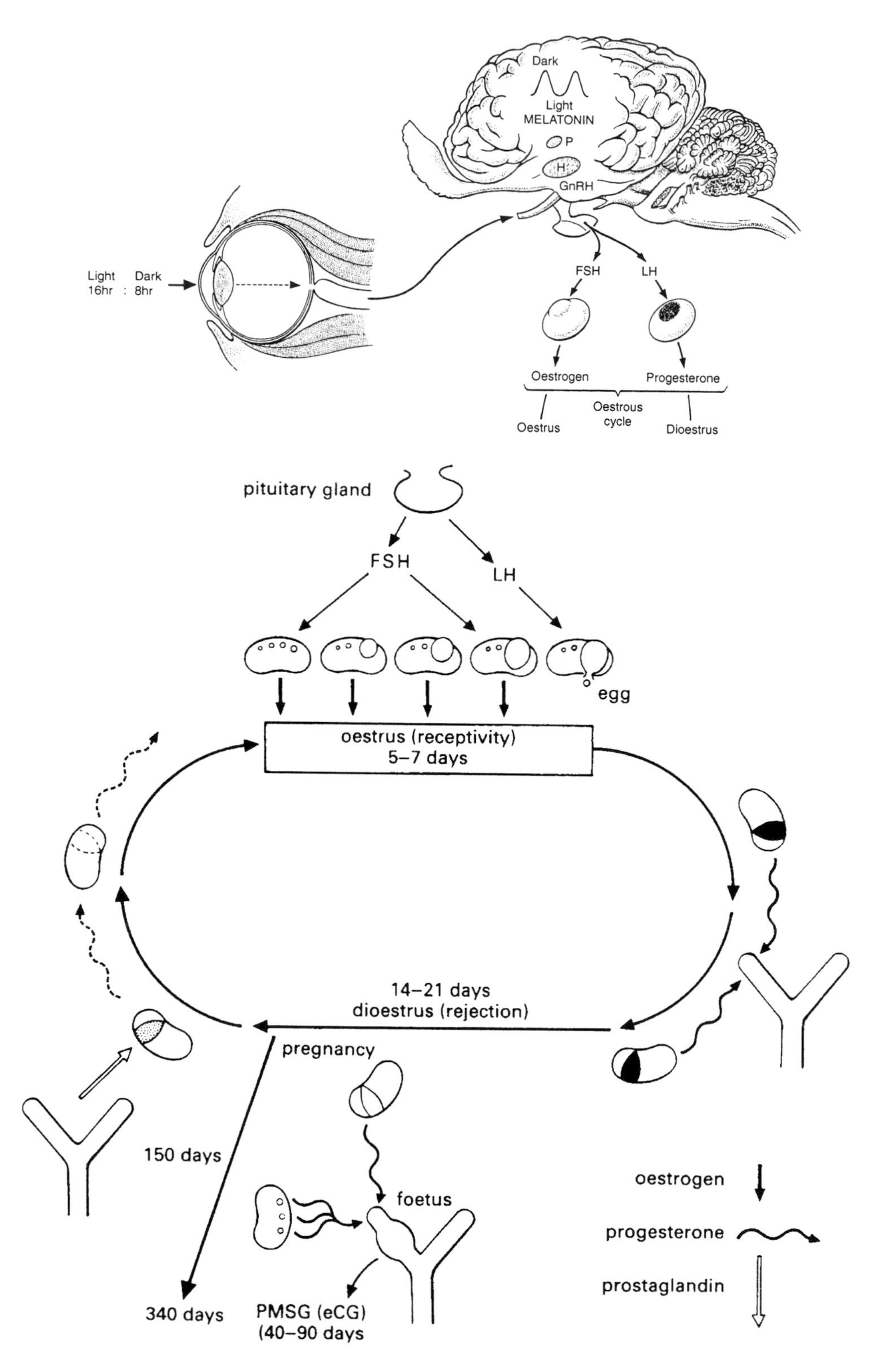
Dark
Light
MELATONIN
P
H
GnRH
Light 16hr : Dark 8hr
FSH
LH
Oestrogen
Progesterone
Oestrous cycle
Oestrus
Dioestrus
pituitary gland
FSH
LH
egg
oestrus (receptivity)
5–7 days
14–21 days
dioestrus (rejection)
pregnancy
150 days
340 days
foetus
PMSG (eCG)
(40–90 days
oestrogen
progesterone
prostaglandin

Figure 2.5 (opposite)

The effect of daylight hours, via the eye to the hypothalamus and pituitary gland, on the oestrous cycle of the mare:

FSH	follicle stimulating hormone;
LH	lutenising hormone;
P	pituitary gland;
GnRH	gonadatrophin releasing hormone;
PMSG (eCG)	pregnant mare's serum gonadatrophin (equine chorionic gonadatrophin).

The circles in the ovary represent follicles, one of which enlarges and ruptures to release an egg at the ovulation fossa. The black wedge is the yellow body that secretes progesterone until it is broken down (or affected) by the hormone prostaglandin

with the behaviour of dioestrus (between oestrus) and to which we attach the phrases off, out of heat and rejection.

For practical purposes, these descriptions reflect the logic behind the practical management of broodmares. The fact that these changes are reflected internally by changes in the hormone patterns is of less consequence to studfarm management than it is to the veterinary surgeons whose point of view we will come to later.

The cycle is typically one of five days in heat and fourteen days out of heat, that is, five days oestrus, 14 days dioestrus. However, this typical pattern is not always present although it tends to conform more in late spring and summer than at other times of the year, when oestrus may last for two or even three weeks and dioestrus even longer.

As the cycle is the springboard and mechanism by which the male and female horse come together for the purpose of achieving conception, oestrous cycles occur naturally in the months of late April to September. This corresponds to the needs of the eleven month length of pregnancy in order to achieve the birth of a foal during late spring and summer. This is when the grass is at its most plentiful and thereby provides maximal opportunity for nourishment of the mare during the later stages of gestation and during the period of suckling.

Outside of these months, it is best that conception does not occur and, therefore, the oestrous cycle is restrained or abolished. This situation, of course, refers to the natural state. We have selected, especially in breeds such as the Thoroughbred, mares which are genetically capable of cycling at other times of the year and modern management techniques support this change to an unnatural state by ensuring that adequate food is available at all times.

Let us now define, in physiological terms, the background to the mare's changing behaviour. In oestrus, the hormone oestrogen, produced by the follicles in the ovary, dominates (Figure 2.6). Oestrogen not only causes the psychological change in the mare's behaviour towards the stallion, but prepares the genital tract for the

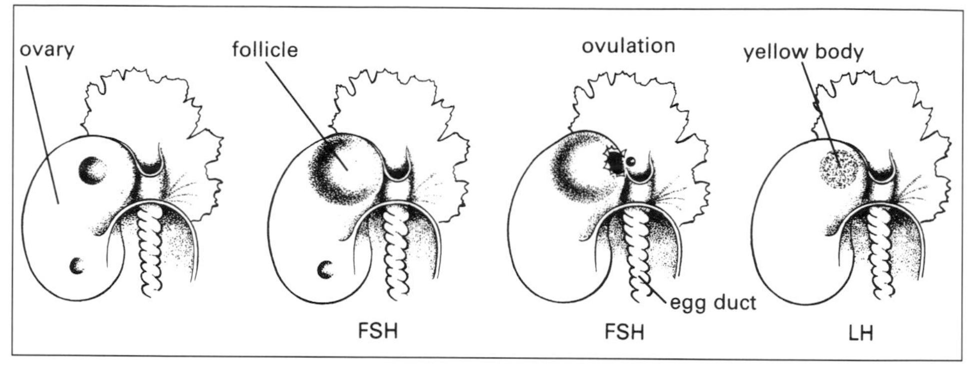

Figure 2.6

The influence of pituitary hormones FSH and LH (from left to right): the ovary in dioestrus; follicle development; oestrus with ovulation; and development of the yellow body

introduction of the stallion's penis from which sperm are delivered at the time of ejaculation. The hormone causes lubrication by changing the mucous secretions in the vagina and uterus to a watery, slimy consistency from its sticky, tacky nature in dioestrus when, as we will see, the dominant hormone is progesterone.

Oestrogen causes lengthening of the vulva and relaxation of the cervix. The period of oestrogen dominance comes to an end following rupture of the follicle (ovulation) and release of the egg (ovum). This occurs typically at the end of oestrus, although it may be up to two days before the mare actually goes out of heat or, as sometimes described, out of season. It is this timing of ovulation in relation to the length of oestrus that determines the success or otherwise of our mating plans. As we will see later, the egg becomes resistant to fertilisation very soon after it is shed and mating following ovulation has, therefore, markedly less chance of resulting in conception than if mating takes place before ovulation. However, the stallion's sperm may not live or retain their own capacity for fertilising the egg for more than two or three days once they enter the genital tract of the mare. Mating may therefore take place too soon as well as too late.

The hormones FSH and LH cause the follicles to increase in size within the ovary during oestrus and eventually to rupture and shed the egg. These two hormones are driven by the release of GnRH from the hypothalamus of the brain. Further, as oestrogen increases in concentration in the bloodstream, so this is interpreted by the pituitary as the time to release the LH that helps to bring oestrus to an end. This is opposite to the situation when progesterone is present in high concentrations, as at the end of dioestrus. High concentrations of progesterone help to raise the storage of FSH in the pituitary pending its release at the end of dioestrus. The response of a gland to its own hormone level is known as feedback; for example, FSH levels rise causing secretion to diminish.

During dioestrus, the hormone progesterone dominates the physiological state. Psychologically it causes the mare to be refractory to the advances of the male, physiologically it causes constriction of the cervix, drying up of the mucus in the genital tract and shortening of the vulva. The source of progesterone is the yellow body or corpus luteum which forms following rupture of the follicle and shedding of the egg (see Figure 2.7). A yellow body has a lifespan of about 14 days during which it actively produces progesterone. However, the lining of the uterus is responsible for secreting prostaglandin and, at about the 14th day, this enters the bloodstream to cause dissolution of the yellow body so that this stops producing progesterone.

Falling levels of progesterone trigger the release of FSH from the pituitary, thereby causing the follicles to increase in size and mature in preparation for ovulation as FSH levels rise, as indicated earlier in this account.

Let us now summarise the changing scenario of hormone production described above. We may start at any point in the cycle, but that of the beginning of oestrus is as convenient for description as any. At the start of oestrus FSH levels are increasing, thereby stimulating growth of follicles in the ovary and their production of

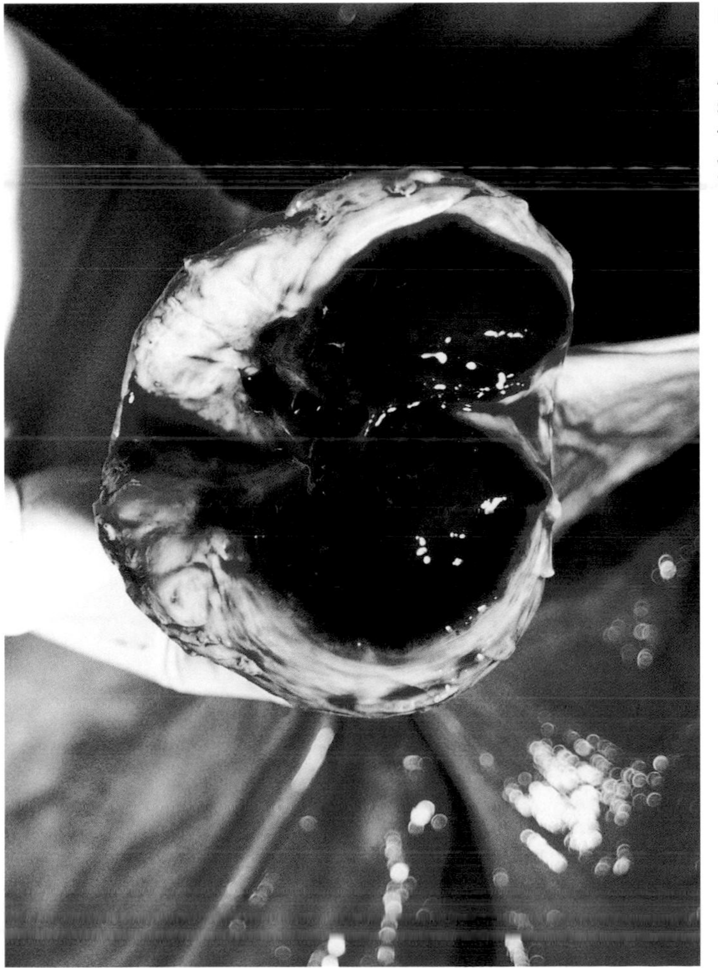

Figure 2.7

A dissected ovary showing a ruptured follicle where the yellow body will form oestrogen. Increasing levels of oestrogen eventually result in the release of LH from the pituitary as a direct stimulatory effect. This, in turn, results in ovulation and the formation of the yellow body.

The lining of the follicle has special cells (luteal) which proliferate and grow into the blood clot that occupies the centre of the ruptured follicle. The cells produce progesterone and the mare goes out of heat. The consequence of the period of progesterone dominance is to cause the build up of FSH in the pituitary and, when the uterus releases prostaglandin that 'kills' the yellow body, this FSH is released; and so we return to the point in the cycle at which we started this account. This intricate interrelationship of rising and falling levels of hormones may be likened to a series in which switches are triggered, one switch related to another; however, we should not think of this sequence in mechanical but in biological terms.

Hormones may be likened to keys (produced by the gland in one part of the body) that fit into a lock in the target tissue; for example, the pituitary produces the keys of FSH which fit into the locks in the lining of the follicles of the ovary. The biological aspect of this relationship is that, however many keys are produced by the gland, they cannot function in their action on the tissue unless an equivalent number of locks are present. Therefore, we may have situations where there are an insufficient number of keys to fit the number of locks present, or conversely, more keys than locks.

Again, taking the analogy of the action of FSH on the follicle, the pituitary may produce an insufficient quantity of keys, whereas the locks on the follicle are sufficient for action to take place should the FSH increase. The locks on the tissue are known as receptors and most hormones have the capacity to increase the number of receptors. Therefore, if FSH levels increase they may also increase the number of receptors (locks) present in the lining of the follicle.

Other hormones, such as LH, may also affect the number of receptors present by diminishing or increasing their numbers, thereby influencing the response of the particular tissue to the hormone that controls its action. Progesterones and oestrogens both operate in this way with respect to the receptors to LH and FSH.

The oestrous cycle is, therefore, based on changes not only of hormone concentrations in the bloodstream, but of the receptor status on tissues such as follicles, yellow body, uterine lining and, in the brain, nerve cells responsible for the psychology of behaviour. The clinical message of this complex interrelationship is that we cannot rely on single measurements to provide us with an answer to the physiological status of the individual at any given time. For example, if we measure the level of FSH or progesterone in the bloodstream, we can form a judgement of how much of the hormone is being released by the gland, but we cannot necessarily interpret its action because we do not know the receptor status on the target organs concerned.

Cyclic and Non-Cyclic Periods

We have already recognised that the period of oestrous cycling is seasonal, related to spring and summer months under natural conditions. This situation is based on the evolutionary development of the horse and represents the basic reproductive behaviour of the glands and organs involved. The arrangement is based upon daylight length so that as the number of hours of daylight increases in spring so the cycles are initiated, whereas in autumn when daylight hours are reducing, the cycles are correspondingly stopped.

The pathways involved are those which start at the retina of the eye where light is first interpreted in physiological terms by the neurones that convey the message of light to the pineal body in the brain and thence to the hypothalamus. Lengthening daylight increases the production of GnRH and, via the action of GnRH on the pituitary, an increase in FSH and LH. Since these two hormones drive the cycle the relationship between daylight and the onset of cycling, or conversely, in autumn, the arrest of cycling, is evident.

Of course, the complexity of the biological process entails a transitional state from no oestrous cycle in the winter (anoestrus) to cyclical activity. This transitional phase may be experienced from management's viewpoint as irregular length of components of the oestrous cycle (for example, prolonged oestrus and oestrus occurring without ovulation). However, this transitional state usually lasts only a few weeks in early spring or late winter and is then replaced by normal, regular cyclical periods.

As already mentioned, selection of individuals for the aims of racing and/or foaling early in the year, as well as additional nutrition, has resulted in many mares exhibiting oestrous cycles in winter and/or late autumn. In fact, some individuals may cycle throughout the year.

Another influence which has been brought to bear, particularly in Thoroughbreds, where foals born early in the year are required for commercial reasons, is the use of artificial lighting. This entails subjecting mares to increased periods of daylight during December and January. The pathway from retina to pituitary is then activated artificially with the result that mares start cycling in February/March. In achieving these ends we are, of course, manipulating the basic physiological makeup of the mare's reproductive system. We return to this subject later.

Anoestrus or lack of cycling may be the consequence of low levels of production of the hormones FSH and LH in the pituitary or the presence of what is known as a prolonged yellow body; that is, a yellow body which is not subject to its production of progesterone being terminated by prostaglandin, either because no prostaglandin is produced by the uterus or because the yellow body is resistant to the action of the prostaglandin. The latter may be because of a scarcity of receptors in the yellow body so that the body fails to respond to the prostaglandin being secreted from the uterus.

The other period when cycling is abolished is, of course, during pregnancy. Progesterone is the dominant hormone which maintains pregnancy within the uterus.

The sequence of events from the time that the conceptus reaches the uterus on the sixth day following fertilisation in the fallopian tube is as follows:

- The conceptus moves actively over the surface of the uterine horns and body and, in so doing, releases a

signal which prevents the uterus from producing prostaglandin.
- The yellow body formed at the time of fertilisation therefore continues its life of production beyond the 14-day period of dioestrus.
- At about day 35, the membrane surrounding the fetus which is destined to become the placenta releases cells which invade the uterine lining and produce the hormone known as equine chorionic gonadotrophin (eCG). The areas where the cells are invaded are known as the endometrial cups, the endometrium being the term used to describe the uterine lining. The cups are active from about day 40 until day 120 of pregnancy and they produce vast quantities of eCG. The hormone helps to produce numerous follicles in the ovary that ovulate and supplement the yellow body of pregnancy established at the time of fertilisation.

Mares in foal do not show oestrus although there are some individuals which appear to do so at times and may even accept the stallion despite the pregnancy. However, these individuals are rare and are often those conceiving for the first time.

Managemental Control of the Oestrous Cycle

As our knowledge of the natural control of the oestrous cycle has advanced, so too has the ability to introduce measures which may be used to augment managerial control. In brief these are as follows:

- The provision of extra daylight has already been discussed. Various regimens have been introduced but the one most commonly employed is to have mares maintained in looseboxes with exposure to low-level lighting (100 w) on a timing system that starts at sunset in early December and continues to 10.00 pm each night.
- Progesterone therapy consists of administering the drug over a period of at least ten days. This activates the feedback effect of progesterone; that is, when progesterone levels are raised the pituitary stores FSH which is released in a bolus amount when progesterone levels fall as the administration of the drug is ceased. This therapy has been augmented in recent years as the synthetic progesterone *allyl trenbolone* has been marketed in a oil preparation that can be administered by mouth. This product is even more powerful in its effect than pure progesterone. It is used when the mare is in anoestrus or in a transitional state between anoestrus and oestrus. It is most effective when follicles are present in the ovary.
- Progesterone and oestrogen combination can be injected daily to mares with the same effect as with progesterone alone. The combination has been found to be useful and was first developed as a means of promoting fertile oestrous periods by workers in Kentucky and California.
- Synthetic GnRH can be injected on a daily basis or administered subcutaneously as a slow-release pellet or implant. This has the effect of raising FSH and LH levels by

mimicking the pathway between the hypothalamus and the pituitary.

Control of the oestrous cycle by artificial means, whether initiating cycles or controlling the time of ovulation, has many advantages in a commercial world where early foals and increase in the likelihood of conception occurring bring commercial benefit.

The problem in practice is to make an exact diagnosis of the hormonal and sexual state of the individual at any given time of a particular case. It is true that we can use the aids of clinical examination, but these fall short of an exact knowledge of the complex mechanism that lies behind sexual function. In applying measures of drug therapy, of whatever form, we are necessarily left with a guestimate of the condition of the individual. It is not surprising, therefore, that therapy to promote or control oestrous cycles fails in a proportion of individuals treated, especially if we expect results in a matter of days or, even, weeks. The most effective and well-tried approach has been the provision of extra daylight; and this therapy takes about two months to be effective.

Applying Veterinary Knowledge to Management of Mares for Breeding

Veterinary and other scientific knowledge accumulates over the years and this leads inevitably to managemental decision-making in what should and should not be applied at any given time to a particular individual or individuals. Fashion plays its part in that a procedure adopted in one country or by one group of breeders may readily be adopted by others on anecdotal evidence of benefit. What are these benefits?

Breeders aim, on the whole, to obtain conception in their mares as early in the year and with as few matings as reasonably possible. Any approach which makes these two aims more likely to be achieved is given ready consideration.

However, the old adage applies that 'if you sup at the devil's table, you must drink the devil's brew'. The advice must always be that every new drug or manipulative procedure aimed at facilitating the getting in foal of mares should be given careful scrutiny. Most of the studies performed which are the basis for scientists and practitioners advocating usage of that particular endeavour are based on relatively small numbers and, importantly, adverse side-effects are rarely if ever assessed, except in the sense of the immediate and obvious (for example, localised generalised reaction). The subtle consequences are rarely investigated. For example, it is well known that we can dissolve the action of the yellow body by injecting prostaglandin; but the follow-up of cases which do not respond has not been nearly so well documented.

If we review the manipulation into the oestrous cycle described above, increased daylight hours appears to be one of the most effective physiological means of inducing oestrous cycles early in the calendar year. The injection or feeding of hormones, such as GnRH, oestrogen/progesterone are quite effective but require a more detailed knowledge of the actual status of the individual in hormonal terms than we perhaps possess in every case. They are, therefore, something of a hit-and-miss procedure which can be recommended, but not with the confidence of success achieved by extra daylight.

The use of prostaglandin is also extremely useful in cases where there is a yellow body which is functioning beyond its normal lifespan of 15 days. It may also be used for short-cycling mares by injection 4–10 days following ovulation. However, in these latter circumstances it is not always effective and this is probably because the individual's ovary either has a corpus luteum which is younger than four days present in the ovary (the yellow body is refractory to the action of prostaglandin in its early stages of development), or there are insufficient receptors present in the yellow body for the prostaglandin to act successfully. Whether or not the injection of prostaglandin in these circumstances is actually harmful and upsets the oestrous cycle is, as discussed above, something which has not been researched perhaps as diligently as it should have been.

The use of HCG (human chorionic gonadotrophin) to cause ovulation is widely practised. On the whole, it is highly successful in mimicking the sharp increase in LH in the bloodstream of the mare which causes ovulation. Again, the use of HCG means that we can, in most cases, predict that ovulation will occur 24–48 hours after intravenous administration of 1,500 to 3,000 i.u. of HCG. This action only occurs if a follicle of more than 3 cm in diameter is present. However, the analogy of lock and keys or quantity of hormone and number of receptors present on the lining of the follicle applies. We cannot, therefore, assume that just because a follicle is greater than 3 cm in diameter that it will necessarily ovulate because we have administered the HCG.

We might claim that the injection is successful in about 80 per cent of cases, while in 20 per cent of cases it does not seem to act in the way we would expect. As far as we can ascertain, injections do no harm, although repeated injections may raise antibodies in the mare's bloodstream. Research workers have claimed that these antibodies are not in fact harmful because they do not cross-react with the mare's natural LH.

The injection certainly assists in helping stud management in reducing the number of matings that are necessary per mare during a stud season; and may be very useful in arranging for a mating to take place close to or just before ovulation occurs, thereby making the period between insemination of the semen and ovulation as short as reasonably possible. This is a helpful way of treating sub-fertile mares or those visiting sub-fertile stallions. In these circumstances, it is probably best to give the HCG 12–24 hours prior to mating taking place.

When mares are in a state of anoestrus, following foaling or early in the breeding season, the use of GnRH implants which provide a slow release of the hormone may be helpful, although reports in the literature and the personal experience of the authors, does not suggest that these implants are highly effective in these circumstances.

The first author (PDR) with many years of veterinary practice experience, concludes that careful lay management and attention to detail in the routine of the breeding season is more important in the achievement of the objective of obtaining conception in mares than the use of artificial aids. The latter should be used in conjunction with, and not as a substitute for, traditional expertise of studfarm managers and personnel. The cooperation of veterinarians in stud-farm management is highly useful, but should not be regarded as essential to a natural process of breeding. There are exceptions to this statement, such as the avoidance of the spread of venereal diseases and in the diagnosis and treatment of sub-fertile individuals.

CHAPTER THREE

Management of the Broodmare

Special management practices are necessary to ensure optimum reproductive success. However, the most important preparation practices should be maintained all year round. These include proper nutrition, preventative medicine, a routine programme of parasite control and exercise as well as many other commonsense management techniques.

Many factors may affect the mare's ability to conceive, maintain a healthy pregnancy and produce a healthy foal at full term. Although infertility, or more correctly, sub-fertility is partly determined by inherent or pathological problems, management practices that influence the environment in which the mare lives can affect her reproductive efficiency significantly.

On a small stud it is easy to give each mare individual attention and to come fully to appreciate her individual behaviour. However, when large numbers of horses are managed, some staying only for a matter of days, this level of individual attention can be difficult to maintain. Specific procedures should be chosen according to the size and type of the studfarm, the number of broodmares and the mares' reproductive status. For ease of management, mares are normally sorted into groups according to their status, such as maiden, barren, pregnant and lactating. Management of pregnant and lactating mares is discussed later.

The Maiden Mare

Managing the maiden mare requires special consideration, regardless of her previous background. She should be introduced to the studfarm in a way that ensures a smooth transition into her new role. Maiden mares are normally grouped together so that careful attention can be given to their oestrus state as they may show erratic oestrus pattern and behaviour during the early weeks of their first breeding season.

As with any other new arrival, if the mare is turned out with the others, she should be carefully introduced to an established herd as she may not mix well with other settled mares (Figure 3.1).

Ideally, maiden mares should be allowed to start adjusting to their new

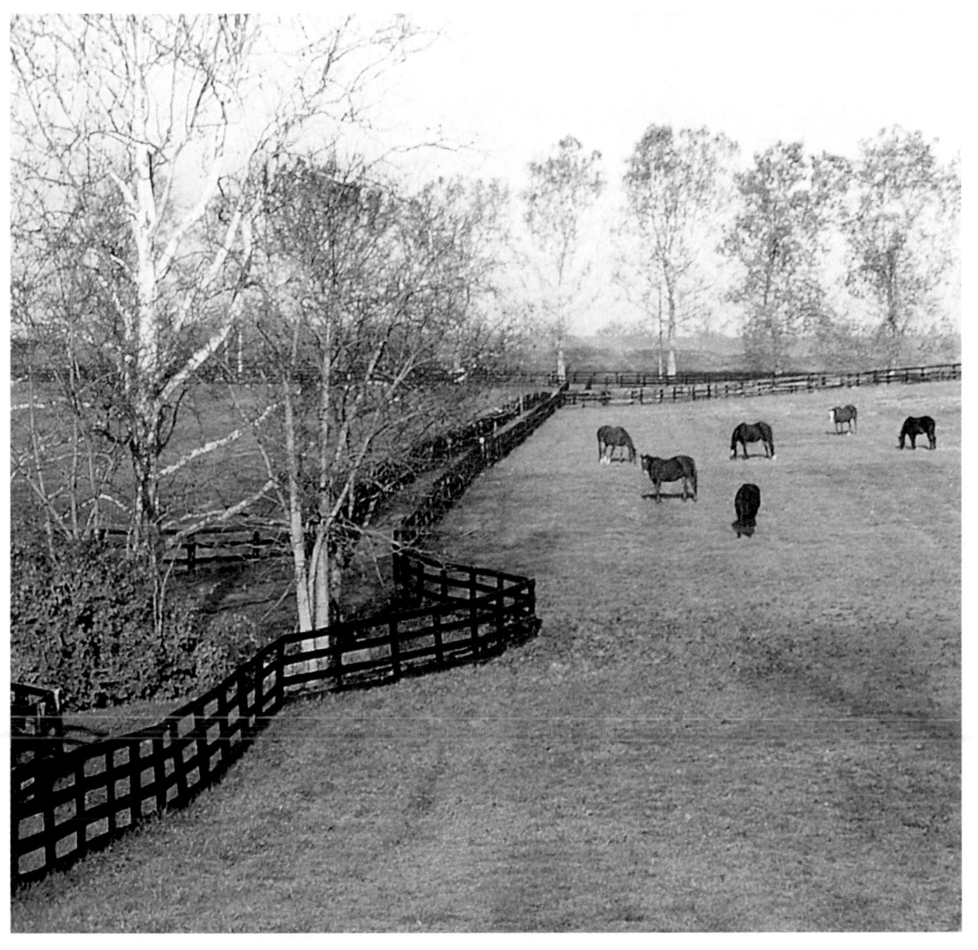

Figure 3.1

A settled group of maiden mares in a well-fenced paddock

role from the late summer/autumn in the year preceding their first breeding season. This gives the mare a chance to adjust to her new surroundings, routine and feeding programme. Maiden mares may take some time to adjust mentally and physically from being, in many cases, a highly-fit athlete to being a broodmare.

However, some mares may take only a short break from training to go to stud and return to training or racing through the early part of their pregnancy; if this is planned then special consideration will need to be given to their needs. Mental and physical stresses associated with high-level performance can cause oestrous cycles to be irregular and some mares may have required medication in training which could affect their reproductive ability for a time. The use of steroids, for example, to treat a lameness, can cause the mare's ability to overcome infection to be impaired; if

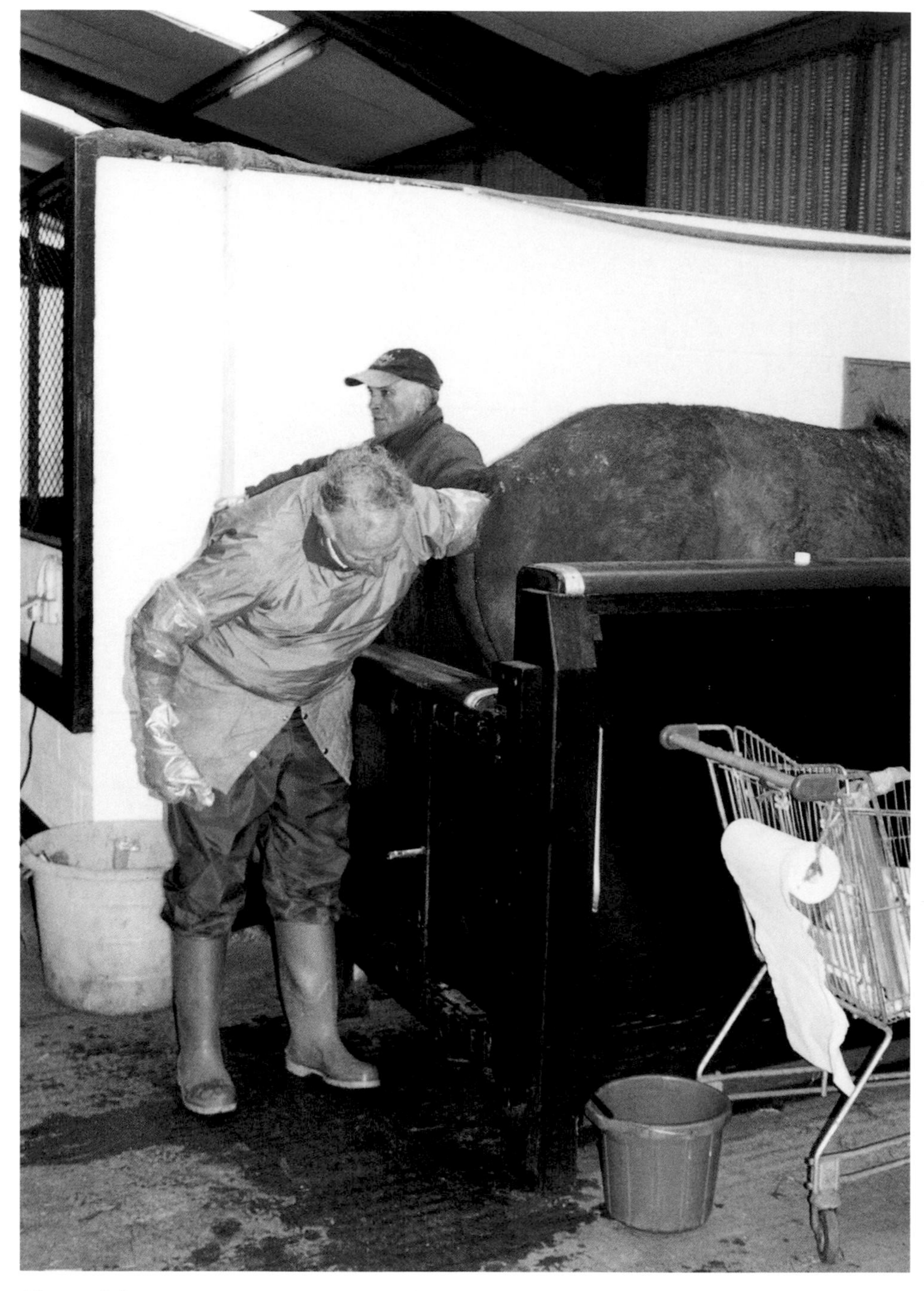

Figure 3.2

A maiden mare being examined rectally to assess the condition and maturity of her reproductive organs

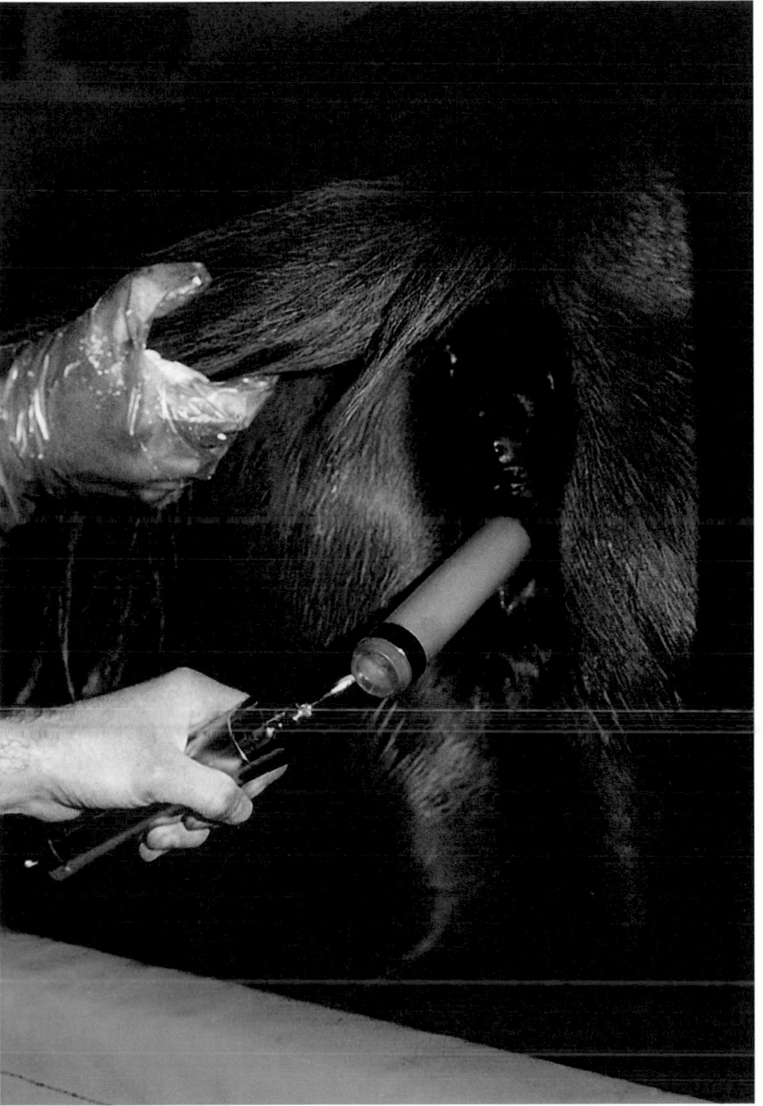

Figure 3.3

The cervix is examined with a speculum

she has been treated over a long period, the mare may be susceptible to genital infections.

Generally, mares going to stud for the first time have an initial reproductive examination (Figures 3.2 and 3.3). This enables her physical breeding ability to be assessed. It is also a common procedure for those mares intended to be sold for breeding purposes.

The genital tract of the mare is examined for serious defects and her reproductive maturity is evaluated. Even though many mares have essentially undergone puberty as early as 18–24 months, at three or four years of age she still may not be physically mature enough to be bred and maintain a pregnancy to term. Individual and breed-related differences in maturity should be considered carefully before a young mare is bred. Some old maiden mares can suffer from long-term genital infections and should be assessed carefully regardless of their seniority in years.

contributing to her condition. Malnutrition can prolong anoestrus and cause further irregularities in the pattern of her oestrus periods when she does begin to cycle. However, being overweight can also affect her breeding ability.

The Barren Mare

It is surprisingly common for barren mares to be forgotten until the breeding season begins. These mares may be barren because of a reproductive problem and, ideally, time should be given to establish any possible cause for this before the breeding season starts. If the mare is cycling regularly, appropriate treatments can be carried out during oestrus – these may include cultures for bacterial infections, uterine biopsies and endoscopy. The high oestrogen levels during oestrus can help in overcoming infection as this hormone increases resistance to uterine inflammation. If the mare has developed an infection during the previous breeding season then treatment should be given to her at that time so that during the winter months of anoestrus, the reproductive tract can have a chance to recover. Overcoming these problems well in advance of the breeding season is essential to give the mare the best possible chance of conception.

The effect of physical condition on fertility in both maiden and barren mares is well documented. Studies have shown that mares that are losing weight going into the breeding season may begin cycling properly up to a month later than mares that gain weight during this period. If a mare is free from genital infection and abnormalities but remains barren, diet may be

Artificial Lighting

The use of artificial lighting to encourage early return to breeding for maiden and barren mares is well known. Cyclic ovarian activity is affected by changes in daylight length. In response to a lengthening daylight period, the hypothalamus secretes more gonadatrophin releasing hormone (GnRH) which, in turn, stimulates release of follicle stimulating hormone (FSH) and lutenising hormone (LH) from the anterior pituitary. By simulating these events the transitional period from winter anoestrus to oestrus may be shortened. Artificially simulating these events has no affect on fertility and does not cause early anoestrus in the autumn. Indeed, if necessary, the end of the breeding season can be prolonged in just the same way. This is not common practice with Thoroughbreds as their breeding season is set to finish at an early date, but may be more useful in pony and performance horse breeds, especially to give more time for infected mares to be treated and bred.

Although the use of lighting varies from stud to stud, there are several important points to be covered. The mare must be stabled at night, although in climates other than that of the UK mares may be kept in floodlit paddocks. To be effective, mares should be under lights for a long as possible prior to the breeding season. Some studies show a minimum of 60 days as a guideline, but most studs start with their maiden and barren mares as early as mid-November. To further mimic the natural events, studfarms may add half an hour on the time the lights are on by December, increasing this every week or so until a maximum total time of 16–18 hours of 'light' is achieved. Recent research has indicated that this time period may not be strictly essential to maintain effectiveness.

By early January, the mare's reproductive system begins to behave as if spring has come early and she will begin to cycle. Normally her first few cycles are irregular and shallow, these being replaced by the short, regular oestrus periods required for the breeding season. Lighting programmes may sometimes be ineffective with a mare in deep anoestrus. However, response to lights can be further enhanced if the mare is on a high-protein diet and is gaining condition. Rugging mares in this state to increase warmth may also be useful, but a definite connection between temperature and ovarian activity has not yet been established.

The light source should be 100 kw and, as with all electrical appliances used in stables, safety is a very important consideration. The lights should be covered with wire or clear plastic and be of the type designed for outside use. Indoor and outdoor lighting systems can be controlled with a variety of automatic timers; however, manual controls work just as well for a smaller studfarm.

Breeding Records

Complete records of the mare's breeding history are vitally important as a management tool and often assist as an aid to diagnosis of a fertility problem (Figure 3.4).

Most studfarms keep a record of the mare's oestrus behaviour, her oestrus patterns and any veterinary treatment she has had. This will be combined with details of her pregnancy and a list of the foals she has produced, information on any problems she may have had with foaling, the general health of her foals, previous genital infections and/or treatments she may have received, etc. All of these records build up an invaluable picture of the mare's reproductive history and can be particularly useful to a stud she may be visiting for just a short period.

Being able to understand an individual mare's normal pattern of behaviour quickly can save both time and money when she is sent away to stud. An accurate record like this can also be useful for management when assessing reproductive efficiency of an individual within a herd, or for a prospective purchaser.

Although examination of the mare for reproductive purposes is carried out by the veterinary surgeon, the first step in a pre-breeding examination is evaluation of the mare's apparent physical condition. Does she reflect good health? Will she require any special treatments before becoming an addition to the broodmare band? Examine her closely, even lifting her tail and examining her external genital conformation and hindquarters. Does she have desirable pelvic and vulval conformation? Has she been stitched?

In older mares, or those with poor conformation, the anus and vulval lips may sink inwards; this can present a problem as faeces collect around the vulva and will predispose to infection.

Name: **ANY MARE**
1995 ches. by Sharpo ex
Princess Rosananti by Shareef Dancer

Passport: 100000

Status: IF Flying Spur LSD: 23.03.99 *First Foal*

Owner: J. Dean

Last Vacc: Duvaxyn IET+ 16.01.00
Last Vacc: Duvaxyn EHV 1,4. 08.09/01.11/02.01.00
Additional Information: In from Italy. Rapido Transport.

01.02.00	**Arrived**. Copy passport. CEM & EVA & Coggins supplied
03.02.00	WEC -ve. Wormed Strongid P
17.02.00	Farrier
15.03.00	**Foaled bay colt**
16.03.00	Newborn exam + I/D. 4ml tribrissen + TAT. *Mare farrier & wormed Strongid P.*
17.03.00	Foal blood for IgG>800
18.03.00	Foal 4ml tribrissen.
24.03.00	L0 U3+ Involution fair R4f Endo swab & smear.
13.04.00	C3+ L4.5f U3+ R0 *Mare farrier and wormed Equest. Foal farrier and wormed ½ Strongid P.*
14.04.00	2 vials chorulon (JRC) **COVERED** Mare DNA sample and foal microchip, I/D and blood kit.
16.04.00	Lov U2+ Ract
30.04.00	C1 U2 **Sc+ve** left horn Good picture. BFP = 7.0
03.05.00	C1 U2 **Sc+ve** left horn Good picture 19 days.
11.05.00	*Mare and foal farrier. Foal wormed ½ Furexel*
12.05.00	C1 U2 **Sc+ve** left horn Good picture and development 28 days.
24.05.00	C1 U2 **PD+ve** left horn All good 41 days.
26.05.00	Foal inject i/v Gentaject + Crystapen. BFH.
27.05.00	Foal inject i/v Gentaject + Crystapen.
28.05.00	Foal inject i/v Gentaject + Crystapen.
29.05.00	Foal inject i/v Gentaject + Crystapen.
30.05.00	Foal inject i/v Gentaject + Crystapen.
31.05.00	Foal inject i/v Gentaject + Crystapen.
01.06.00	Foal inject i/v Gentaject + Crystapen.
02.06.00	Foal inject i/v Gentaject + Crystapen.
05.06.00	Examine foal re: respiratory condition. Congested.
07.06.00	Foal: upper respiratory tract infection - worse. 5ml Ventipulmin i/v 8ml Tribrissen.

Figure 3.4

Detailed record of a mare's gynaecological and routine management during a breeding season

Any discharge around her hindquarters may also indicate reproductive infections. Examine the area around the anus and vulva for signs of scars or previous damage from mating or foaling. External scars can be important clues of internal damage.

Answering these basic questions can assist when the veterinarian examines the mare internally.

Detection of Oestrus

The need for management to detect signs of sexual behaviour in mares stems from the fact that we separate the mare from the male of her species. In the feral state, the stallion assesses the sexual state of his mares by smell and sight, accentuated by taste and sound. Detection of oestrus in the mare is, perhaps, one of the most important aspects of stud management. Although mares display characteristic behaviour to show that they are receptive to the stallion, this behaviour can vary dramatically dependent on time of year, the status of the mare and the way in which she is being observed.

Broadly speaking, when the mare is in oestrus she will be receptive to the stallion and permit herself to be approached and mounted. When she is in dioestrus, she will react aggressively towards the male horse and behave violently if approached by a stallion or he attempts to mount her.

Most studfarms nowadays use the terms 'showing', 'in use', 'in season' and 'on heat' to describe a mare that is receptive and 'teasing off', 'not in use' and 'not in season' to describe a mare that is not receptive. This behavioural pattern is controlled by the physiological changes and influences that have already been discussed.

Teasing

There are many methods used for detecting oestrus in the mare, but all are commonly termed 'teasing' or 'trying' (see Figures 3.5 and 3.6).

'Teasers' are stallions; on a Thoroughbred stud, teasers may be pony stallions kept specifically for the purpose, or an older Thoroughbred who has retired.

Rather less common is using a horse which has been vasectomised as a teaser. This has obvious advantages in that the horse can be allowed to run freely with his mares and there is no risk of any mare becoming pregnant. However, there is a very real risk of infection as the horse may mate with many of the mares in the group and pass infection from one to the other.

In the past, it was common for a small stallion, such as a Shetland pony, to be allowed to run with a group of mares – the size difference naturally prohibiting mating in most cases. However, this too can have its problems; having a stallion in with a group of mares can make routine management difficult and if there is any chance of mating being possible, the risk of cross-infection is present. Today, most farms keep their teasers in the same way as their stallions and quite separate from the mares.

A good teaser is invaluable to the stud manager; an experienced horse will respond to mares that may be shy and lack confidence in the presence of a male horse, and ignore those that are on the point of returning to dioestrus although they may still be displaying strong oestrus behaviour. A teaser may also be used to introduce maiden mares to being mounted for the first time – a process termed as 'bouncing'. Although the teaser will mount the mare, he will not be permitted to enter her and may be asked to mount her repeatedly until she relaxes and accepts the procedure.

Although this sounds frustrating for the teaser, many experienced horses switch their sexual behaviour on and off quickly, displaying no distress at being taken away from the mare. A poor teaser is of little use as he shows no interest in the mares and may be reluctant to mount. Careful management of the teaser is essential to retain his interest and confidence. Some teasers are also stallions who regularly cover mares; however, due to the extraordinary value of some stud horses, great

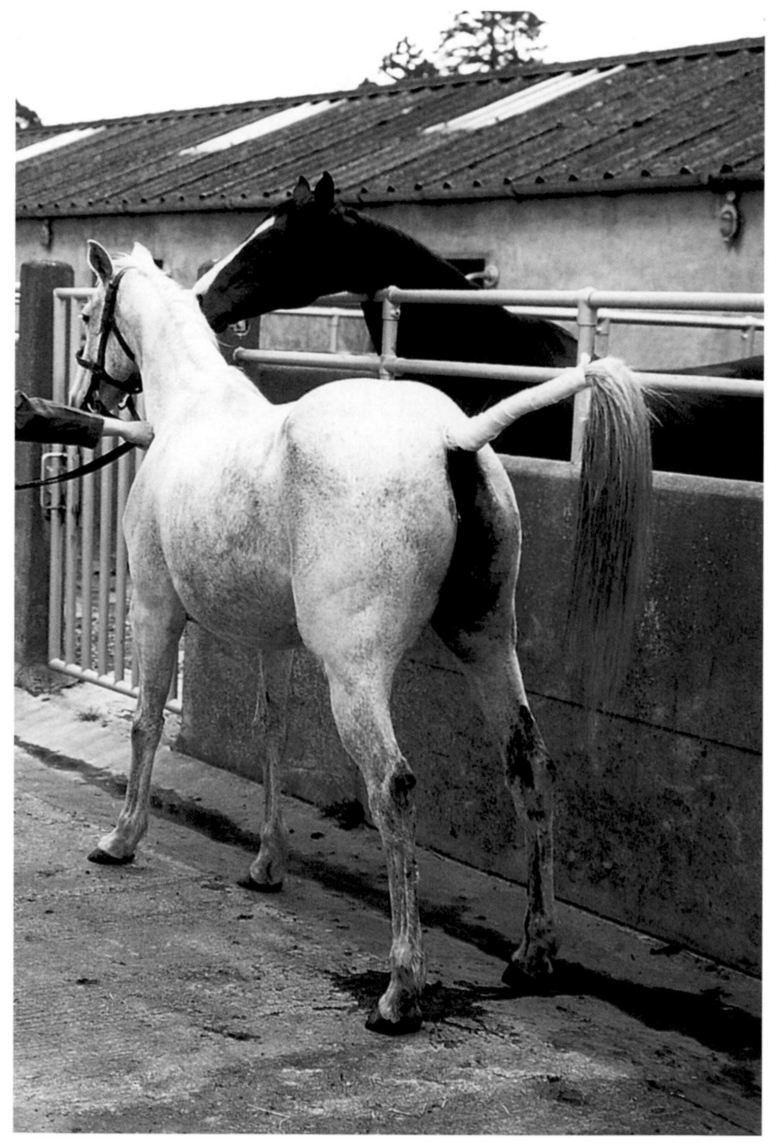

Figure 3.5

Teasing by leading the mare up to the teaser, who is loose in the yard care has to be taken to avoid injury and this may prohibit the use of the main stallions themselves in this role.

The areas used for teasing are varied, but most studs have a specially designed teasing board. This is usually a reinforced and padded gate, or a boarded and padded area within a line of paddock fencing. It is important, due to the violent reaction that teasing can provoke in a dioestrus mare, that the structure is strong enough to withstand the full force of a kick. Conversely, it should also be strong enough to contain the overly amorous teaser!

The mare is brought up to one side of the teasing board and the teaser led up to the other (see Figures 3.7–3.10). They are normally presented head to head initially and then the mare moved until she is standing side on to the board.

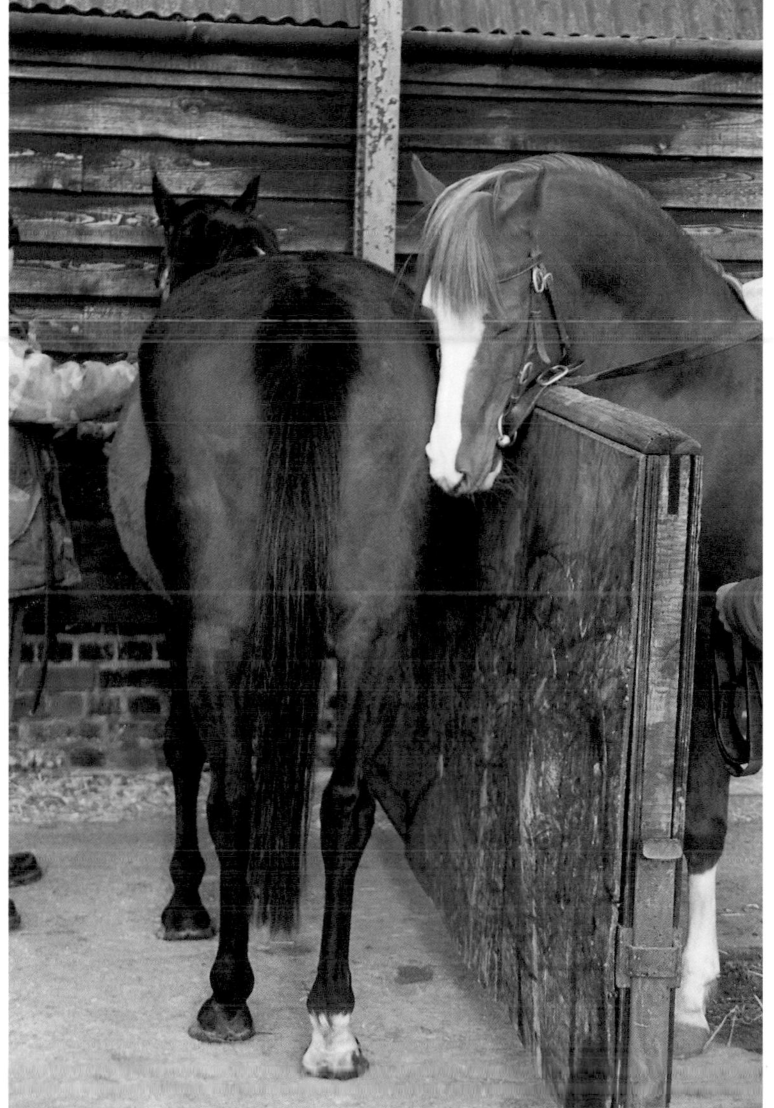

Figure 3.6

Teasing using a pony stallion

The teaser will generally nip and lick the mare down her neck and shoulder, working to her hindquarters. If the mare is in oestrus, she will lean towards the board and straddle her hind legs. She may also squat slightly and produce a stream of thick yellow urine that has a characteristic and strong odour. This urine is full of pheromones to further indicate her sexual receptiveness to the stallion.

The mare will also lift her tail and evert the lips of her vulva exposing the clitoris – a process known as 'winking'. Winking is commonly the first sign that a mare is coming into oestrus – careful observation of the mare may reveal the winking under an only slightly raised tail. By observing the external genital organs of the mare, the vulva appears lengthened and relaxed; sometimes it appears moist and slightly engorged.

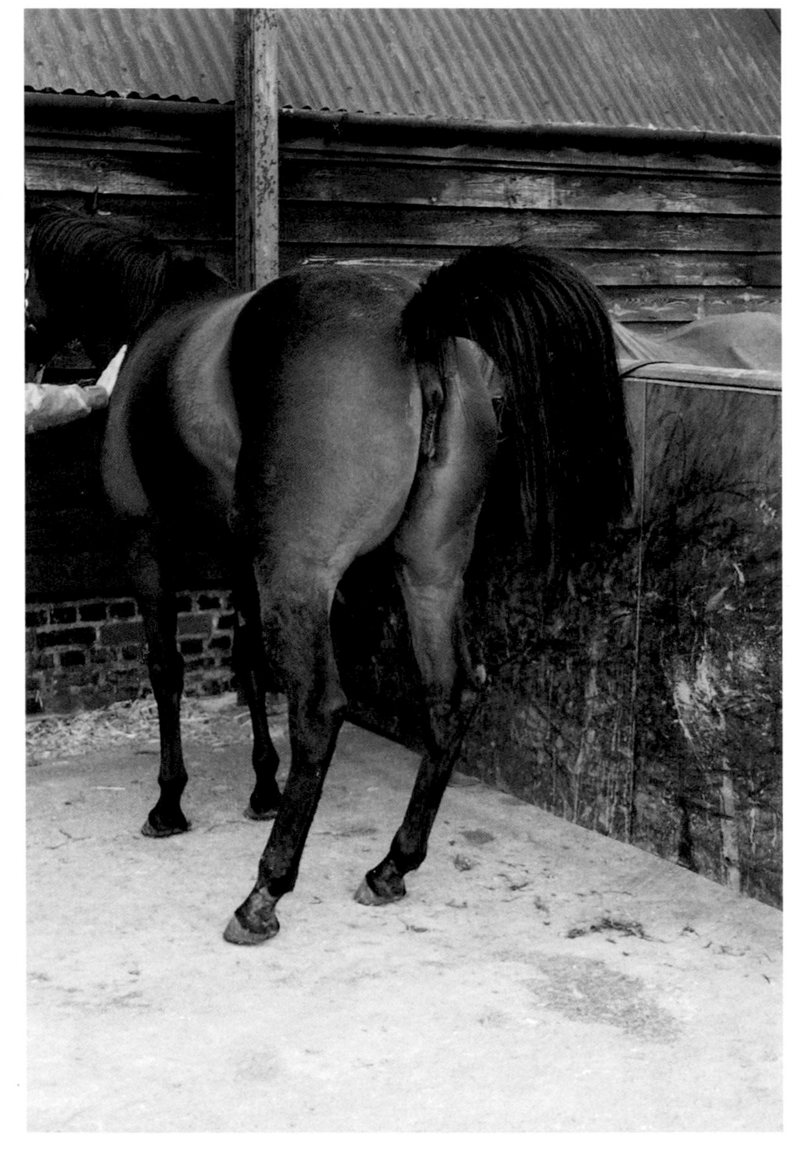

Figure 3.7

A mare showing characteristic oestrus behaviour

The most dramatic change is that of the mare's behaviour, particularly apparent in mares that are normally short-tempered and difficult to handle. The mare may become more placid and easy to handle; for example, a mare that is normally difficult to catch may come to the handler easily. Some mares may also display oestrus whilst being groomed over the hindquarter area by an attendant.

The signs of dioestrus are normally the opposite of that of oestrus. The mare becomes aggressive to the teaser and may be reluctant to approach him. She will clamp down her tail, put her ears back, attempt to bite and may kick with some force at the trying board.

Some mares leave the handler in no doubt as to their status; however, others just become quiet at the board and these mares need careful observation to avoid

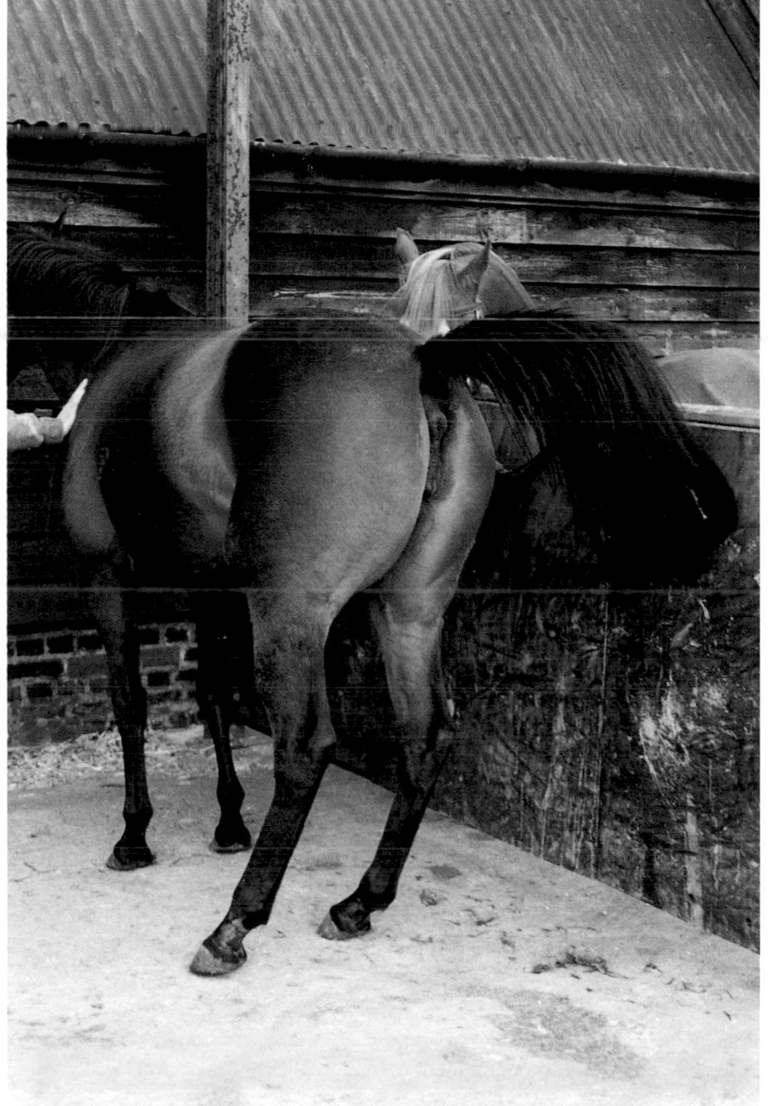

Figure 3.8

This mare is relaxed to teasing, lifting her tail, and leaning towards the teaser misinterpreting their behaviour. With the invaluable veterinary assistance available to many studfarms, such mares can be properly assessed without having to rely entirely on their behaviour with the teaser. Mares that are pregnant or in anoestrus generally show behaviour associated with dioestrus. There are reports of mares displaying strong oestrus behaviour even though they are pregnant and in rare circumstances continuing to cycle and ovulate in early stages. These cases are very rare and not all result in the loss of the pregnancy; however, it should be assumed that a mare that returns to oestrus fol-

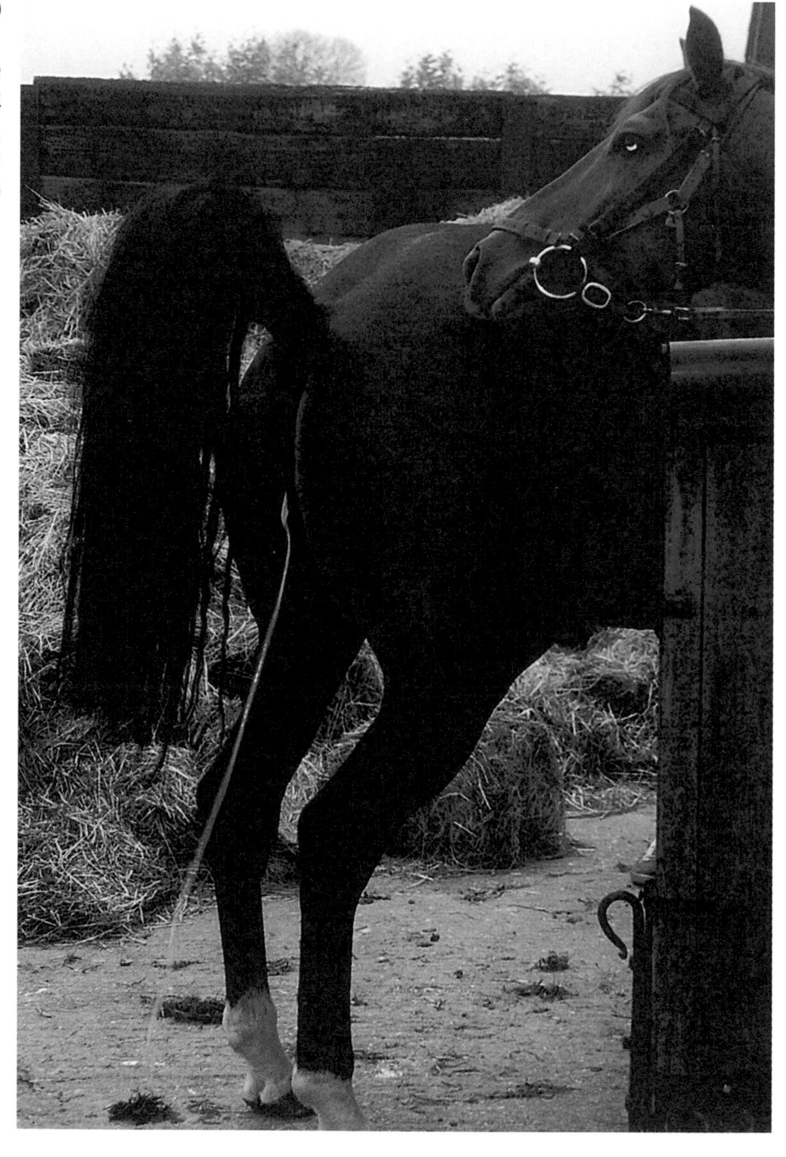

Figure 3.9

Here the mare is passing thick yellow urine, rich with pheromones

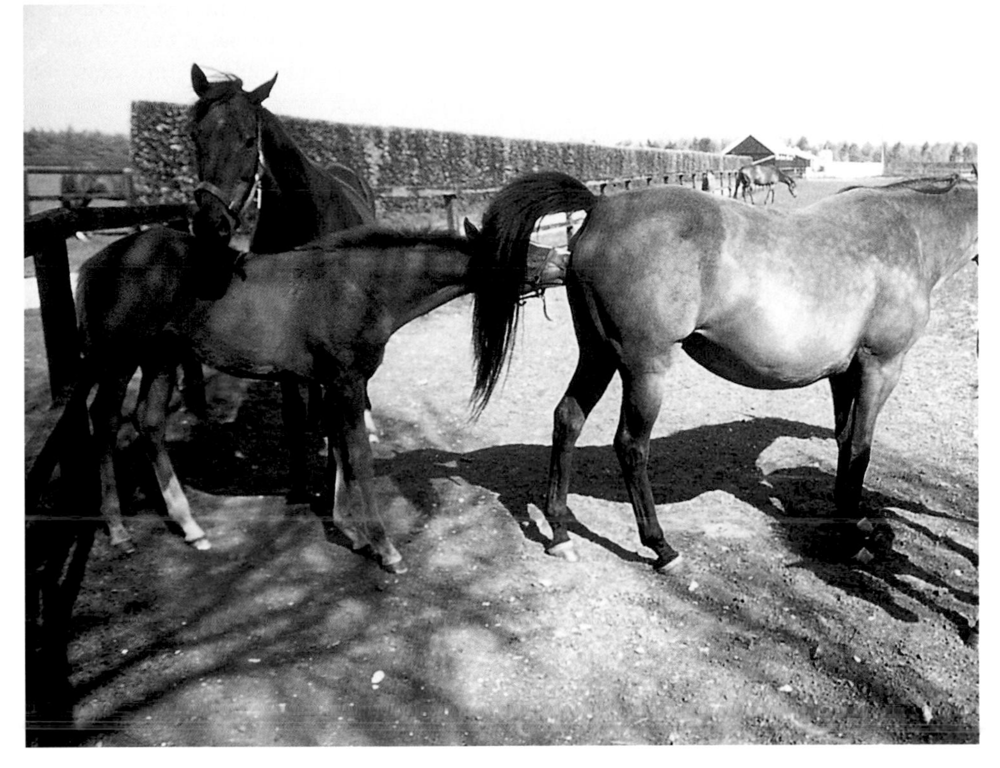

Figure 3.10

A mare displaying oestrus behaviour to other mares and foals in the paddock

lowing mating on a previous heat is unlikely to be pregnant. Observation of the external genital organs will normally show a tight and dry vulva.

Abnormal Behaviour

Mares that are routinely teased during the breeding season come to associate being taken up to the trying board with the stallion.

It is important that this practice is not forced – there are cases of mares that will always react aggressively towards the teaser at the board, only to display strong oestrus behaviour on return to the stable. There are many reasons why this may occur. It is important to remember that the teasing procedure practised on most commercial farms is artificial – many mares have no sight or sound of a male horse except at this time and they may be nervous or shy of him.

Some mares that are over-protective of their foals react in this way when taken to the board alone – especially if they can hear their foals calling from the stable. It is also not unusual for a mare to associate a previous bad experience with the teasing and to resent the procedure. For these reasons careful observation of all the mares should be practised. Watch the mares still in their stables and especially out in the paddock – this is particularly worthy of note with maiden mares having their first experience of stud life. Some mares will display oestrus behaviour in the paddock to other mares and yet remain aggressive or disinterested at the teasing board. For this reason some studfarms also walk the teaser around the farm close to the mares out at grass.

In some countries, such as Australia, where Thoroughbred studfarms tend to be on a larger acreage, a common practice is to have pony teasers in a small enclosure or paddock within the mares' paddock. This can work well as the mares become accustomed to the teaser's constant presence and, when in season, will move to be near him and openly exhibit oestrus behaviour. As normal methods of trying, when mares are led up to the teaser at a board, are labour intensive, this method can reduce dramatically the number of handlers needed and the time taken to tease the mares each day.

Teasing Routine

The mare in oestrus should be at her peak for conception. The physiological and psychological changes that occur prepare her for an optimum chance of a successful pregnancy. The time of year that she is cycling regularly ensures that the foal will be born when climatic conditions provide the best chance of optimum growth and development. The mare ovulates only during oestrus so this will also ensure that only healthy sperm have a chance to fertilise the ovum. From a management point of view, it is, therefore, important to utilise fully this knowledge of the oestrous cycle to give every chance for broodmares and stallions to perform at their full potential and to produce healthy live foals.

Teasing is normally carried out every other day during the breeding season with barren and maiden mares. This means that the stud manager can establish each mare's oestrus pattern. It may be carried out each morning before the mares are turned out. For studfarms that have regular veterinary attendance, this will mean that mares can be assessed and then kept back for examination on the vet's round. Some studfarms prefer to tease in the evening when the mares have been brought in for the night. Either practice has advantages and disadvantages. Teased in the mornings, some mares are keen to go out in the field and may give a false response at the board, teased in the evening and they may be anxious for their feed. A mare teased just a few hours before the vet's round will enable the manager to give the vet a current appraisal of her behaviour – some mares have very short cycles and may have ovulated overnight; a mare that was showing the night before may be completely different in the morning. Teasing is labour intensive so staffing levels may also dictate the best time for this procedure to be carried out. There is no hard and fast rule – what works for one studfarm may be completely wrong for another.

Once the mare has come into oestrus and been mated, she will be teased until she shows signs of dioestrus. This is normally combined with examination by the vet to confirm that ovulation has taken place. The hormone progesterone secreted following ovulation means that the mare will return to dioestrus and becomes aggressive towards the teaser. When this has occurred the mare is usually left un-teased until 12 days from mating when teasing begins again, every other day. This may appear to be a very early stage once the oestrous cycle is fully understood, but a mare who may have a uterine infection following mating will commonly 'break' or return to oestrus as early as 12 to 13 days later. Teasing early allows for quick identification of these mares and, therefore, for the optimum chance of treating and allowing time for the infection and resulting inflammation to subside.

If the mare does not return to oestrus after about 15–18 days following mating then she will normally be scanned to establish if she is pregnant. Some studfarms will continue to tease pregnant mares following the pattern of her oestrous cycle for the first few weeks to attempt to identify cases of early pregnancy loss. However, due to the common practice of regular scanning (see Chapter Four) at 16–18 days, 21–28 days and 40–42 days, this additional teasing is not essential.

Mares who have foaled return to oestrus at about 6–14 days from foaling. This heat is commonly termed the 'foal heat'. It is thought that this oestrus period is designed to allow the uterus to recover fully from foaling rather than for breeding, but many Thoroughbred mares are bred on this heat. Normally, mating on the foal heat depends on the mare's recovery from foaling. The mare will be examined by the vet who will assess the state of her uterus and a swab will be taken to check for any inflammation or post-foaling infection. With today's veterinary techniques, mating on this heat does not normally affect the mare's chance of conception if her recovery from foaling has been good. Once the foaled mare has been covered, she will be teased in the same way as a barren or maiden mare.

CHAPTER FOUR

Management and Veterinary Services

The relationship between management and veterinary science has changed quite considerably over the years. On the one hand, those responsible for management of breeding horses have become more knowledgeable and more highly trained, as a result of educational courses now open to them including those leading to degree status; and on the other hand veterinary clinicians have acquired an extensive range of diagnostic and therapeutic techniques developed by research in both medical and veterinary fields. Therefore, veterinarians have at their disposal such technologies as ultrasound and a wide variety of hormonal and other drugs by which to control the oestrous cycle or treat cases of sub-fertility.

If we look at the evolution of the relationship over the past 50 years, it is possible to discern a trend in which veterinary surgeons have become increasingly integrated with stud management, performing duties which may be described as aids to management in addition to the traditional medical and surgical services provided by the profession.

Before the Second World War, stud management programmes included routine trying or teasing of mares for signs of oestrus, a basic procedure performed to this day. However, veterinary knowledge, at that time, provided insufficient means of assistance to make veterinary attention a routine procedure. The vets were, therefore, involved largely in medical and surgical services which may have included measures to diagnose and treat severe cases of subfertility, or as it would have been termed in those days, infertility. Even in this respect, knowledge was too limited and the means of therapy insufficient for there to be a great veterinary impact.

Breeding programmes, in those days, were based on certain maxims such as limiting the number of mares being presented to the stallion each year, at least as far as Thoroughbreds were concerned. A full book was in the region of 30 mares and first season sires were confined often to about 20 mares.

When mares were determined by the stud groom to be on heat, mating would be arranged on the third and fifth day; maiden mares were not mated until April or, even, May for the first time.

Teasing continued after mating and, if the mare did not return into heat, it was assumed that she was in foal. Pregnancy diagnosis in those days was confined mostly to observation, although chemical tests on blood and urine became available in the late 1930s. However, these tests were not reliable until pregnancy had advanced to 45 days or even more.

In the 1940s, vets began to understand the oestrous cycle of the mare with its peculiarity of ovulation occurring typically two days before the end of oestrus in a way which led to pioneers introducing gynaecological examinations of rectal palpation and vaginal inspection. In the UK, Fred Day of Newmarket led the way, as did Dymmock in the USA. Soon there were many veterinarians experienced in rectal palpation and the means of determining the sexual state of the mare at any given time, including the prediction of when ovulation would occur and the presence of pregnancy from about 40 days from service, onwards.

The close integration between veterinary and managerial expertise practised today started in the 1950s. Routine examinations of mares prior to service and for pregnancy became commonplace. There were limitations to the technique of rectal palpation, at least with respect to interpretation of what was felt. In the early decades of this approach, mistakes of interpretation were quite frequent. It was only when ultrasound was introduced in the late 1970s and 1980s that follicles could be seen, rather than felt, and ovulation identified. Ultrasound provided a much more accurate method for diagnosing pregnancy; and a diagnosis could be made at 14 days after service rather than at about 40 days using only rectal palpation.

Even more important to management was the fact that ultrasound provided a means of diagnosing twins and of eliminating these at about 17–20 days following service. Therefore, twin conceptions, with their poor outcome, which Thoroughbreds suffered at an incidence of about 5 per cent of pregnancies per annum, have become a feature of the past and twins are rarely encountered as a cause of abortion nowadays as was the case prior to the introduction of ultrasonography.

The veterinary contribution to management may be summed up, therefore, as an assistance to control and apply the oestrous cycle in a way which maximises the efficiency of each mating (that is, increasing the chances of conception), limiting the number of matings required for each individual conception and, consequently, the chance of increasing the number of mares in a stallion's book with a minimum of wasted services. Over the years, stallions which were limited to about 30 mares per breeding season now mate with well over 100 in many cases and, even, are now exchanged in order to serve in the northern and southern hemispheres within the same calendar year. In this way, a stallion may mate with over 200 mares a year using less than 300 matings.

Veterinarians, therefore, play a dual role in providing an essential element to management while applying their veterinary expertise in cases of mares that are sub-fertile (have difficulty in conceiving). Refinements of technology and its application to breeding programmes has been a feature over recent years. As well as ultrasonography, laboratory analyses of blood hormone levels, microscopy of specimens from the uterus and visual inspection of the uterine lining through endoscopy have become commonplace in the diagnostic approach.

Therapies have also developed from antibiotics to hormonal treatments to treat the various abnormal states that may be encountered in any given individual.

Veterinarians have, rightly, become increasingly involved in the education of stud personnel, students and established staff. This programme helps to raise standards and, importantly, to give management and personnel an understanding of the use that can be made of veterinary services, thereby augmenting the collaboration that has so successfully developed during the last half century.

In non-Thoroughbred breeds, the employment of artificial insemination (AI) and embryo transfer are well established; and techniques of genetic manipulation are currently being contemplated. In the Thoroughbred, these techniques are taboo. It is perhaps ironic that one of the arguments used against the employment of AI is that it will result in huge increases in the number of progeny from certain selected families. The irony is that the use of stallions to mate with more than 100 mares in each of the northern and southern hemisphere breeding seasons may be described as a natural means of artificial insemination! There is, at present, no limitation to the number of mares that may be mated in this fashion so long as the transfer of semen to mare is not performed artificially.

Artificial insemination could be used with great commercial benefit if measures were taken to limit its use to the transfer of whole ejaculates, rather than in split form. Splitting the ejaculate, as is commonly practised in other species and in non-Thoroughbred breeds of horses, provides an added advantage when used with sub-fertile mares because it enables spermatozoa to be deposited in the uterus on a daily or even twice daily basis. Further, there is evidence to suggest that by depositing the spermatozoa close to the fallopian tubes, the chances of conception in sub-fertile mares may be raised.

It should be noted that Thoroughbred stallions tend to have rather poor quality semen compared with many other breeds and that splitting the ejaculate in some instances may not, therefore, provide adequate numbers of live normal sperm to achieve conception.

Imaging Techniques

One of the most exciting developments during the past decade, for veterinary surgeons, has been the introduction and development of ultrasonography. This technology has enabled vets to diagnose events such as follicle development and ovulation in the ovaries, early pregnancy and various states of the uterus with far greater accuracy than was previously the case when it was necessary to rely on palpation per rectum alone. Management has gained the benefit of these improvements both in terms of providing them with the means of better control of mating plans as well as furthering their understanding of mares (and to a lesser degree stallions) that suffer sub-fertility problems.

Echography

First, the reader should understand the basic features of the subject. Echography literally means the study of echoes. Ultrasound describes the fact that the technology is based on the use of a certain ranges of soundwaves, that is, wavelengths that are not audible but are nonetheless of a character similar to sound. The wavelengths employed range between about 2 and 9 MHz. Hence they are ultra short compared to soundwaves; thus the term 'ultrasound'.

The technique is similar to that used for the detection of submarines or other underwater objects. The ultrasound waves are emitted from a source, travel outwards until they meet a change in surface, as in the case of the submarine between water and the wall of the vessel where the sound becomes reflected and returns to the source of emission (Figure 4.1).

In medical practice the principle is such as described but the soundwaves are passed through different tissues and some of the waves penetrate and go further while others are reflected at each surface through which the beam passes. Contours of this multiple fractional return of parts of the original beam are interpreted electronically by the receiver and converted thereby into what we recognise as an echogram or ultrasonogram; that is, a picture of the tissues through which the beam has passed (Figure 4.2).

Figure 4.1

Illustrating the function of ultrasound, first used for the detection of submarines. Beams of ultra-short soundwaves are emitted from the ship and when they strike an object (that is, the submarine) they are reflected back to the ship

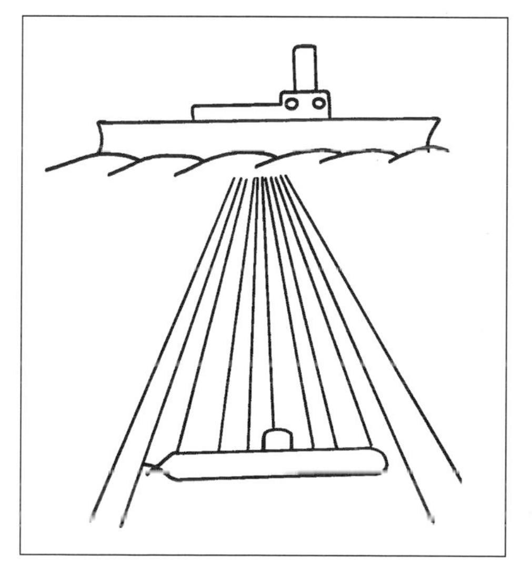

Figure 4.2

Echogram or ultrasonogram of a foal in utero obtained via the abdomen, that is, a picture of the tissues through which the ultrasound beam has passed and been reflected at different interfaces of tissue. From top to bottom, the white line is the peritoneum below which are the two converging lines of the fetal foal's rib cage. The aorta can also be seen as a dark channel running horizontally from left to right

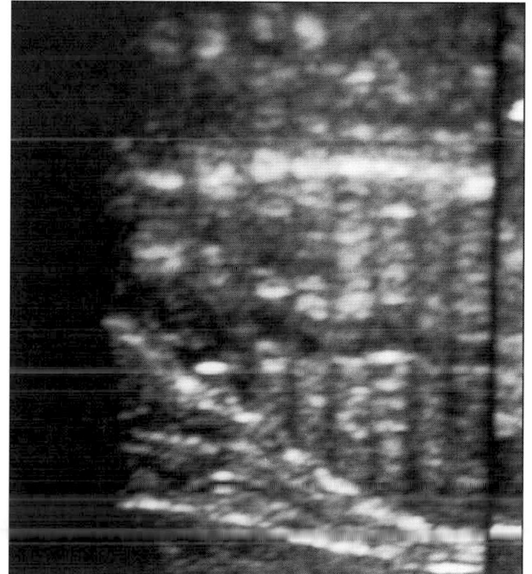

The picture is built up from a sequence of beams each returning to its source, thus the term 'scan' has been introduced to depict the composite arrangement providing a linear (straight) or sector (wedge-shaped) section of tissue or organ that lies in the pathway of the sound beams. The point of emission of the beams is usually called the probe and the machine that controls the probe the scanner.

The shorter the soundwave (for example, 2 MHz) the greater the penetration (perhaps 30 cm into the body); and the longer the soundwave (for example, 7 MHz) the less penetration (for example, 4–5 cm) but the greater the clarity of the picture.

There are a number of technical matters which are the responsibility of veterinarians to interpret such as the facts that ultrasound does not penetrate air, is mostly absorbed by bone and may be reflected in such a way as to produce artefactual shadows.

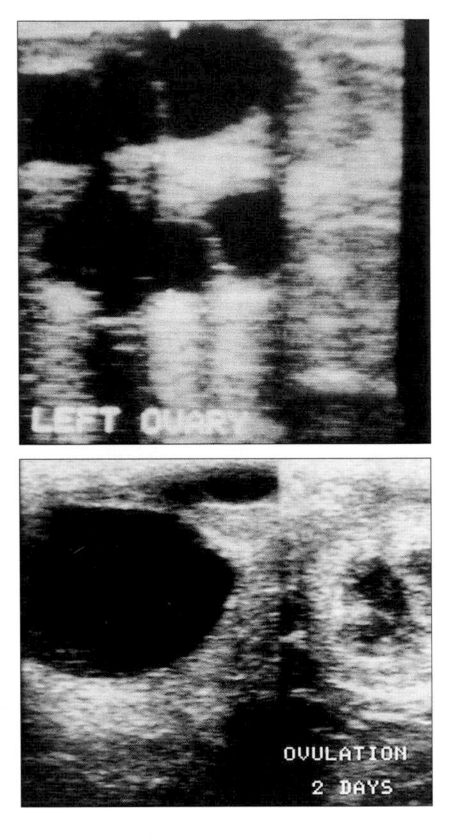

Figure 4.3 (top)

Ultrasonogram of ovary showing numerous follicles of about 3 cm in diameter

Figure 4.4 (bottom)

Split screen of ultrasonogram showing mature follicle (4 cm diameter) in left ovary and recent ovulation (yellow body) in the right ovary

Echography in Equine Reproductive Practice

Now let us consider how ultrasonography has assisted veterinarians in their diagnosis and interpretation of events of the oestrous cycle.

Ovaries

The examination per rectum consists of moving the probe over the surface of the ovary in order to diagnose the presence of follicles, their size, shape and consistency (Figure 4.3) and the presence of the corpus luteum, yellow body (Figure 4.4), together with its approximate age if present.

Both ovaries are scanned in this way and a determination made of the ovarian status in relation to the oestrous cycle (see Chapter Two) at any given examination.

In addition to the normal structures of the oestrous cycle, the examination may reveal an absence of follicles (anoestrus) or states of pathology such as ovarian tumours (see Chapter Seven).

Uterus

The state of the uterus may be visualised by the scan and recorded on echograms (Figure 4.5) in terms of thickness of the wall, presence of oedema (water) in the uterine lining or fluid in the lumen. The degree and nature of the oedema or fluid may also be determined as may the quantity. In addition, the presence of abnormal features such as tumours, cysts or haemorrhage may be visualised and their presence correlated with clinical signs of disease or conditions of subfertility.

In the pregnant mare, the presence of a conceptus may be viewed in the uterus as early as ten days following conception, but at this stage it is only a few millimetres in diameter and routine pregnancy examinations are not usually performed before about 14 days following conception (perhaps 16 days following the last mating) as discussed earlier.

The conceptus is, at first, viewed as a black hole (see Figures 4.6, 4.7, 4.8) but by 21 days the first outline of the fetus itself may be viewed and within a day or two more a heartbeat recorded within the fetal body.

From this time onwards the fetus becomes increasingly visible, with greater detail recorded from a 7 MHz than a 5 MHz probe as per the sequence of views from early pregnancy to day 60 (see Figures 4.6, 4.7, 4.8). The benefit to management and veterinary diagnosis of these means of pregnancy examination are discussed later. Here, let us consider the benefit related to

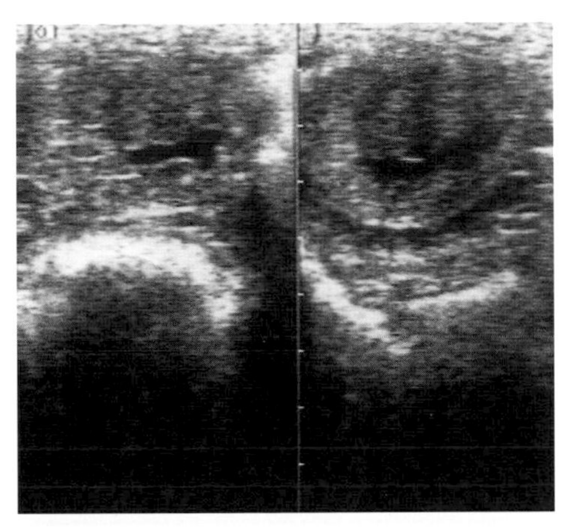

Figure 4.5

Two views of the uterus: (left) the body; and (right) one of the two horns. A small amount of fluid (dark areas) is present in both

Figure 4.6
A conceptus at 16 days after mating

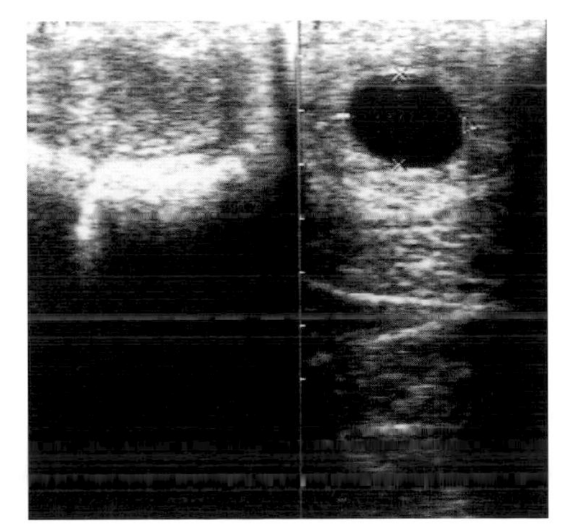

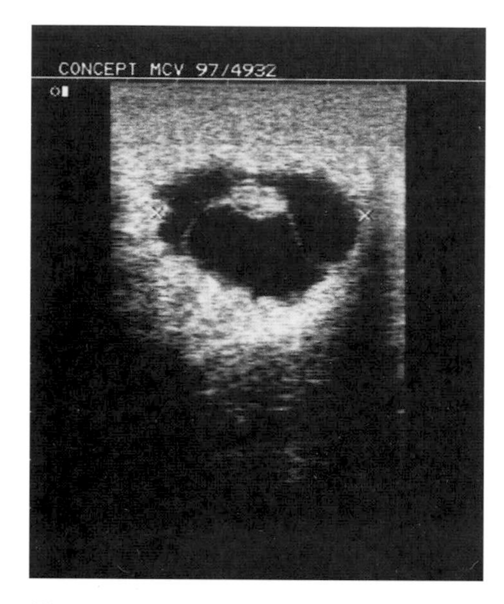

Figure 4.7

A conceptus at 33 days after mating

Figure 4.8

A conceptus at 41 days after mating

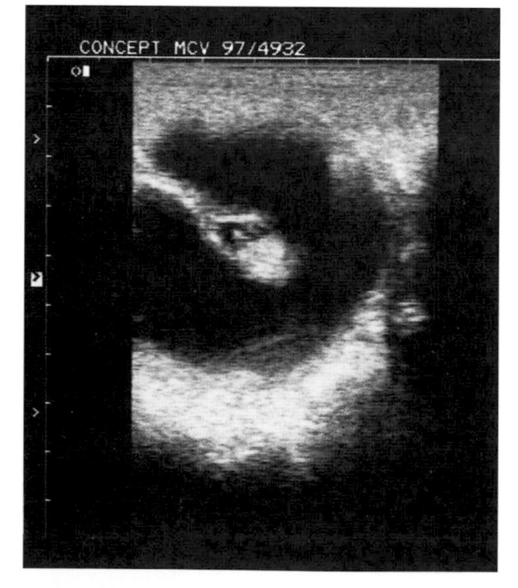

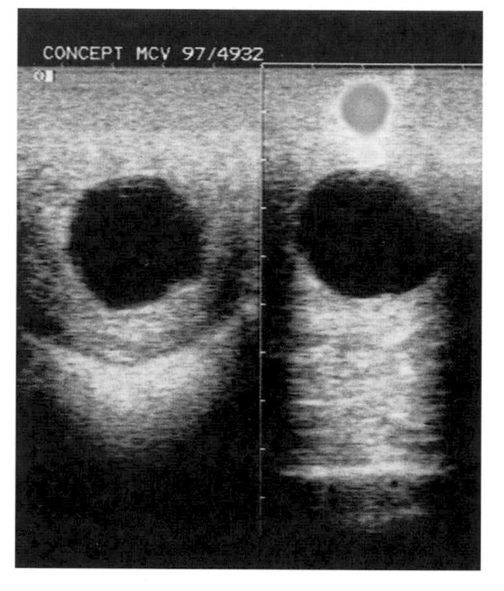

Figure 4.9

Twins present in the left and right horns of the uterus 16 days after mating. The dense object above that of the right horn is an artefact

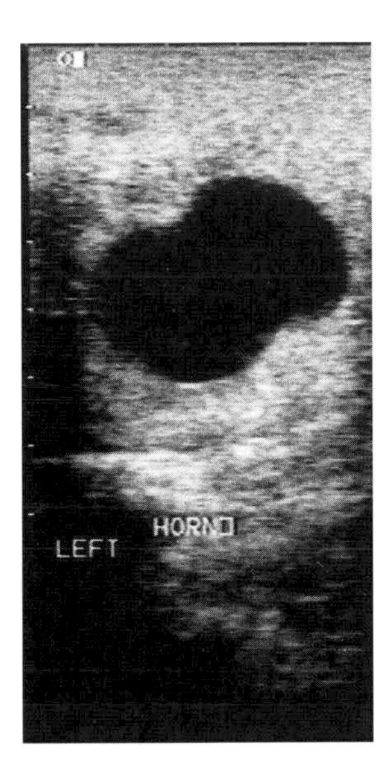

Figure 4.10

Twins lying together in the left horn of the uterus at 17 days after mating. These twins were successfully separated, one being eliminated by squeezing

avoidance of the problem of twins (see Figures 4.9 and 4.10).

In the days before echography was available for these examinations, 5 per cent of pregnancies recorded in Thoroughbreds involved twins; and these pregnancies ended in abortion or in foals that were undersized and frequently died at or shortly after birth.

With echography, the presence of a second fetal sac can be detected in the early stages (15 days from conception) and one or other of the fetal sacs eliminated by squeezing, in most cases. This has resulted in the elimination of the problem of twins and only very few are now carried into the later stages of pregnancy providing that their presence is monitored in the early stages by echography.

Of course, as with all measures of diagnosis and therapy involving biological systems, the situation is not entirely black and white or, in the case of twin avoidance, as simple as the statement just made. It is not always possible, for example, to distinguish the presence of twins at 15 days from conception. The major difficulty at this stage is the fact that the conceptus moves around the uterus (see Chapter Eight) and therefore one, or even both, fetal sacs may be missed during the scan, particularly in view of the fact that the sac is extremely small at this stage. It is therefore prudent to re-examine mares if they have been checked for pregnancy at 15 days, once or even twice more during the period 15–35 days of pregnancy. The larger sac and fetus itself, together with the presence of a heartbeat, make the re-examination increasingly accurate during this period.

The reason that 35 days is cited as being the upper end of the period is so that, in the breeding season, a mare may be re-mated if necessary before endometrial cups have formed (see Chapter Eight).

At 15 days pregnancy, the fetal sacs become fixed either in one of each uterine horns or both together in one horn (Figure 4.10). The approach to eliminating one or other of the sacs is the same for all circumstances of positioning; however, there is more risk of eliminating both if they happen to lie together and cannot be separated. The usual method of elimination is to squeeze the uterus between two fingers or to press the organ against the pelvic girdle over which the uterus lies.

The elimination is performed by the veterinary surgeon in a manner based on individual experience and preference both as to how the procedure is performed and the day or days on which it is attempted. When the fetal sac is mobile it may be possible to follow it to the tip of the uterine horn, otherwise it may not be possible to rupture the sac. When it becomes fixed it is much easier to perform this procedure, although on occasions it is necessary to repeat the attempts at 24 hour intervals as the tone and thickness of the uterine wall may play a role in the ease or otherwise of being successful; and conditions, in this respect, change quite considerably over a period of 24 hours.

CHAPTER FIVE

The Stallion

Breeding Organs

The genital organs (Figure 5.1) consist of two glands (testes) which are responsible for the male gametes (spermatozoa). To each testis is attached a structure, known as an epididymis, in which the sperm are stored. The epididymis is connected with a single tube (ductus or vas deferens) which in turn joins with its opposite number to form the urethra. This is a single duct providing a common outlet for urine and semen. Semen consists of spermatozoa together with fluids and substances secreted by the accessory sex glands.

Testes

The two testes are oval structures contained in folds of skin (scrotum). Each has flattened sides presenting two surfaces, two borders and two extremities. The free border is below and convex. The upper border is the one by which the testis is suspended in the scrotum and to which the epididymis and spermatic cord are attached.

In a mature stallion the testes measure about 10 cm x 5 cm x 4 cm in length, depth and breadth and weigh about 300 g. There is, however, considerable variation in testicular size between individuals. Size is roughly related to the capacity for producing sperm in any individual, although there is, in this respect, quite a wide variation and most stallions produce sufficient numbers of sperm to achieve good levels of fertility. It is only with respect to artificial insemination, where the ejaculate is split several times, that the size of the testis and its capacity for producing sperm becomes particularly important.

The left testis is usually larger than the right but not to any significant degree.

Each testis is covered by a strong fibrous capsule and the gland substance is soft and reddish-grey in colour. It is sub-divided into lobes by fibrous tissue and muscle and composed of minute tortuous tubes which, as they unite with other tubes of similar kind, form larger, straighter tubes (Figure 5.2). These converge toward the front part of the gland and pass through the tough fibrous coat to enter the epididymis.

The spermatozoa develop from round cells lining the coiled tubes of the gland. These round cells become elongated as they grow towards the central lumen of the tube in the centre of which are the fully-formed mature

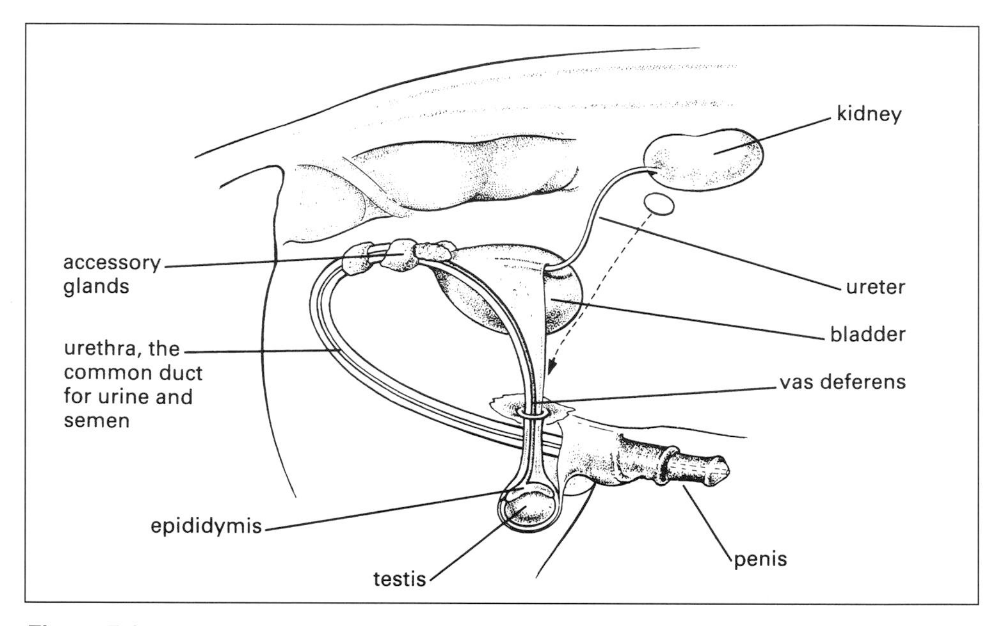

Figure 5.1

The stallion's genital organs (seen from the right side). The dotted line indicates the route taken by the testis in its descent from the abdomen to the scrotum

Figure 5.2

The testis, showing divisions into areas containing coiled tubes in which the sperm develop. Straighter tubes eventually enter the epididymis

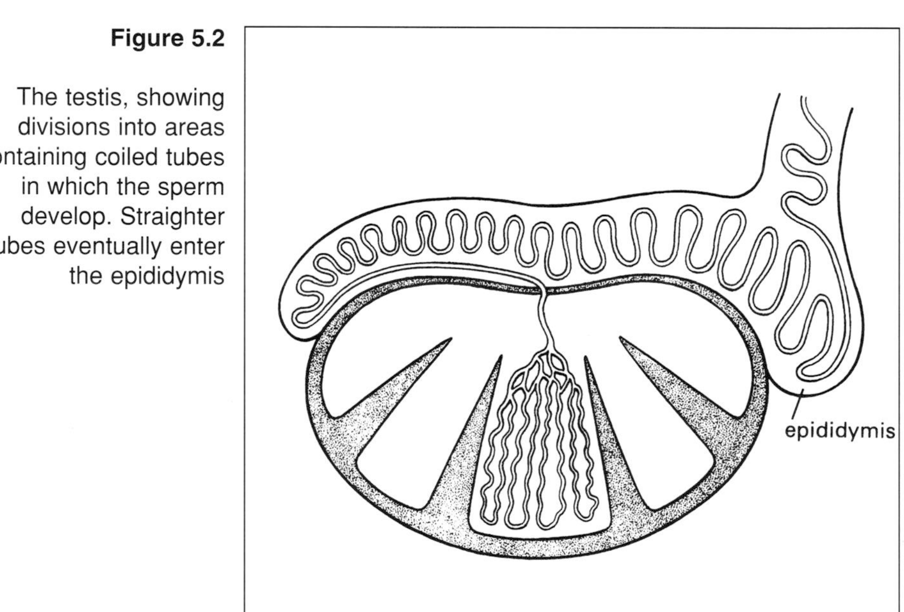

spermatozoa. On the outside of the tubes there are special cells (interstitial) which are responsible for the production of the hormone testosterone (Figure 5.3).

Descent of the testes

In the fetus the testes are found close to the kidneys but towards the end of pregnancy they migrate and pass through an opening in the abdominal muscles – the inguinal ring – and from there through a canal into the scrotum. The mechanical factors which bring about migration of the testes are largely unknown but increasing pressure of the abdominal contents may play a part.

In some cases one or, more rarely, both testes may fail to pass through the abdominal opening and are left inside the abdomen. Such a horse is known as a cryptorchid – colloquially, a 'rig'. The retained testis is usually small, thin, soft and not productive of sperm. However, the retention of one testis in the abdomen does not prevent the individual from being fertile, although it may be associated with aggressive behaviour. In some cases of hind limb lameness, the testis retained in the inguinal canal may be blamed and the individual therefore subjected to castration.

A testis frequently remains in the inguinal canal until the horse is three or four years of age, after which the testis completes its descent into the scrotum. This latter condition is not true cryptorchism but one of relatively late maturity. Once the abdominal ring closes, as it normally does soon after birth, only those testes which are already below the ring can enter into the scrotum. They otherwise become retained in the abdomen.

Epididymis

Each epididymis attached to the upper border of the testis stores the sperm

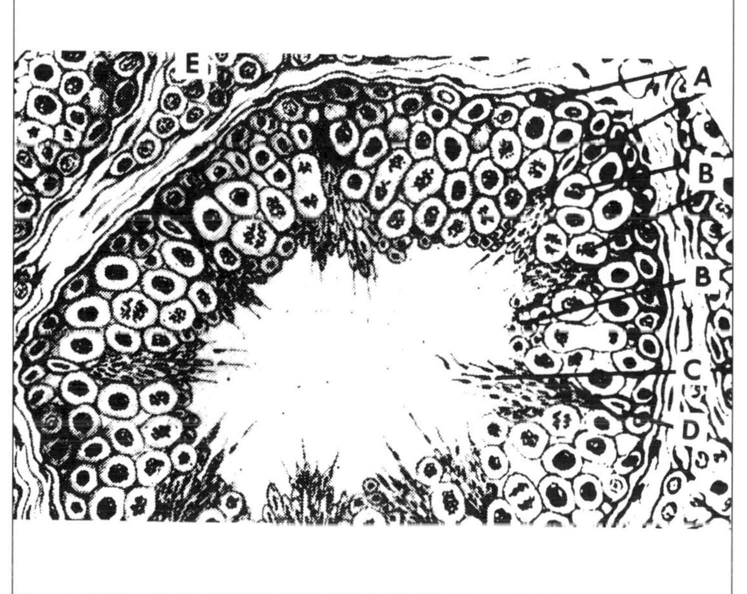

Figure 5.3

A section through the coiled tube of the testis. A and B are cells which are the precursors of sperm, C; D is a special cell (Sertoli) to which the sperm become attached before breaking loose and travelling in the tubes leading to the epididymis; E are intestinal cells which produce testosterone and consists of a head, a body and a tail. The head is composed of a dozen or more coiled tubes which unite to form a single tube known as the duct of the epididymis. This duct, with its complex coils, forms the body and tail of the epididymis and terminates in the ductus deferens along which the sperm are eventually transported to the urethra at the time of ejaculation.

Ejaculatory ducts

The ductus or vas deferens extends from the tail of the epididymis to the urethra. It ascends in the spermatic cord enclosed in the inguinal canal to the opening (inguinal ring) in the abdominal muscles. Here it runs backwards and towards the midline of the abdomen to the pelvic cavity. Each duct opens into the urethra close to its origin with the bladder and at a point beneath the prostate gland.

The urethra is a long tube which extends from the bladder to the glans penis. The duct can be divided into the pelvic and extra pelvic parts. In addition to the vas deferens it receives openings from the accessory sex glands. The urethra is enclosed in a layer of muscle which plays an important role in the ejaculation of semen and evacuation of urine.

The penis

The penis is the male organ of copulation, composed of erectile tissue enclosing the extra-pelvic part of the urethra. The glans penis is the enlarged free end of the organ and its base is surrounded by a prominent margin, the corona glandis, through which the end of the urethra projects for about 25 mm. The penis becomes erect when its veins become engorged with blood. The veins are arranged as relatively large spaces forming a network of vessels in the dorsal part of the penis.

The prepuce

The prepuce, popularly known as the sheath, is a 'pocketing' of the skin which covers the free portion of the penis when it is not erect. The skin of the prepuce contains a double fold so that there is an internal and external portion. The internal layers are hairless and supplied with large numbers of sebaceous glands which produce a fatty smegma, a continual secretion with a strong, unpleasant odour.

The spermatic cord

The spermatic cord consists of structures carried by the testis in its migration from the abdominal cavity to the scrotum. The cord contains arteries, veins, lymphatics, nerves, the vas deferens and the cremaster muscle which is capable of lifting the testis from the scrotum into the lower part of the inguinal canal.

The accessory glands

The accessory glands are the seminal vesicles, the prostate and bulbo-urethral glands.

The seminal vesicles

These two elongated sacs lie on either

side of the urethra close to its origin at the bladder. They are about 15 cm long and some 5 cm in diameter and each has a duct which opens into the urethra.

The prostate gland

Placed at the junction of the bladder and beginning of the urethra, into which it opens through about 15 ducts. The secretion of the prostate gland is milky in appearance.

The bulbo-urethral glands

There are two, situated one either side of the urethra. They are about 5 cm in length and each has about six to eight ducts which open into the urethra. The function of the accessory glands is to secrete seminal plasma.

Semen

Semen consists of spermatozoa and seminal plasma (see Figure 5.4). The average volume of ejaculate is 40 ml to 120 ml, containing some 100–150 million spermatozoa per cubic millimetre.

Spermatozoon

The spermatozoon (*pl. spermatozoa*) is the male sex cell (gamete). It is very different in character from the egg because it is a highly motile cell capable of swimming relatively great distances in

Figure 5.4

The constituents of semen (asterisks denote average values)

Volume of semen	40–120 ml
Number of sperm	100–150 million per cu mm
Abnormal spermatozoa (coiled tails and protoplasmic drops)	about 16%
pH	average – 7.330 pH units
Seminal plasma	
Specific gravity	1.012
Ergothioneine*	7.6 mg/100 ml
Citric acid*	26 mg/100 ml
Fructose*	15 mg/100 ml
Phosphorus*	17 mg/100 ml
Lactic acid*	12 mg/100 ml
Urea*	3 mg/100 ml

Figure 5.5

Diagram of a spermatozoon

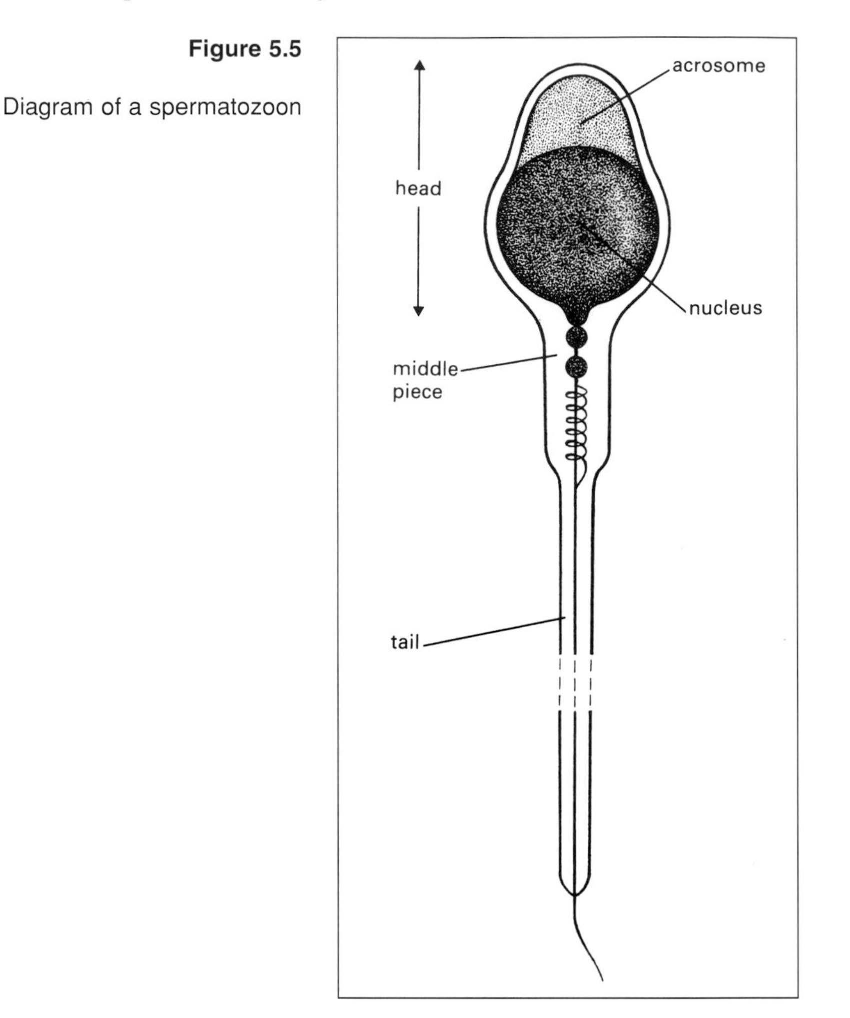

the female genital tract, seeking the egg and combining with it to achieve fertilisation. The spermatozoon is made up of a head, middle piece and tail (Figure 5.5). Its size is about one-hundredth that of the egg which is no more than the size of a grain of sand.

The head contains the nucleus which forms the greater part of this region and which is capped by the acrosome.

The sperm are formed by the multiplication of cells which line the coiled tubes in the testis. During this process of multiplication the number of chromosomes contained in the cell nucleus is reduced by half, the mature spermatozoon containing, therefore, half the amount of inherited material present in each body cell. At the time of fertilisation the egg supplies the other half to the new individual. Body cells are said to contain the diploid number of chromosomes and sex cells the haploid number; in the horse that is 64 and 32 chromosomes, respectively.

Seminal plasma

The exact function of seminal plasma is not known. It certainly provides a vehicle in which sperm may be carried into the uterus but once in this organ it is thought that the sperm separate from the plasma as they make their way to the fallopian tubes. It has been suggested that the plasma nourishes the sperm and even that it may eventually kill them off to prevent them from ageing. Sperm age rapidly, and it seems that the longer sperm reside in the female's genital tract before conception the greater the proportion of fetal abnormalities. This phenomenon has not been demonstrated in horses but is known to occur in other species.

The characteristic components of equine semen are fructose, ergothioneine, citric acid and sulfhydryl. The fructose content, considered so important in the semen of many species, is, in fact, scarce in that of stallions. The significance of this is not known. Some work has been carried out on the sulfhydryl content of plasma because this substance, present in highest concentration in the last portion of the ejaculate, is known to be toxic to sperm. Attempts have been made to correlate fertility with sulfhydryl content but the results have been inconclusive.

Seasonal variations in semen quality can be judged from the fact that citric acid, ergothioneine and the numbers of spermatozoa decrease from February to June and then show an increase. Ejaculate volume is low until April and increases greatly in May and June during which months the concentration of sperm may be increased.

Once in the uterus the spermatozoa (Figure 5.6) are moved passively, through uterine contractions, and actively swim to the opening of the fallopian tubes at the tips of each uterine horn. From here they travel up the tube to meet the egg which one of them will enter and fertilise.

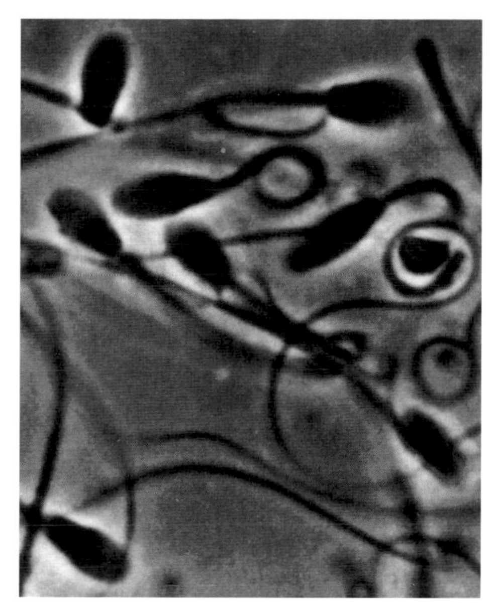

Figure 5.6

Highly-magnified equine spermatoza, some of which have straight and some coiled tails

The capacity of any semen sample to fertilise the egg decreases with the age of the sample. In practice it is reckoned that two days is an average period during which a horse can be fertile from a mating. Cases have, however, been recorded where fertilisation has occurred seven days after coitus.

In general the more dilute the semen sample, in terms of numbers of spermatozoa per millilitre, the less fertilising capacity it possesses and there is a critical point below which it entirely loses its fertility. It is curious that, although many million spermatozoa are placed in the uterus, there may be too few for the one that is required to achieve union with the egg. The reason may be that conception is a cumulative effect. For instance, spermatozoa are retained at the junction of the uterus and fallopian tube and travel up the tube in relatively small numbers. Then, before fertilisation can occur, the spermatozoa must remove the debris around the egg by secreting an enzyme known as hyaluronidase; the number of sperm required to achieve this is not known. In addition, the sperm have to go through a process of ripening (capacitation) before they are capable of fertilising the egg. If for any reason they do not undergo this ripening process the number of live active sperm in a semen sample is not related to their fertilising power.

Some stallions' semen seems to lose its fertilising power more quickly than others. A great deal more research is necessary before we can understand why this is so or whether there are measures we can take to improve matters in any particular case.

As far as individual mares are concerned, conditions in the uterus are likely to influence the fertilising power of the semen. Infection and perhaps immune reactions between the mare's cells and spermatozoa are two major considerations. Again, more research is required before we can understand and overcome these problems.

Hormonal Control

The production of sperm and the sexual behaviour of the stallion are controlled by hormones secreted by the pituitary and testes. The pituitary hormones (FSH and LH) are similar to those produced by the same gland of the mare. FSH stimulates the growth and formation of spermatozoa in the testes while LH causes the interstitial cells to liberate testosterone into the bloodstream. Testosterone promotes the male characteristics and sexual drive (libido).

The activity of the pituitary tends to vary with the seasons and it is affected by the amount of daylight just as is the case with the mare. The quality of semen and sexual drive of the stallion is thus greatest during late spring and summer which coincides with the natural breeding season.

Management of the Stallion

Stallions are the heart of any public stud and the quality of their progeny directly affects the profitability and reputation of the studfarm itself. The stabling and care they receive is of the highest level; often they are housed in purpose-built stallion units and have individual paddocks.

All stallions regardless of their breed, their background, or the number of mares they are to cover, require individual and experienced care. The performance and fertility of a stallion is affected directly by the way that he is managed both before and during the breeding season, especially as the stallion that is housed and handled during the mating procedure is subjected to a very artificial environment; this alone can affect his sexual behaviour to a variable degree. Reducing these effects on each individual stallion is an important part of stud management. On Thoroughbred studfarms, the stallion is often cared for by a full-time handler.

In such cases a considerable rapport can be established – in some cases a stallion handler can care for his/her stallion for upwards of 15 years.

Thoroughbred breeding is restricted by Jockey Club regulations to natural service only. The ruling states that the foal must be conceived by natural mating of the mare with the stallion and not by any other means, otherwise the resulting offspring cannot be registered as a Thoroughbred. Performance and pony breeds are not restricted by such rulings so the use of artificial insemination, as well as embryo transfer, is becoming increasingly commonplace. These methods are discussed in more detail later.

In the case of the non-Thoroughbred stallion, it is quite common for competing and other activities to continue throughout the stud career. However, due to the structure of racing and the extraordinary value of most Thoroughbred stallions, it is more normal for the horse to be retired to stud and not to continue to race.

Seasonal Breeding

As with the mare, the stallion is known to be seasonally active. Most stallions show some interest in mares out of season; however, they are generally slow to arousal and may produce reduced quantities of sperm and require several mounts before ejaculating. The stallion may be required to start mating during a period of reduced libido and when the mare is subject to erratic oestrous patterns. The use of lighting as discussed with regard to the management of mares can be effective and is commonly practised by most studfarms that have to start the breeding season early.

Stallion Evaluation

There are many important factors that affect the stallion's value as a sire. Perhaps the most important factor is that of genetic potential. Most breeders are looking for a sire that can pass on his own ability ideally to produce offspring that maintain or improve the quality of a breeding herd. This might be athletic ability, performance or conformation. A stallion that is able to fulfil these criteria with the majority of his offspring is not only valuable to the breed, but also valuable to the studfarm for economic reasons. Breeders often judge a stallion by his phenotype (physical appearance), but it is the genotype (genetic conformation) that is most important as it is the genes that are transmitted that dictate success, or otherwise, of his progeny. This is best judged as the conformation and performance of his offspring.

The stallion's ability to perform well at stud is governed by his physical condition, most importantly the condition of his reproductive organs. All stallions that are being assessed with a view to a career at stud will be examined by a veterinary surgeon, particularly those that are being sold as stud horses.

With Thoroughbreds the purchase price of the horse is such that careful and detailed physical evaluation of the stallion is carried out – sometimes by more than one veterinary surgeon and nearly always also by a practitioner for an insurance company. It is common today for a stallion to be insured against such risks as first-season infertility; this would provide cover for the new purchasers against the stallion being unable to cover in his first season due to factors such as injury or disease. The financial losses that could potentially be incurred to the purchaser, as an individual or as a syndicate, normally outweigh the enormous premiums attached to such policies.

Physical examinations include assessing the stallion's genital organs in detail – the size, shape and symmetry of the genital organs is evaluated and an experienced practitioner can soon identify possible congenital defects that would preclude the stallion from stud duties. For example: the penis will be examined, normally by stimulating the horse to become aroused with a mare. External signs of injury, growths or sores will be checked for, as well as the horse's ability to produce and maintain an erection. However, it is not common for the stallion's fertility to be checked by taking a semen sample at this stage and, generally, the stallion is sold with the proviso that no guarantee is made or inferred regarding fertility – hence one of the reasons for the provision of first-season infertility insurance if desired. For a stallion who has not been at stud before and, therefore, not mated before, a semen sample would not necessarily be indicative of his fertility potential. The ejaculate produced would contain many 'old' sperm and this could provide a false negative; also some stallions have excellent fertility levels and yet have a relatively high degree of defective sperm in each ejaculate.

During the assessment of the stallion, careful note is also taken of his physical ability to cover a mare – if he is to retire to stud following an injury, it is possible that this may affect his long-term physical health and mobility. If he has suffered a spinal injury or has a long-term lameness or limb weakness, then he does not have long-term potential as a stallion.

Physical fitness is essential for a breeding stallion. Although most stallions retire from active competition when going to stud, it is still important that the stallion is kept fit and physically active.

The stallion's temperament should also be evaluated, remembering that in a natural state the stallion would have to behave in a very masculine way to ensure maintenance of his herd and his status. However, temperament alone may be a vital factor on certain studfarms – if the stallion is to be used for mainly artificial insemination then he must be tractable enough to permit samples to be taken regularly, perhaps also to mate using a 'phantom' mare. A stallion that is savage with his mares and/or with his handler is a liability to all concerned and, although horses like this are very rare, consideration would have to be given to his usefulness at stud.

Training for Breeding

It is important that the stallion is correctly prepared for his role in the breeding shed. Poor or rough handling will result in a horse that may be reluctant to behave appropriately with his mares, costing the stud not only a great deal of time but also a great deal of money if he is unable to get his mares in foal.

Even though the horse has been domesticated for many years, the artificial environment on most studfarms can cause management problems if consideration is not given to the stallion's instinctive behaviour. Experienced stallion handlers generally establish a combination of respect and quiet discipline with their charges. For a young stallion during his first season there may be several problems to overcome. Take the young colt who has been in training as a racehorse since he was a yearling; he will have been trained not to be distracted by the young fillies stabled or ridden near to him. Sometimes colts are disciplined for displaying sexual behaviour when in training and this can be a problem to be overcome. The first few times the stallion is brought to his mares he should be encouraged to behave as a stallion, although he may be nervous of the handler's reaction. Rough handling at this stage will only serve to confuse the horse further. Experienced stud staff will tend to allow the young horse to tease mares regularly for the first few weeks to gain confidence and they will also endeavour to choose a quiet matronly mare for the stallion's first cover.

Any horse going to stud for the first time, whether male or female, benefits from a period to 'let down' prior to the season's start. This is of particular importance with a horse retiring from high levels of performance such as racing or eventing as there is a significant difference between breeding condition and that required for top-level performance. The stallion has a chance to adjust to his new surroundings and daily routine – stallions tend to thrive on the security of a daily routine.

Exercise for the Thoroughbred stallion will normally be in the form of free exercise grazing in a paddock, lungeing and walking in-hand and ridden work. Walking in-hand on a daily basis can be very beneficial for a young stallion if he is led around the stud itself and becomes accustomed to the sight of mares around him. Properly exercised stallions tend to be more relaxed with their mares and more consistent in the breeding shed. The amount and type of exercise will depend on the stallion's temperament and physical condition. Some stallions, when turned out to graze, relentlessly pace their boundaries and become quite distressed – weight loss can be as damaging to fertility as obesity. A horse like this needs to be turned out for only short periods each day – although some will settle if provided with a companion in a paddock nearby. Whichever form of exercise is chosen it should most importantly suit the stallion as well as the routine of the studfarm.

One of the most significant aspects of routine stud management is reducing the risk of infection to all the horses and, due to his role, particularly the stallion. The annual tests and examinations for each stallion are discussed in more detail later, but high standards of hygiene are essential. A successful stallion may mate directly, or indirectly, by insemination, in excess of 100 mares on a commercial studfarm – any illness will significantly affect his fertility as well as that of any mare that he may cover if he is infectious. As the breeding season in many cases is very short, any period of time that the stallion is unable to mate can precipitate considerable losses to a commercial farm.

Safety and Housing

As already mentioned, most studfarms have specially designed areas for their stallions. Although the natural environment would be one of spacious plains to graze and lush vegetation, this has to be compromised for the domestic horse. In the wild the horse would graze continually, moving to new areas that would be relatively uninfected and clean – such provision is nearly always impractical or impossible to provide. Stables are unnatural to any horse; however, with a good level of stable management, most adapt well to this environment. Some studfarms have a large stable for the horse with an adjoining paddock that can be accessed directly from the stable. This provides perhaps the best compromise for the horse and is normally possible on most studfarms. Other studfarms have a stallion unit away from the stallion paddocks and the horses are led to their grazing each day. High-class Thoroughbred studfarms provide palatial housing for their stallions. The units are designed specifically to ease the management of the stallions at all times of the year and to make a high level of stable hygiene possible. There may be covered walkways to the breeding shed, rubber-floored display areas for visitors to view the stallions and security cameras to monitor the wellbeing of each individual housed there. Stallions spend much time in looseboxes and it is essential that these should have high standards of air hygiene – that is, good ventilation and first-class, dust-free bedding. The same need for minimal dust applies to hay fed to the horse. Poor air hygiene may increase the risks of asthmatic type conditions developing, followed by infective bronchiolitis.

As with all housing and fencing, the environment itself should be as safe as possible for the horse. Stallions may be more active in their boxes than mares and the stable itself should be large enough to reduce the risk of injury. Strong fittings and locks are essential to avoid the risk of the horse accidently escaping from his stable. The fencing for stallion paddocks is generally higher than that for a gelding or mare, again to avoid the risk of escape. As stallions tend to be territorial, the paddock designated for each should be kept ungrazed by other horses. Stallions have a very highly-developed sense of smell and scenting is an important part of their behaviour. The smell of other horses in his paddock can cause him to become upset and possibly aggressive if he feels that his territory has been infringed.

Safety when handling a stallion is of prime importance. A handler who is afraid of the horse is as damaging as one who is overly rough. An experienced handler will spend time with each new stallion getting to know him and what to expect from him. It is important not to forget the potential of a stallion and not to be blasé about his temperament. Stallions react much more strongly and quite differently from geldings or mares in a variety of situations and it is vital that the safety of the horse and his handler is not forgotten at any time. Specific reference to safety when teasing and breeding is discussed later.

Whether the stallion costs just a few hundreds of pounds or several hundreds of thousands, his needs as a horse are the same. Care and consideration at all levels of his management will help to produce a horse that is relaxed, secure and successful at his job.

Mating

There are three main methods of breeding horses: free, or paddock, breeding; in-hand; and artificial insemination.

Each studfarm will have its own breeding methods and each will have advantages and disadvantages. It is important to consider certain factors, such as the breed of horse, the number of mares to be mated each year – both visiting and permanent residents – the number of stallions and the facilities that are available on that particular studfarm.

Most breed societies permit the use of artificial insemination and embryo transfer. This allows completely different procedures to be used and presents a total contrast in management techniques to those demanded by natural conception methods.

The Thoroughbred, however, must be conceived by natural methods and the use of artificial insemination or embryo transfer has always been completely prohibited. This ruling, made for both political and economic reasons, makes managing a Thoroughbred stallion somewhat more complex, but the traditional methods practised are successful and the fertility percentages remain as high as those achieved by current artificial techniques.

The economics of most commercial studfarms demand the most efficient and effective use of the stallion in order to maximise production and minimise cost and risks. However, the artificial environment in which stallions are kept may not always guarantee the same rates of fertility as those achieved by horses breeding in the feral state, even in this time of advanced veterinary care and procedures, if not carefully monitored.

Free, or paddock, breeding

In the wild, horses would mate in a completely natural environment. By allowing a stallion to run free with a group of his mares in a large paddock, the domestic version of the wild state can be produced. It is important that the area is large enough to allow natural breeding behaviour. Ideally, the grazing should be of sufficient quality so that concentrate feeds are not required. The paddock should be situated so that the stallion is not too close to other horses in different paddocks and access to and from the paddock should be carefully considered.

If the mares are to remain in the paddock all year round then it must be suitable for foaling as well. If the mares are to be moved to another area for foaling, then this too needs consideration. This method is commonly used with pony breeds, such as New Forest and Welsh Mountain. These ponies run wild for the majority of the year and are rounded up and penned only for very short periods. The stallion observes the mare's behaviour and periods of courtship are common before mating occurs. The stallion appears to be aware of the optimum time for mating the mare and high levels of fertility can be maintained. The importance of using healthy horses for such a form of breeding cannot be over-emphasised. If one mare has a reproductive infection then it will be transmitted to the whole herd. This may not only affect the health of the horses, but also, in the long term, affect fertility rates.

Introducing a young stallion to this type of breeding can be time consuming, especially if he is nervous. There are many ways to overcome this, but if time allows, putting him in a paddock with just one mare and then gradually increasing the numbers can be of assistance. He must learn that he cannot approach every mare as she may not be receptive; there will be times when he will need to learn this the hard way. Even with an experienced stallion there is a risk of serious injury during the initial adjustment period.

Careful observation of the herd should be practised regularly to try to establish which mares may be in foal. Some stallions may resent this and, although rare, aggressive stallions can be unsuitable for such a breeding programme.

The number of mares that can be safely kept with a stallion varies with the individual stallion's fertility and libido. The production rates from this form of breeding may not vary that much from those produced by breeding in-hand, but in a truly wild state the fertility rates are normally close to 100 per cent.

The studfarm that practises this form of breeding may find that visiting mare owners are reluctant to allow their mares to join the herd as the risk of injury is so high. As with any other group of horses, the social structure is strong and new members being introduced can result in quite aggressive behaviour. The submissive mare that is likely to have a low status in such a herd can be badly injured by more dominant mares; dominant mares are perhaps unsuitable for such management practices.

There are many disadvantages with this form of breeding; most significantly, it is impossible to protect the stallion and/or mare from injury. This factor alone makes this method impracticable for most studfarms. The enormous value of stallions means that risk of injury must be reduced by every means possible. Most studfarms would not have the facilities to run a stallion with their mares, especially if they stand more than one stallion. This type of breeding, therefore, remains common only with wild herds such as the New Forest and with some types of pony studfarm.

Furthermore, it is also almost impossible to be certain about when the mare was mated and most breed societies require a date of mating for registration purposes. However, although the disadvantages are many, there are advantages to this method of breeding. When the correct environment is established, the behaviour and interaction of the mares and the stallion without management related stress can reduce the number of normal problems with breeding such as irregular oestrous cycles in mares. The economic advantages are also obvious. There is no need for extensive stabling and enclosed breeding areas and the necessary maintenance costs are also eliminated. If the horses are of a type that can live out all year without supplementary feeding and the grazing is of sufficient quality, then massive savings can be made on feed and forage costs. The other immediate saving is that of labour costs. There is no need for large numbers of staff to care for and handle the horses, as all of the usual procedures of teasing, vetting and stabling are removed.

The significant advantages of such a breeding programme, over closely managed practices, may be particularly useful for a studfarm that is breeding small numbers of mares each year and if those mares are of a breed type that permits registration on such a basis.

Breeding in-hand

Breeding in-hand is by far the most common breeding method used on commercial studfarms. This involves the stallion being led on a bridle to his mare and being held the whole time that he is mating with the mare. The mare is also held by one or two attendants. Normally the mating is performed in a specially designed area or breeding barn.

The immediate advantage to this method is that the risk of injury to either mare of stallion is reduced dramatically. The stallion is brought only to mares that are in full oestrus and usually the mare is at the optimum point in her cycle for conception to occur. Accordingly, any problems with fertility, mare or stallion, can be closely monitored and dealt with accordingly.

With this method, the management of each stallion can be fine-tuned and special practices can be developed for each individual as required. However, it should be remembered that, as already mentioned, this method is extremely artificial and fertility rates can sometimes be dramatically affected by poor management. In-hand breeding allows for more efficient use of the stallion and avoids 'wasted' matings, which cannot be avoided with methods such as paddock breeding; also, the exact date and status of the mare when she was mated can be recorded. This means that she can be examined early for pregnancy and mated again if this was unsuccessful.

However, without proper management, breeding in-hand can result in the over-use of a stallion, especially if he is bred from early in the season. In-hand breeding does limit the number of mares that a stallion can cover during the breeding season, compared to insemination. However, this rarely presents a problem unless he is in very high demand and/or if he has a low libido.

Artificial insemination

Artificial insemination is becoming more common as the method of breeding. The ejaculate from the stallion is collected using an artificial vagina and the sample is used either whole, or split into 10–20 separate samples, for insemination into the mare or several mares. Artificial insemination and embryo transfer are discussed later.

The main advantage of using this method is that collections can be made at any time of the day and stored for later insemination. The mares do not need to travel to the stallion and can be kept on their home studfarm. It is now common for semen to be shipped globally for use anywhere in the world. This extends not only the availability of stallions but, therefore, also extends the gene pool available for selection by breeders. With competition horses, this method is particularly useful. Stallions do not have to stop competing for a period each year and many become so used to the collection procedure that it can be performed quickly either weekly, daily or whenever required with minimal interruption to their training programme.

Carefully managed, this procedure eliminates the risk of injury to both the stallion and the mare and, most importantly, it should eliminate the risk of disease. The stallion should be subject to the same tests as if he was to mate with each mare naturally; this ensures that the ejaculate he produces is free from pathogens that could be transferred to the mare.

Breeding Facilities

There are many types of facilities used for breeding in-hand, but there are several factors that should be considered when designing an area for such a purpose.

If the breeding area is to be enclosed, most commonly an indoor school or barn-type structure is allocated for breeding, it is important that it has two entrances, one for the stallion and one for the mare. It should be reasonably dust-free to minimise contamination of the mare's or the stallion's genitalia. The flooring should be non-slip. Many studfarms use rubber flooring which has many advantages; it is totally non-slip, dust-free and it can be thoroughly washed. The use of wood chip is also common, but this tends to need regular damping to avoid becoming too dusty. The flooring should also cushion a fall.

The location of the breeding area should be away from the heart of the studfarm so that distractions are kept to a minimum. The proximity of the stallion's box should also be considered.

On many studfarms, the breeding shed is located close to the stallion yard and special loading ramps are kept for mares being boxed in for service only (walking-in).

Ideally there should be an area set aside for the preparation of the mare. A set of veterinary stocks is very useful with hot and cold water also supplied to the area, ideally with a shower attachment which enables quick and efficient preparation of the mare.

The surface of the breeding area should provide for a size difference between the stallion and his mares as this can cause considerable difficulty. Normally there is a pit, a mound or platform to help the stallion if he is mating with a mare that is much taller or shorter than he is.

Preparing the Mare and Stallion for Mating

The stallion is brought to the breeding area in his usual bridle and a long lead rein. Some stallions become more boisterous when going to the breeding barn and a stronger bit may be necessary to ensure adequate control is maintained at all times (Figures 5.7–5.8).

It used to be common for the stallion's genitalia to be washed extensively prior to mating. This practice is now considered unnecessary and, in fact, it can be detrimental. Washing the genitalia can remove the natural protective bacteria that are present and allow a secondary infection to proliferate. It can also cause soreness of the sensitive skin covering both the penis and the testes. Some types of soaps and washes are also known to be spermicidal.

The most important factor of all when preparing the stallion for mating is safety. Each attendant present in the breeding barn should fully understand the covering procedure and should be experienced enough to carry out each step calmly and attentively. If problems occur, carefully planned emergency procedures can prevent horses and handlers from being seriously hurt. Appropriate actions should be studied as carefully as that of the covering procedure itself. The area used for breeding should be safe for this purpose with adequate space for both the horses and their handlers, especially in case of an emergency. For this reason, only the stud staff involved with mating should be permitted into the breeding area; on most high-quality studfarms there is a

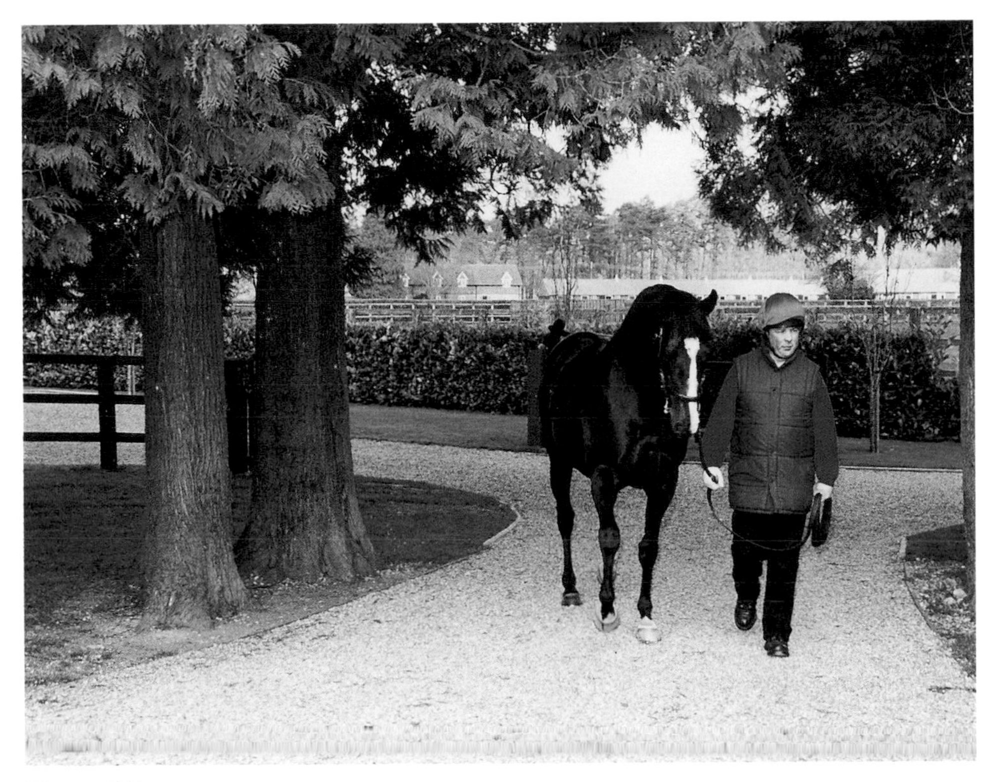

Figure 5.7

A stallion being led to the breeding area. The stallion is led using a bridle and long rein. Note also the handler's hard hat – an essential item of safety equipment in the breeding area

specially designed breeding barn with a viewing area or gallery for visitors.

It is normal for a stallion to be allowed to tease his mare for a brief period prior to the actual mating. This encourages him to 'draw' – extend the penis and produce an erection. Most breeding barns have a teasing board for this purpose, normally of the type that can be folded back out of the way for mating, although some managements may like to tease the mare prior to entering the breeding barn.

The length of time required for each stallion to produce an erection varies enormously. Some need no time at all and others may require as long as ten minutes. Normally it will be the young stallion that requires a longer period of stimulation. Treating each stallion as an individual is very important at every stage in his management, but at no time more so than in the breeding barn. Some stallions can be permanently affected by thoughtless actions during this time. A stallion that is slow or reluctant to arousal can be a frustration not only to the stud manager and his staff, but also to the mare owner. Stallions with this type of problem,

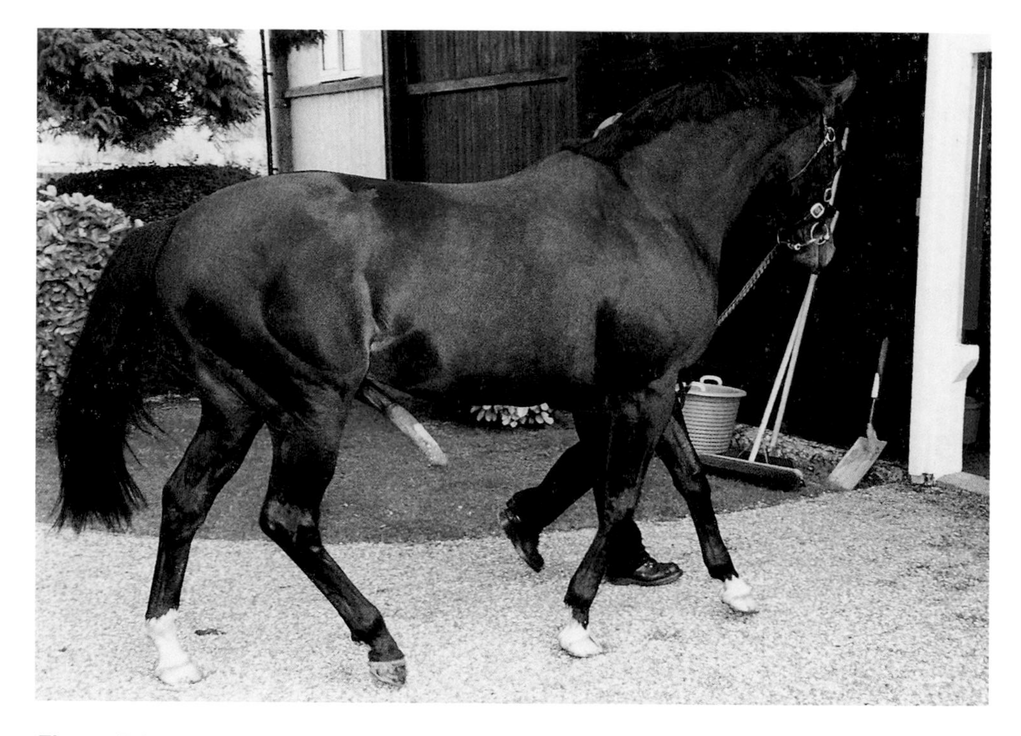

Figure 5.8

Stallions often become aroused just by being brought towards the breeding area

whether it is physical or psychological, are very time consuming and may produce very poor fertility rates each season.

In the wild state, the stallion has a period of courtship with his mares, which can be quite extended. This allows him to be certain of her sexual state and to mate with her only at the correct time. In the domestic environment this behaviour is removed and the stallion is only allowed to be near to mares that we have chosen for him – no wonder that commonly there are problems at this time!

The mare is normally prepared prior to her being teased by the stallion (Figure 5.9). She will also be led in a bridle with a long lead rein or reins. Mares are washed with plain water before mating; this helps to remove any faeces that may have contaminated her vulval area. She will then have a tail bandage put on to keep her tail hairs away from the stallion's penis (Figure 5.10).

Once she is led into the breeding barn and positioned correctly, she will have hind kicking boots put on. These boots are specially designed for this purpose only and are normally made of thick felt or leather. The boots completely cover her hind feet and should fit securely so that they do not slip or come off should she kick. Maiden mares being covered for the first time may become upset at the sensation of these boots and may need to be walked

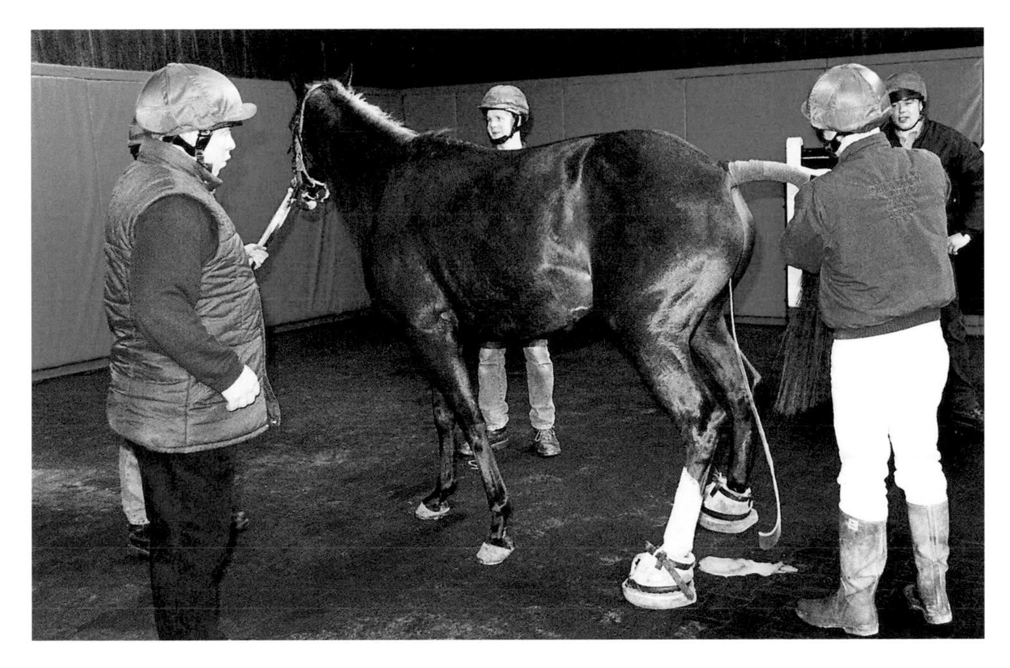

Figure 5.9 The mare is prepared for mating. The breeding area is designed specifically for mating and has a non-slip rubber floor, padded walls and a teasing area

Figure 5.10 The mare has a tail bandage put on and wears thick felt covering boots. The tail bandage is disposable for hygiene

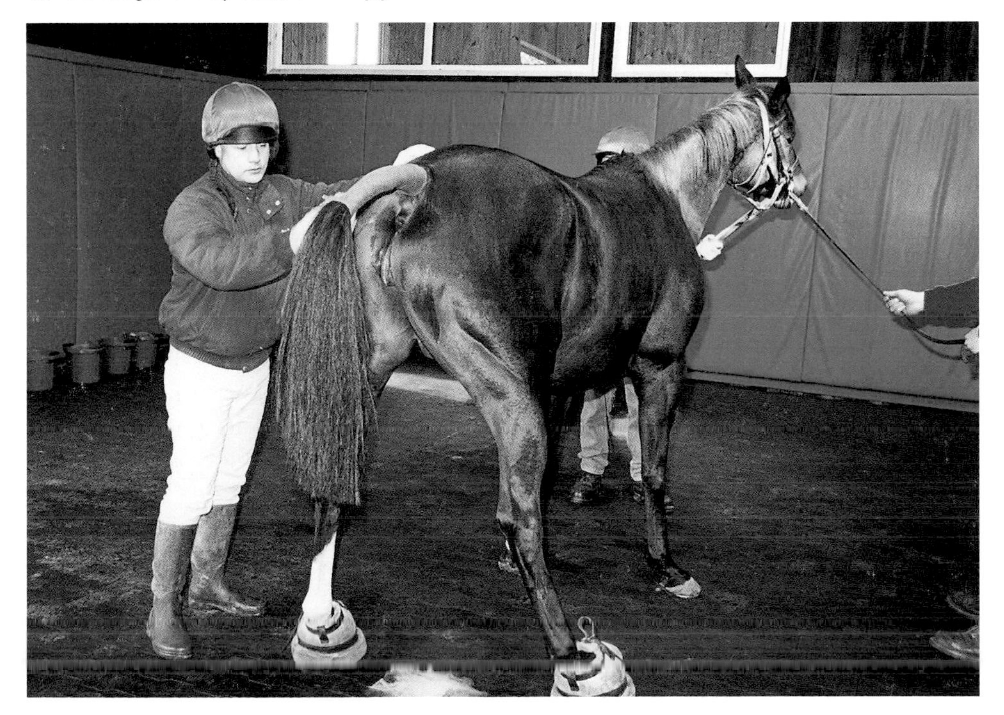

around a few times to accustom themselves. A point to mention here is that no mare should be covered with hind shoes except in exceptional circumstances, as even with the boots on she can inflict considerable, possibly permanent, damage to a stallion.

Some studfarms like to use a cape or neck rope for their stallions. The cape covers the mare's neck and fastens underneath. This is normally made of leather or thick canvas. Generally, neck capes are used with stallions known to bite or savage their mares during mating – the cape is purely protective but can be useful to give further grip to a young inexperienced stallion. The neck rope is used for similar reasons; basically, it is a thick padded neck strap that some stallions like to catch hold of with their teeth during mating. The use of equipment like this will vary depending on the needs of each individual stallion and may not be necessary at all. Again, some young nervous mares may need a little time to become used to the feeling of a neck cape.

It is common for a mare to be twitched during mating to ensure that she remains calm and still. Twitches should really only be applied at the last minute before the stallion approaches, especially if the stallion is known to be slow to cover and they should be removed as soon as it is safe to do so once the stallion has dismounted. The mare's attendant normally holds both her reins and the twitch, but if two attendants are used then one can hold the twitch handle and the other the reins (Figure 5.11).

The use of hind leg hobbles is not

Figure 5.11

The mare ready for mating, with attendants at either side of the head. The attendant to the mare's hindquarters will hold her tail out of the way when the stallion mounts

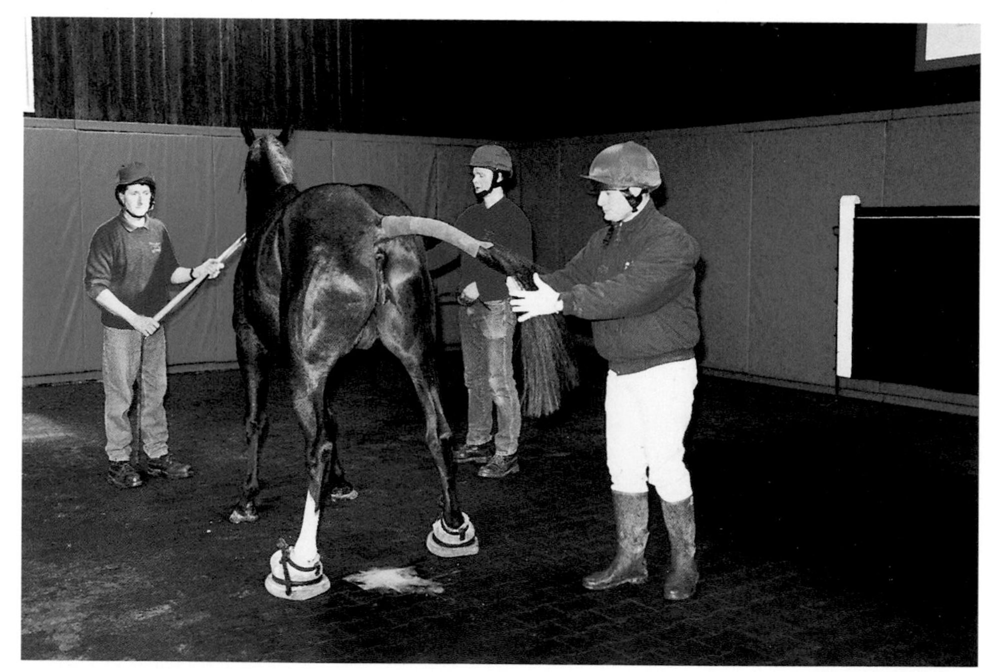

nearly as common as it once was. If a mare is correctly prepared and is in full oestrus, the use of hobbles is unnecessary. Hobbles can be dangerous if used by inexperienced handlers and can cause the mare to fall. However, a strap to hold up one front leg is common. This is generally used to stop the mare from moving forward when the stallion is mounting. Once the stallion has penetrated the mare, her leg should be released to allow her some movement with the stallion. If the stallion has a large penis, the mare should be permitted to take a few steps forward as he thrusts into her, as this will help to avoid her cervix becoming bruised during mating.

A breeding roll may be used when a large stallion is mating with a small mare. This breeding roll is a large, normally leather covered, padded cylinder with a handle at one end. It is held between the buttocks of the mare and the stallion's hind legs to stop him from thrusting too deeply into her. It is essential to avoid the mare's cervix being damaged in any way during mating as this can directly affect her chances of conception, possibly permanently.

Tranquillisers may be used in the case of a particularly difficult or nervous mare. However, this may lead to a deceptive state in which an apparently tranquil individual wakes up with the movement of the stallion resulting in traumatic consequences.

Mating

Once the stallion is stimulated, it is important that he is allowed to mate with the mare as soon as possible. If brought to her too early he may not have managed to produce enough of an erection to penetrate; if he is brought to her after too long a period, he may have lost interest.

The stallion handler normally brings the stallion up to the mare's left side at an angle of about 45° (Figure 5.12). Inexperienced horses may sometimes try to mount immediately from the rear, but mounting from slightly to the side reduces the risk of the stallion being kicked. The stallion should be encouraged to approach the mare as calmly as possible. Stallions that rush and jump at their mares will nearly always end up being injured by a kick from the mare, as well as terrifying the handlers. If the mare is aware of the stallion's approach, she will usually show her receptiveness by squatting and 'winking', as well as leaning towards him as he mounts her.

The mare handlers should stand to either side of her head and just in front of her shoulders, although sometimes only one handler is used for the mare. This handler is responsible for restraining the mare and must ensure that the mare can see the stallion approach. The mare's handler must be ready to move out of the way should the mare or stallion strike; he should also be ready to move the mare if necessary.

The stallion handler should stand to the stallion's left side and must maintain control of the stallion at all times. Once the stallion has mounted the mare, his handler will stand to the side and ensure that the lead does not become caught in the stallion's legs as he moves on the mare.

There is normally another attendant, usually the stud manager or stallion manager, who stands to the right side of the mare and holds the mare's tail out of the stallion's way as he mounts. This attendant may also need to guide the stallion's penis at the time of penetration. This should always be done with

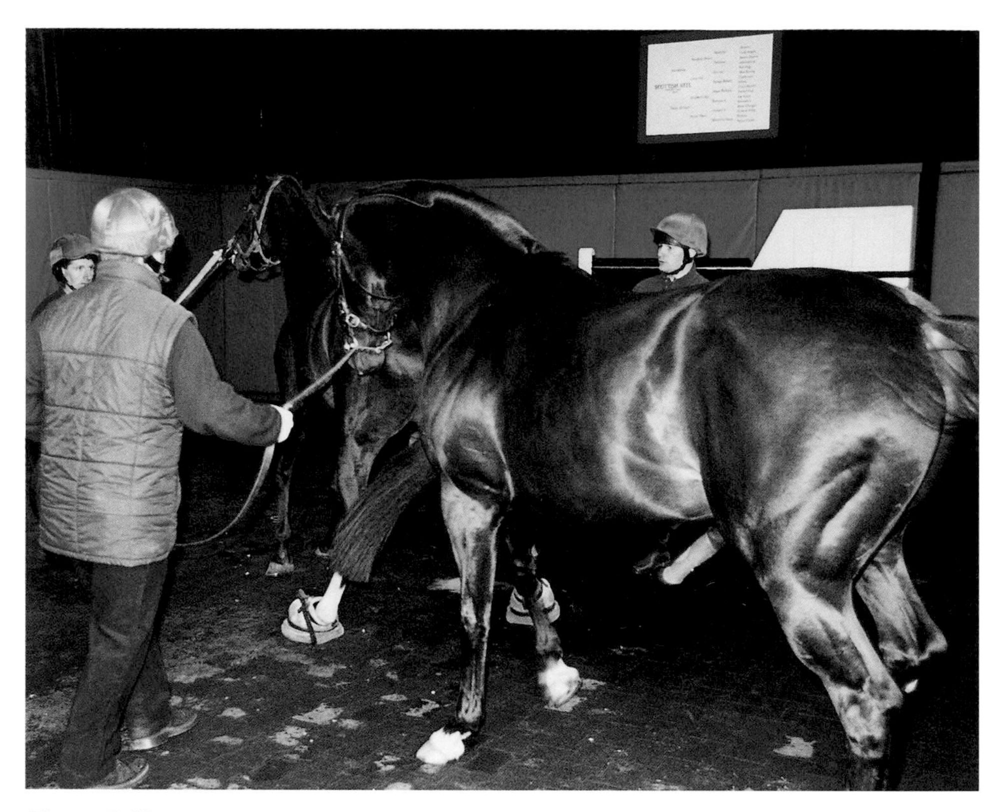

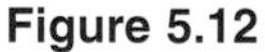

Figure 5.12

The stallion is led up to the mare's left side at an angle of about 45 degrees

gloves on for hygiene. This attendant is also responsible for feeling the pulse along the base of the penis when the stallion ejaculates. It should be noted that excessive handling of the stallion's penis or legs at this stage may cause the stallion to become discouraged and nearly all stallions resent too much interference.

The number of thrusts required before ejaculation is reached varies between stallions and may also be dependent on the time of the breeding season. The actual mating lasts on average about one minute but it may be as short as 30 seconds, or as long as five minutes. Ejaculation occurring causes the stallion's tail to flag and can be assessed by an attendant placing a hand along the base of the penis (Figure 5.13); pulsing of the fluid can be felt along the urethra (at the base of the underside of the penis).

Once ejaculation has occurred the stallion should be allowed to remain on the mare for a few seconds; normally he will dismount when he is ready to do so. The mare should be turned to her left to prevent her from possibly kicking out at the stallion as he dismounts. The stallion should be backed and turned away from the mare. A quick dismount

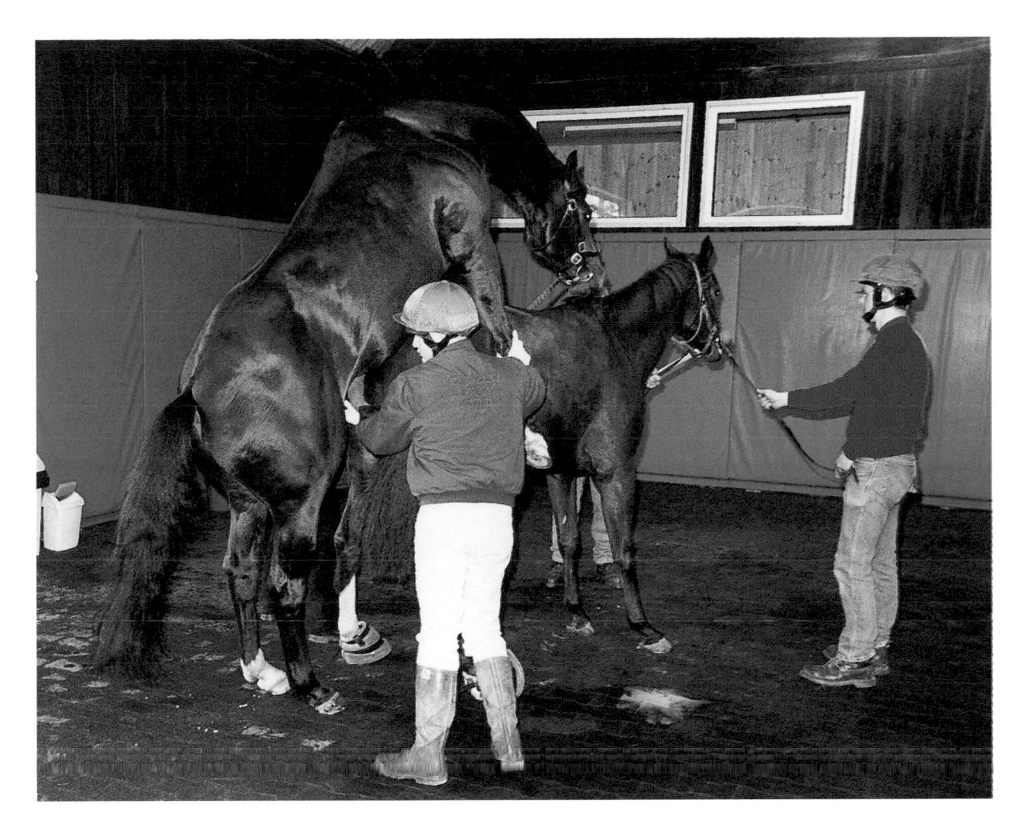

Figure 5.13

The stallion mounts the mare and the attendant at the mare's hindquarters feels for the pulse of semen along the penis as the stallion ejaculates

can cause injury to the mare's vagina or vulva as the head of the penis is considerably enlarged at ejaculation. It may also allow large amounts of air to be sucked into the mare's reproductive tract.

After mating, the stallion's penis is normally washed with plain warm water (Figure 5.14). His front legs and belly may also be washed to remove the smell of the mare and any sweat (Figure 5.15). The mare will have her boots and tail bandage removed, as well as the neck cape if this has been used.

Some breeders like to walk the mare for 15–20 minutes following covering to stop her straining and expelling semen. However, this is not necessary, as the semen will have been ejaculated directly through the cervix into the uterus in a proper mating and little, if any, should be present in the vagina. Any that is expelled at this stage is of little use to the mare.

The question of whether or not foals should accompany their dams into the breeding barn is a contentious one. Some studfarms will not permit the foal to be with the mare and others always bring the foal in. There are many reasons for and against the foal being present and, ideally, there should be

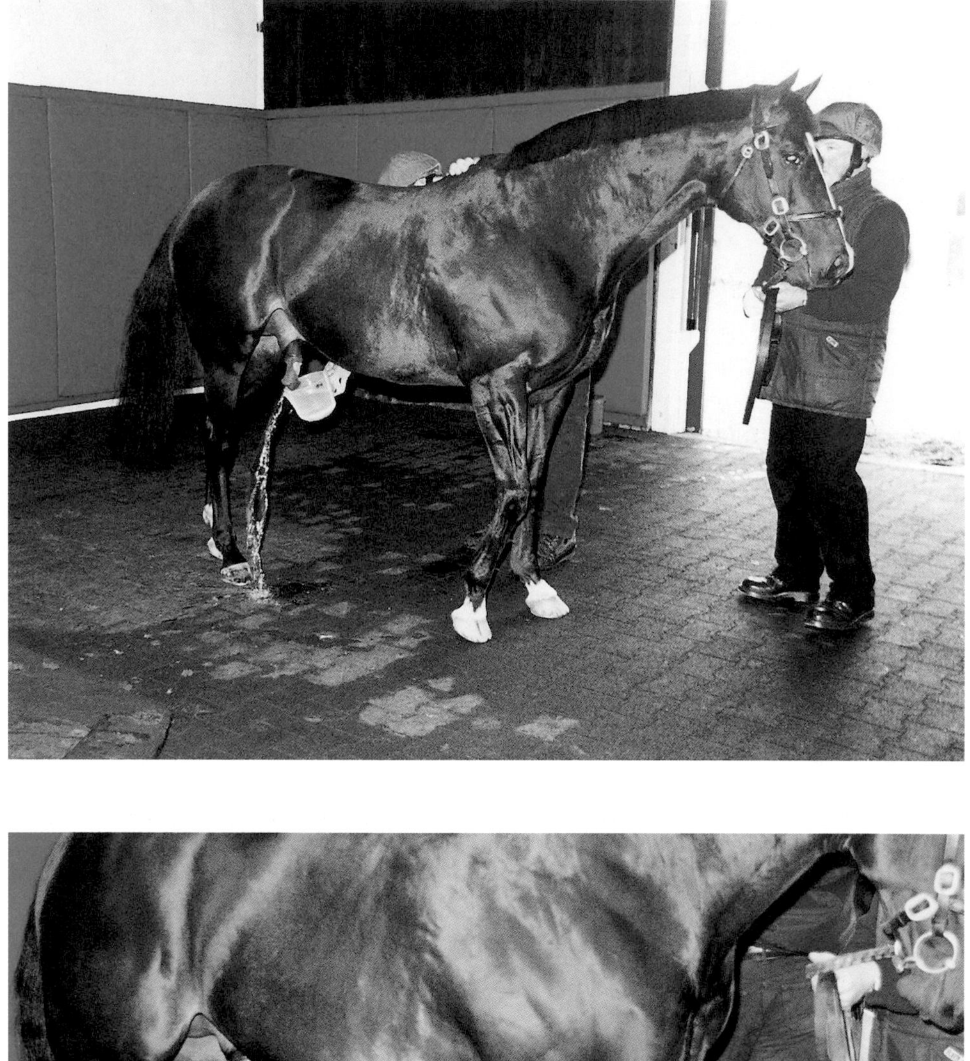

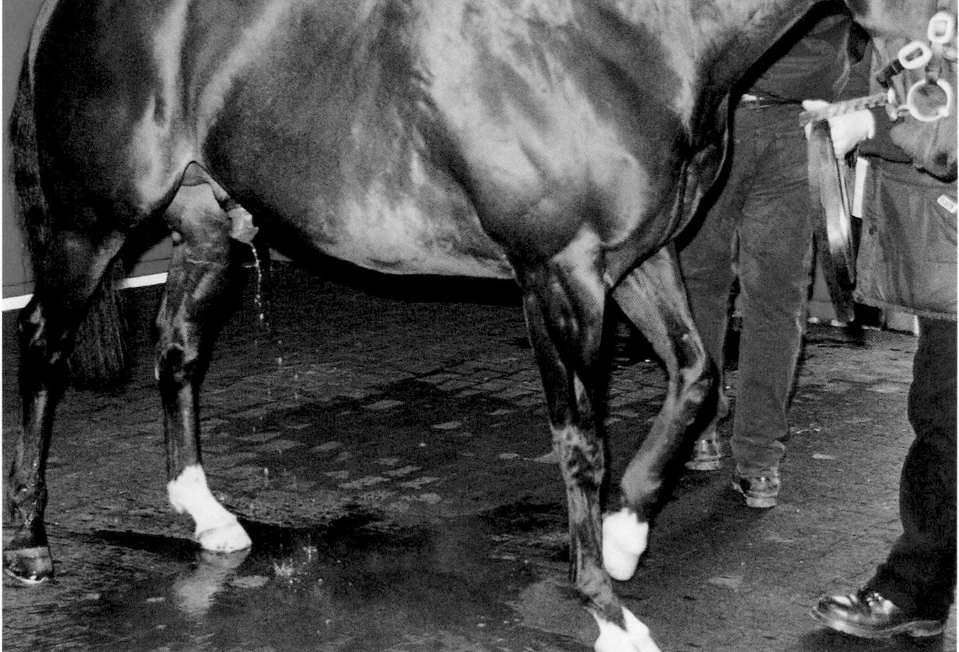

Figure 5.14 (opposite, top)

The stallion's penis is washed off with plain, warm water water after mating

Figure 5.15 (opposite, bottom)

It is common for the front legs and belly of the stallion to be washed after each mating to remove the smell of the mare

some flexibility if the particular mare warrants it. Some mares become distraught if taken from their foals and will not permit the stallion to approach without behaving aggressively. Other mares show no concern at all about being separated. If the mare is particularly foal proud, then allowing her foal to accompany her to the breeding shed can help to keep her calm. The most important factor is the safety of the horses and the handlers. Is there sufficient space to allow the foal to be held in a safe place away from, but still within sight of the mare? Is the mare more relaxed with the foal present? The majority of mares do not mind being away from their foals for such a short period but each situation should be dealt with individually on its own merits.

The Young Stallion

Whichever breeding method is planned for the stallion, in-hand, paddock or artificial insemination, it is important that his first few matings are in-hand. This helps to ensure that he is not injured and that he can be correctly introduced to his new role. It can often be overlooked but this is a sensitive and somewhat difficult time for a young stallion and he has much to learn. If he learns to be afraid of his handler he may become aggressive or overly anxious during the covering procedure. This can have long-term effects on his stud career and may shorten it dramatically.

The stallion's first attempts can be frustrating for all concerned and the key point to remember is patience. Some studfarms allow their young stallion to watch another stallion mating, if this can be done in absolute safety, and this is reported to be beneficial.

When preparing a stallion for his first covering it is important to make sure the area is as safe as possible. He may get over-excited and falls from mares are common with a young stallion. The first mare chosen should be a gentle and experienced mare that is a little smaller than the stallion. She should be well in oestrus and willing to stand still for the stallion, even after three or four attempts.

Any unpleasant experience during this training period may cause many psychological problems for the stallion, such as an aversion to certain mares, refusing to acknowledge the presence of a mare in oestrus and inability to produce and maintain an erection.

When the stallion is brought in to his

first mare, he should be guided firmly to her left side and allowed to sniff and lick her. He should be moved away if he tries to bite or strike at her. Some stallion handlers teach their stallions to back on command and this can be particularly useful in the breeding barn. Once the stallion is sufficiently aroused he should be encouraged to mount the mare. Care is needed to avoid allowing him to mount too early, although as mounting is difficult to maintain he will nearly always dismount of his own accord. Care should also be taken to avoid him becoming too aroused or the glans of the penis will become too large to allow penetration. Some young stallions may attempt to mount the mare sideways or sometimes on her neck, careful guiding of the stallion towards her rear may help with this. As mentioned before, the mare may take one or two steps forward; this does actually help the stallion so, in most instances, should not be restrained.

The first mating is often unsuccessful. The stallion may lose interest or fall. The stallion handler should deal with this calmly in order to avoid further injury to the stallion or making him feel further anxiety. Although it is essential to teach the stallion good manners when in the breeding barn, the first few covers should allow him to establish for himself what goes where and what is expected of him. Any behaviour such as biting should be discouraged carefully so that the stallion does not misunderstand what he is being reprimanded for. The young horse may also make several mounts before ejaculating – this too should be discouraged and a longer period of teasing before mounting may be helpful.

Rough or cruel handling at any point in a stallion's life may cause permanent damage. The stallion that fears or resents his handler will concentrate on him alone and not his mares – he will watch every movement and expression. Correction of behavioural problems is time consuming and some may never be completely solved; emphasis must therefore be placed on prevention.

It should always be remembered that stallion handling is an important part of stud management and one that affects every aspect of the horse's and the stud's productivity.

[The information in the following Figures 5.16 to 5.21 is supplied by Professor S. W. Ricketts, FRCVS, and shows improvement in live foal percentage and a decrease in percentage of barren mares over the period 1970–1999.]

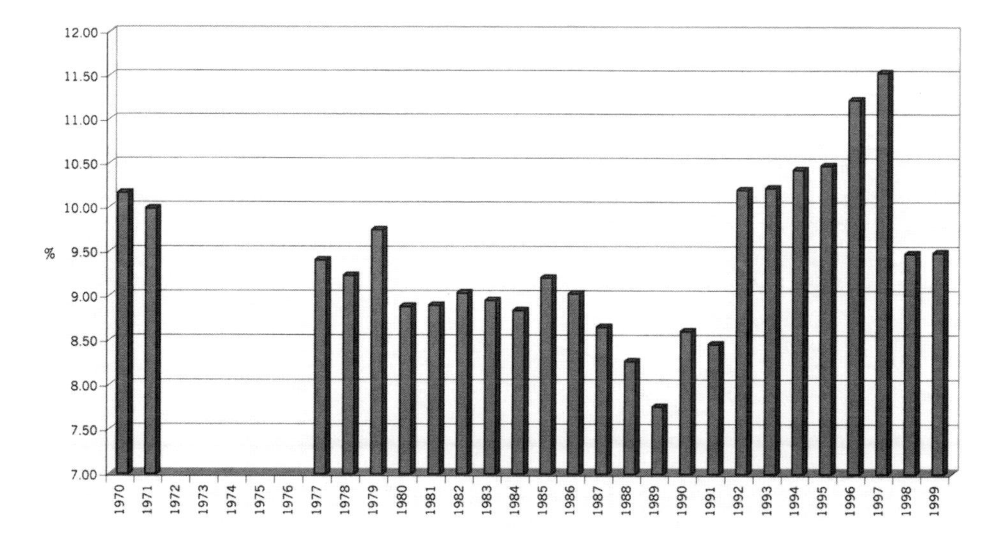

Figure 5.16

Weatherbys returns for UK and Irish TB mares: gestational failure percentage

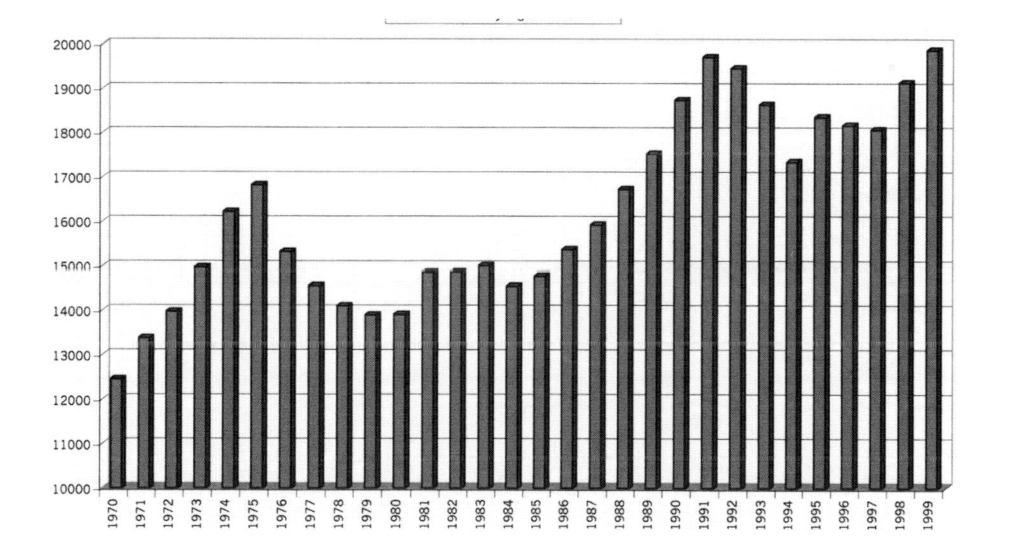

Figure 5.17

Weatherbys returns for UK and Irish TB mares: mares covered by registered stallions

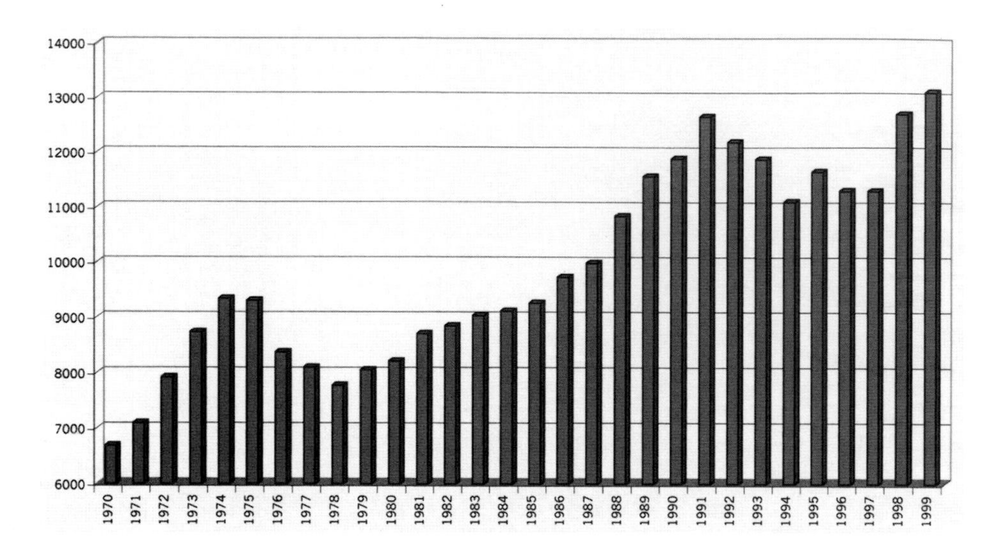

Figure 5.18

Weatherbys returns for UK and Irish TB mares: live produce

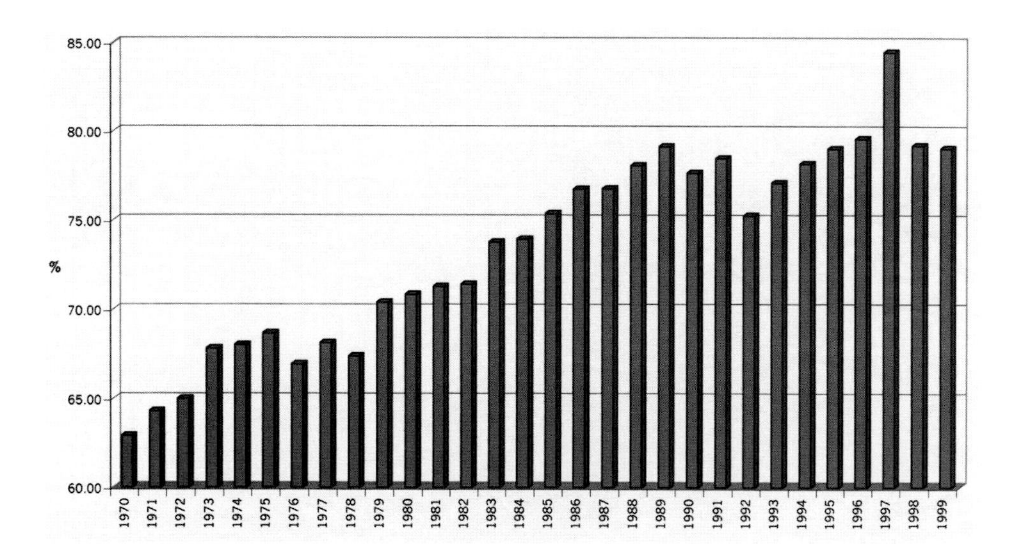

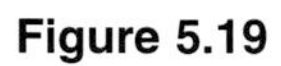
Figure 5.19

Weatherbys returns for UK and Irish mares: live foal percentage

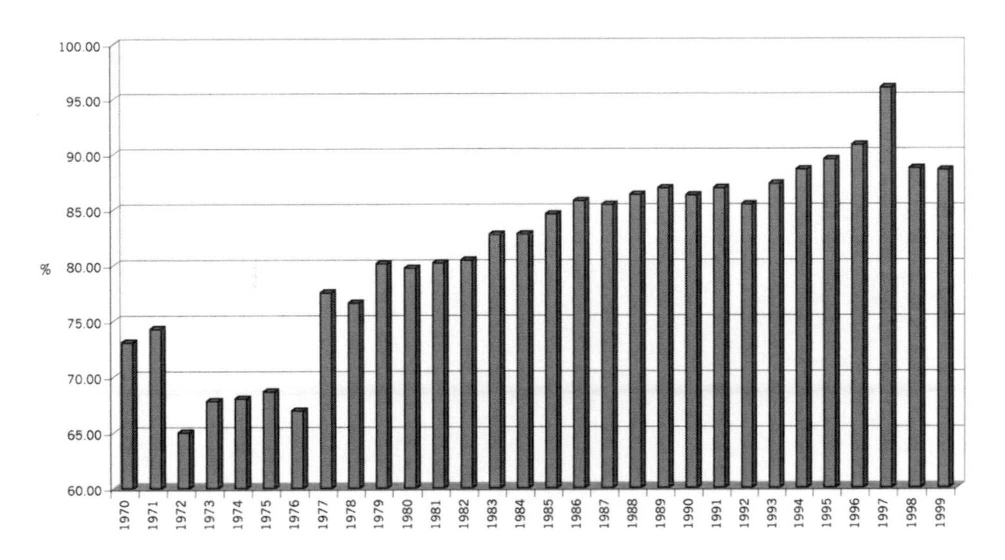

Figure 5.20

Weatherbys returns for UK and Irish TB mares: conception percentage

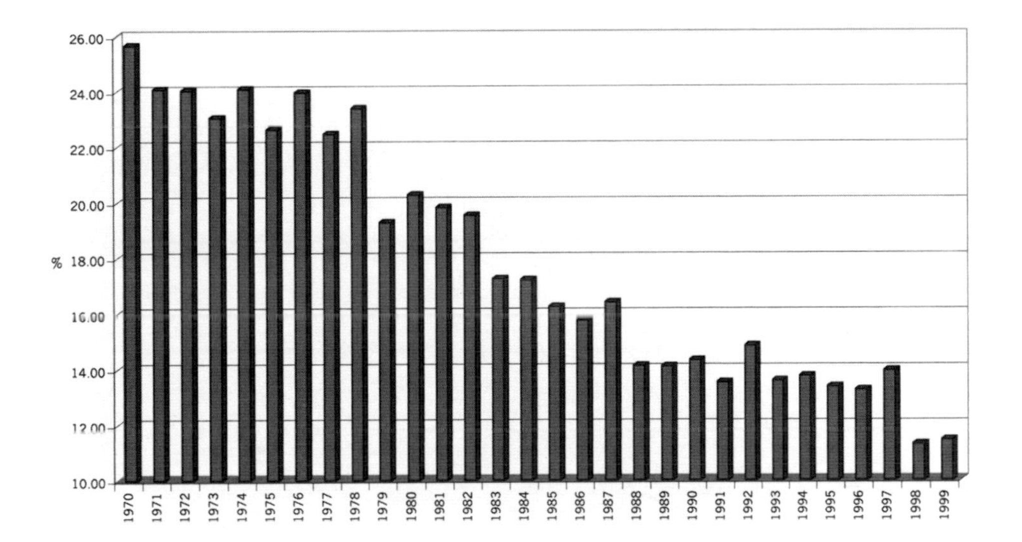

Figure 5.21

Weatherbys returns for UK and Irish mares: barren percentage

CHAPTER SIX

Artificial Insemination and Embryo Transfer

Artificial insemination (AI) is a commonly used reproductive technique with most domesticated animals, particularly cattle. It is now also increasing as a technique for breeding horses not being produced for Thoroughbred racing. To date, the use of any artificial conception method for Stud Book registered Thoroughbreds is prohibited.

AI was reportedly used as early as the 1300s in Arabia through to the 1800s in Italy and, by the turn of the twentieth century, the technique was used in the USA with horses that failed to conceive to natural service. The Russians were also involved and developed techniques for inseminating a wide species range from birds to sheep. The early techniques were very crude and fertility rates were poor; however, techniques are improving at a startling pace and the transfer of embryos as well as insemination are now relatively routine methods of conception.

Regardless of arguments against the use of AI, this technique is becoming an important part of the performance horse breeding industry. If properly used, AI is efficient, maximises production and allows total control over breeding hygiene and safety. However, it is wise to remember that artificial insemination is not the answer to all breeding problems and it may not be the best technique for most breeders.

The main advantages are as follows:

- It minimises the spread of infection by doing away with the need for contact between the mare and stallion, or for travelling horses to different premises for breeding.
- It is possible to reduce the number of naturally occurring bacteria in an ejaculate for insemination into susceptible mares – or even treat the ejaculate with antibiotics prior to insemination.
- AI reduces the risk of injury to mare or stallion. AI can be a particularly useful technique for stallions that have a tendency to savage or reject their mares.
- AI is useful in optimising conception rates if properly managed. It cannot be stressed too much that AI is not a simple procedure to manage and requires skilled operators. In the first year of using this technique, a farm may actually report a marked drop in conception rates.
- AI can eliminate the physical and psychological stresses associated

with natural service. It is common for an injured mare to be safely inseminated during her convalescence when natural service would be impossible. Some elderly stallions or those with a disability can be trained to use an artificial vagina without the need of a jump mare or dummy mare. However, there are strong ethical arguments against using inherently weak or unsound horses for breeding.

- Careful evaluation of each ejaculate means that each stallion's fertility can constantly be assessed. This not only aids management decisions, but also alerts managers to a problem before it becomes too severe.
- In most cases, each ejaculate can be split safely many times for insemination. AI can therefore be used to prevent over-use of an individual, especially if several mares require mating on one day. However, the reverse can also be true when a popular stallion can potentially produce a very high number of foals. Any commercial breeder will endeavour to ensure that the market is not flooded, as the price realised for each offspring will be affected adversely.
- With performance horses, it may be that a very large stallion is chosen for a smaller pony type mare – AI does away with the practical problem of size difference between mare and stallion.
- AI requires very careful management and recording. It may be that the increased level of records, paperwork and registration required for each insemination will actually improve the quality of registration and record keeping outside of the Thoroughbred breed.
- Semen can now be shipped globally, widening the availability of bloodlines to other countries and reducing the previous prohibitive costs involved with using foreign bloodlines.

Although it seems, on the face of it, that AI has more than enough potential completely to revolutionise the breeding industry, there are as many, if not more, disadvantages to using it as a routine reproductive management tool. Some of these are as follows:

- Human interference with the breeding process of all horses has been shown repeatedly to produce negative effects on fertility rates. A technique as far from the natural method as AI requires very careful management. Human error and management problems can cause a high level of sub-fertility in both mares and stallions.
- Artificial methods of conception are not permitted by some breed organisations, such as The Stud Book for Thoroughbreds.
- If a breeding operation is to use AI regularly, it will require specialised facilities – the initial costs involved with setting up can be very high. The staff involved with the procedure will need to be experienced in the handling and collection procedures, and it is common for a relatively high level of veterinary backup to be required.
- AI can improve conception rates in some individuals that suffer from inherent reproductive problems but there are always arguments against breeding from such horses. Horses are rarely selected primarily for fertility and the natural occurrence of low fertility in some individuals reduces the reproduction of some abnormalities.

- Any form of artificial breeding needs to be very carefully regulated to reduce the risk of malpractice and fraud within breeds. Recently, breed authorities such as Weatherbys, who hold The Stud Book for Thoroughbreds, have begun a programme of DNA sampling every registered Thoroughbred, in addition to the routine blood sampling of all foals and new registrations. As well as establishing a DNA library for all the horses in the Stud Book, all registered foals are now required to have a microchip inserted in the muscle of the neck.
- The use of AI reduces the risk of some infections being transmitted, but all stallions should be screened in the same way as those used specifically for natural covers. Serious diseases such as equine viral arteritis (EVA) can be transmitted from stallion to mare through insemination alone.
- There are strong financial disadvantages with the use of AI, unless it is very carefully regulated. For example, as each ejaculate can be split to be used in several mares, a popular stallion's offspring may actually reduce in value due to increased availability.

Facilities

The layout of the AI facility can affect efficiency and safety; therefore, it requires careful consideration. For a studfarm setting up such a facility for the first time, it is well worth visiting established studs and finding out what equipment works best in a range of practical situations.

The first requirement is for a safe semen collection area. Many AI farms use phantom or dummy mares for collection as stallions can easily be trained to use them and it immediately does away with the need for a mare in oestrus for each collection. If a dummy mare is to be used, it should be very securely sited in a safe area with a non-slip floor – some studs site the dummy mare in its own area set up with a rubber floor and, as temperature control is vital for success, close to a laboratory area so that the collection does not have to be transported too far. Once the dummy mare is in use it should not be moved, as the stallions will associate it with a certain place and may be reluctant to use it elsewhere. Many stallions quickly become used to the dummy and become aroused when just being led towards its area, just as those that are used to natural services become aroused when being taken to the covering barn.

Dummy mares (Figure 6.1) should be slightly smaller than the stallion using it (most dummy mares are adjustable on large AI farms), well padded and some have a 'neck' to afford the stallion extra grip. The dummy should be securely bolted to the floor and should be strong enough to withstand even the most vigorous stallion's movements. The material used to cover the dummy mare should be easily washed to avoid any risk of contamination between stallions.

The laboratory area should, ideally, be sited close to the area used for collection. Many studs, even those using traditional methods for conception, routinely evaluate semen production and areas designated for this can normally be adapted as a laboratory for AI use. The laboratory should be set up so that it is easily cleaned and there should be at least one door between the lab area

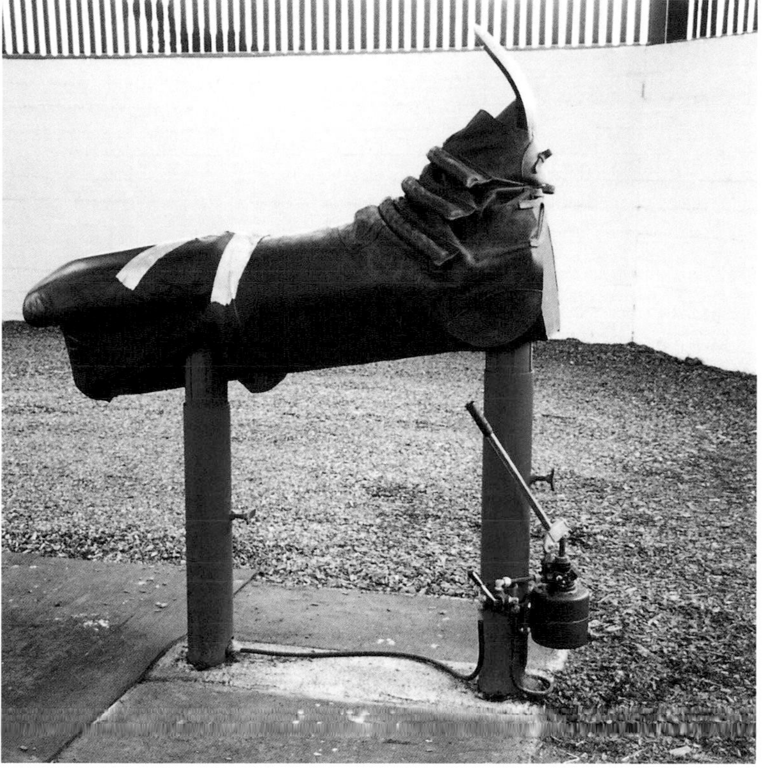

Figure 6.1

An adjustable dummy mare. The height and angle of the dummy can be adjusted hydraulically. Note that the dummy is situated in a safe area, with rubber matting directly behind it to provide a non-slip surface

and the mating area to avoid too much dust being brought in. Power supply, hot and cold water and good lighting are the next essentials, as well as work surfaces that can be kept spotlessly clean. Specialised equipment is discussed in detail later in this section, but the standard equipment required includes an incubator, fridge, autoclave (or similar facility for sterilising) and sealed storage for keeping equipment dust-free – although the size of this type of equipment depends on the size of the AI facility and routine collection rates.

Many specialised farms have veterinary stocks for the mares next to the laboratory (Figure 6.2). These can be of the simplest design or more complex in a larger set up. The stocks need to provide a safe, non-slip area for the mare to be restrained during insemination, with facility for those mares with foals at foot. Again, power supply and good lighting are essential and sufficient doors to reduce the dust levels during insemination.

Equipment

AI equipment forms a major part of the setting up expense within a studfarm. Studs that use a combination of natural service and AI can reduce the transition expenses by using the same areas for mating or collection, etc., but much of the specialised equipment needed for AI is expensive to buy and needs regular routine replacement.

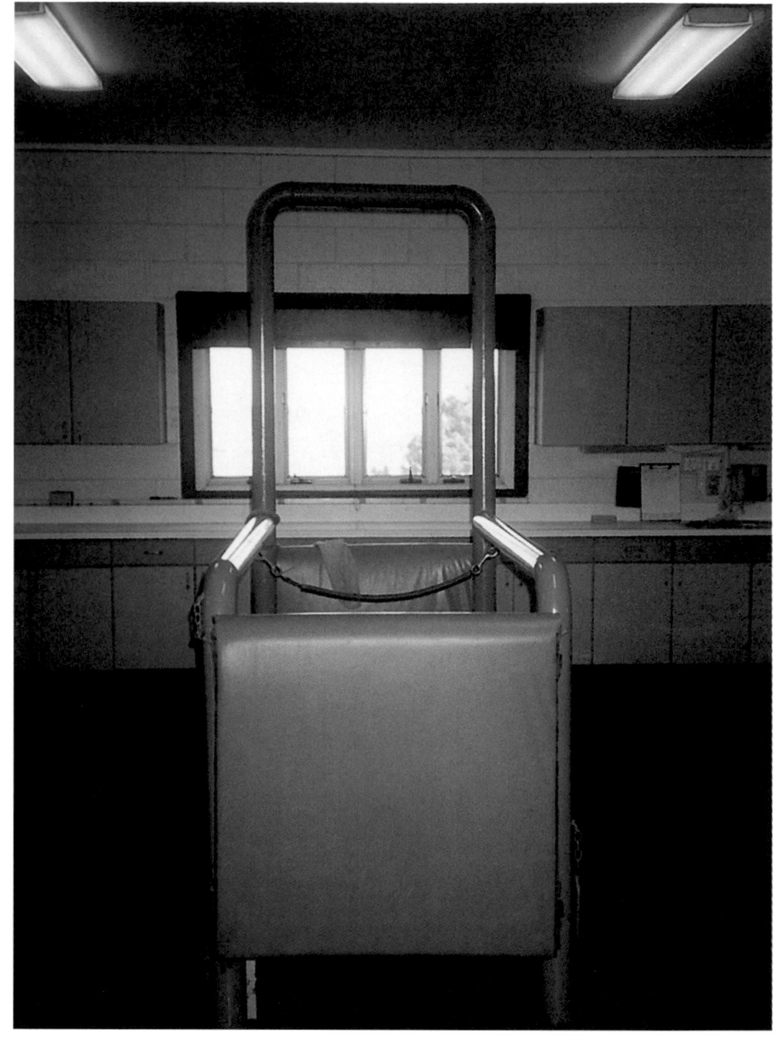

Figure 6.2

Examination and insemination stocks in the laboratory area

A studfarm that aims to operate as a specialised AI station will normally have more than one stallion and will have facilities for all procedures associated with insemination. This will include collection and insemination areas kept just for this procedure, as well as extensive laboratory facilities to enable treatment of the semen. For a studfarm to operate at this level, it requires a high level of veterinary attendance. Many such farms, particularly those outside England, have a resident vet on staff to enable the whole procedure from collection to shipment to be carried out successfully. Some studfarms can also offer non-surgical embryo transfer on the premises as well as AI.

Smaller farms may offer insemination in addition to traditional breeding methods and the amount of inseminations performed may not warrant specialised facilities. Such studfarms generally work closely with their veterinary practice to provide the collection and storage equipment on each occasion rather than invest in their own.

The availability of a dummy mare, for example, is not essential for collection, whereas most farms would invest in their own artificial vagina. In the UK there are also studfarms who offer assistance with AI to other studfarms on a contractual basis.

Artificial vagina

Many methods have been tried for semen collection, but the artificial vagina (AV) is the most effective and essential piece of equipment in any artificial insemination (AI) operation.

There are many different types of AV in use but each is essentially a rigid tubular cylinder with a plug leading to an inner sheath liner which is filled with warm water prior to collection (Figure 6.3). There is a carrier handle on the outside, which may be formed by part of the insulative protective outer cover, or by a separate leather cover – it is obviously essentially that this handle

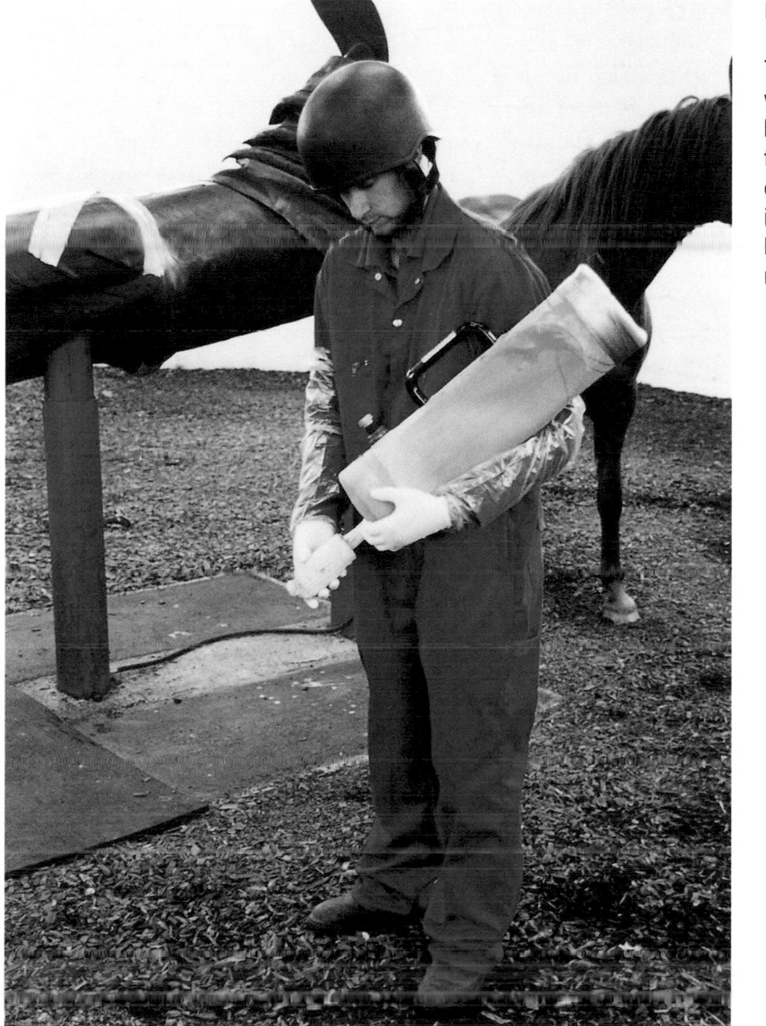

Figure 6.3

The prepared AV with collection bottle fitted. For the purposes of illustration, the insulation cover has been removed can be gripped firmly by the attendant during the collection procedure. The AV is additionally lined with an outer rubber sheath that is usually held in place with rubber bands over each open end. This sheath will provide a smooth passageway for the stallion's penis through the AV. Another liner is added which is fitted at the end the stallion will penetrate and used to attach the collection bottle to at the other end.

The AV is normally filled with warm water at this stage. The amount of water and its temperature is critical in AV preparation and for successful collection. The temperature used is normally between 50–60°C; this temperature is slightly higher than the ideal and allows for some degree of cooling while the final preparations for collection take place. The amount of water will affect the feel of the AV around the stallion's penis. Some stallions prefer the AV to be well filled, others will not use the AV if this is the case – initially adjustments will need to be made to suit the individual stallion's preference. When filled with water the average weight of the AV will be about 9–11 kg.

The AV may now also have another disposable, sterile inner sheath added which helps to avoid contamination of the rubber inner liner, but this is not always the case. Either way, careful monitoring of the internal temperature of the AV should now begin – the final temperature is ideally between 44–48°C.

A collection bottle is fitted to the end of the sheath to allow the ejaculate to be collected without risk of contamination or loss due to external temperature. This bottle is usually pre-warmed and may have a filter inside to separate the gel fraction of the ejaculate from the semen.

In the UK, external temperature is an issue and many AVs have additional padded covers for insulation. These should completely cover not only the main AV cylinder itself, but also, importantly, the collection bottle. Inadequate protection from cold will cause the collection to be damaged, as the majority of sperm will quickly die. In some climates, particularly those with high environmental temperatures, collections are sometimes done without the need for any insulation.

Collection Procedures

As with natural service, the need for an experienced team of handlers who have a calm and professional approach is essential to ensure that the collection is successful and safe for both horses and handlers. If a jump mare is used, the stallion will normally go through the same routine of stimulation as that of natural service. With a phantom or dummy mare, stallions may require the presence of an oestrus mare close to the dummy to become sufficiently aroused (Figure 6.4). Those stallions that are trained to use a dummy mare routinely normally become so responsive to the dummy that they need no further stimulation (Figure 6.5).

As collection is a very unnatural breeding situation, it is important that the handlers are all familiar with the procedure and are able to react quickly in the event of a problem.

The choice of a jump mare should be based on temperament and oestrous state. Some large AI operations artificially synchronise oestrus in jump mares to ensure that there is always a mare available for use; however, with a smaller operation this may not be practical. It is

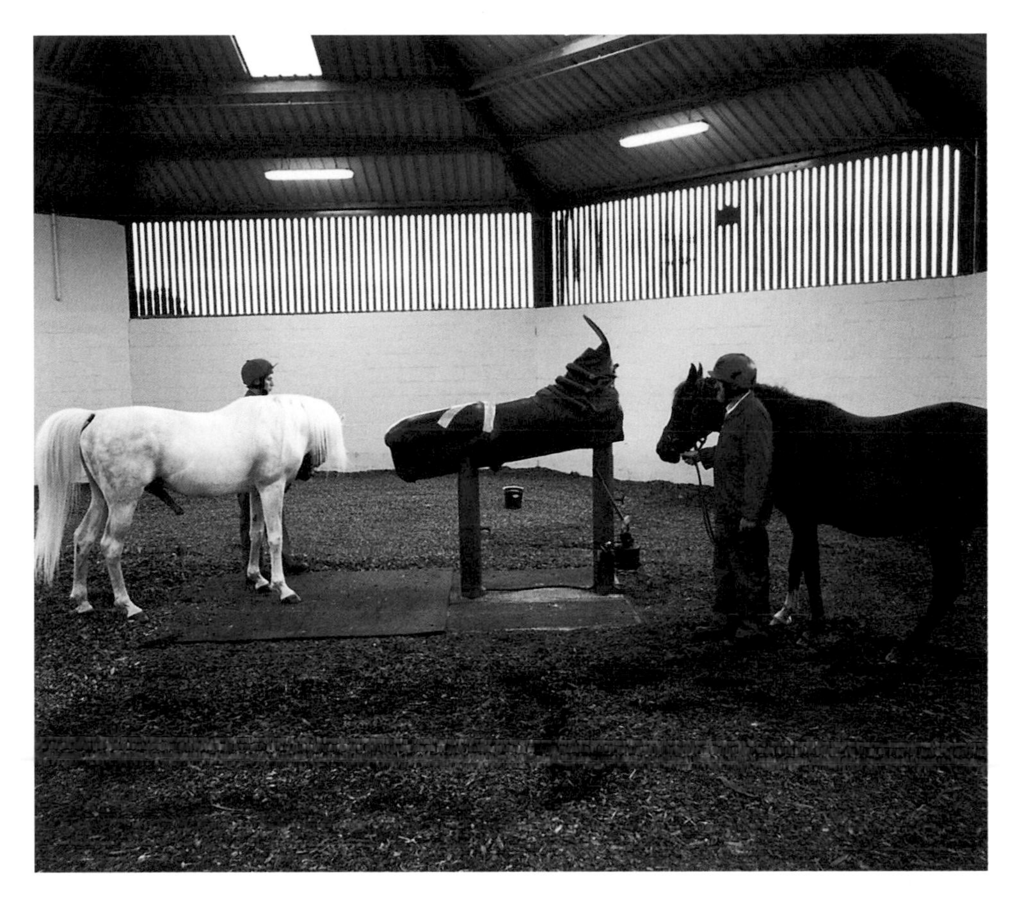

Figure 6.4

The stallion is led behind the dummy mare and is further stimulated by the presence of an in-season mare in front of the dummy

important that the mare is in full oestrus, calm and quiet, as well as adequately restrained. She is normally prepared in exactly the same way as she would be for natural service; this ensures that risk of contamination is kept to a minimum.

Dummy or phantom mares reduce the risk of injury to the stallion during collection, but the dummy mare should be carefully designed and sited to avoid any unnecessary risk of accidents.

Almost all stallions can be trained relatively quickly to use a dummy mare. Normally this is started with the additional presence of an in oestrus mare positioned near to the dummy itself. Some handlers like to mark the dummy mare with urine from an in oestrus mare – this works to arouse the stallion as well as masking any 'false' smells on the padded structure. Some specially designed dummy mares have a 'holder' for the AV to be placed into, which reduces the number of handlers required for each collection and assists

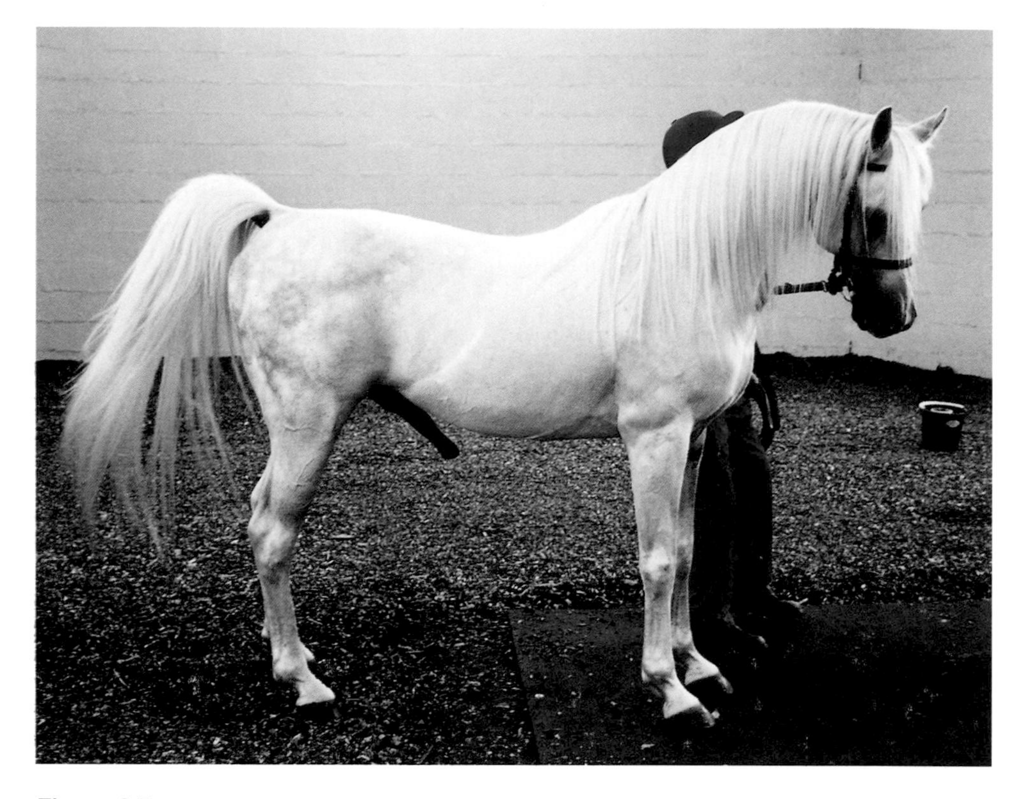

Figure 6.5

The experienced AI stallion will become conditioned to be aroused when led towards the dummy mare. As with traditional breeding, the stallion is equipped with a bridle and long rein

with some sensitive stallions as the AV is always at the same height and is held firmly within the structure of the dummy mare during collection. The stallion is held on the left as this means that his head can be safely brought towards the handlers in the event of a problem.

If a jump mare is used, she too can be turned, moving her hindquarters away from the stallion.

As the stallion mounts the mare, the handler responsible for collection should move along the stallion's flank and deflect the horse's penis into the AV (Figure 6.6). Most experienced handlers allow the first pre-ejaculatory fluids from the stallion to be lost as this is noted to contain the most contaminants and does not contain any sperm. It is important to allow the stallion to thrust into the AV rather than forcing his penis into it. Stallions quickly recognise any abnormal sensation and may refuse to continue.

Avoiding any force is vital with an inexperienced stallion that may become anxious about the whole procedure. Once the stallion has entered the AV, it is usually held close to the mare's thigh

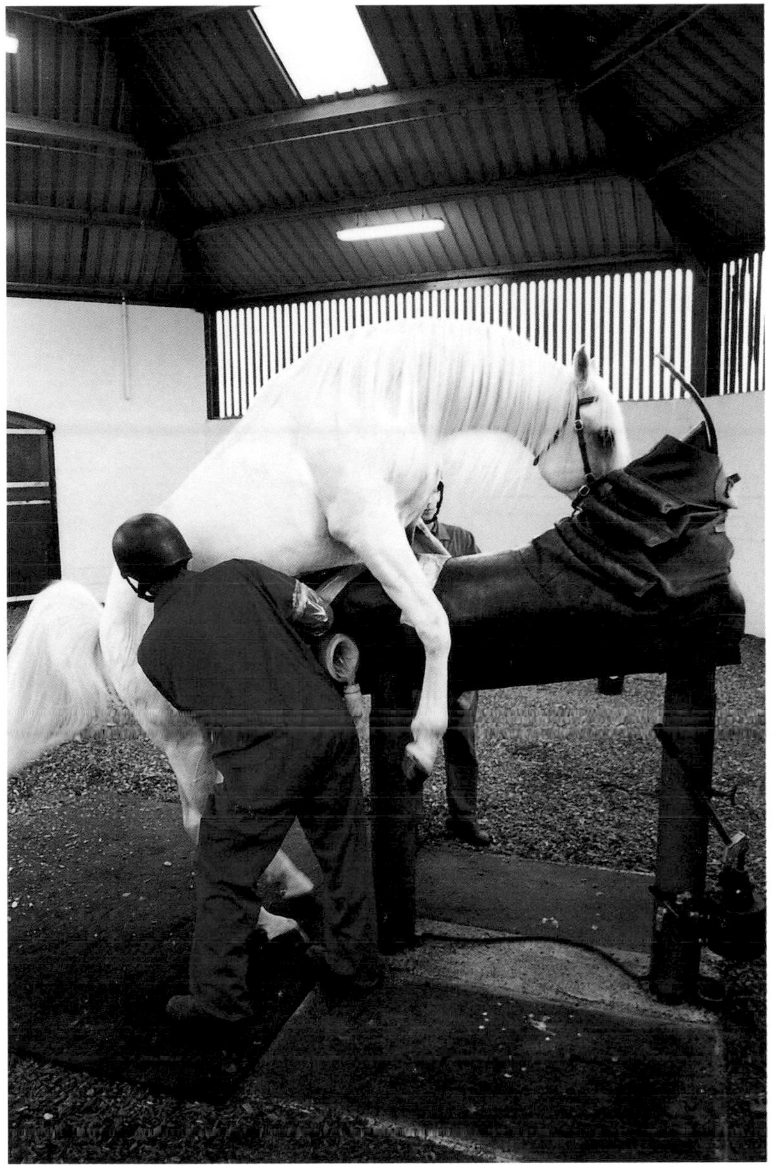

Figure 6.6

The attendant deflects the stallion's penis into the AV

at an angle of about 30 degrees from the horizontal with the collection bottle hanging down. It should be held as steady as possible which, in some cases, means holding the cylinder with both hands; however, experienced handlers are also able to feel for the pulse of ejaculation along the base of the stallion's penis, as is commonly practised by handlers during a natural service. If the stallion attempts to dismount, the handler should not try to follow him with the AV, as this will further reinforce any anxieties that the stallion may have. Once the stallion has ejaculated, he should be allowed to dismount in his own time and should not be hurried (Figure 6.7).

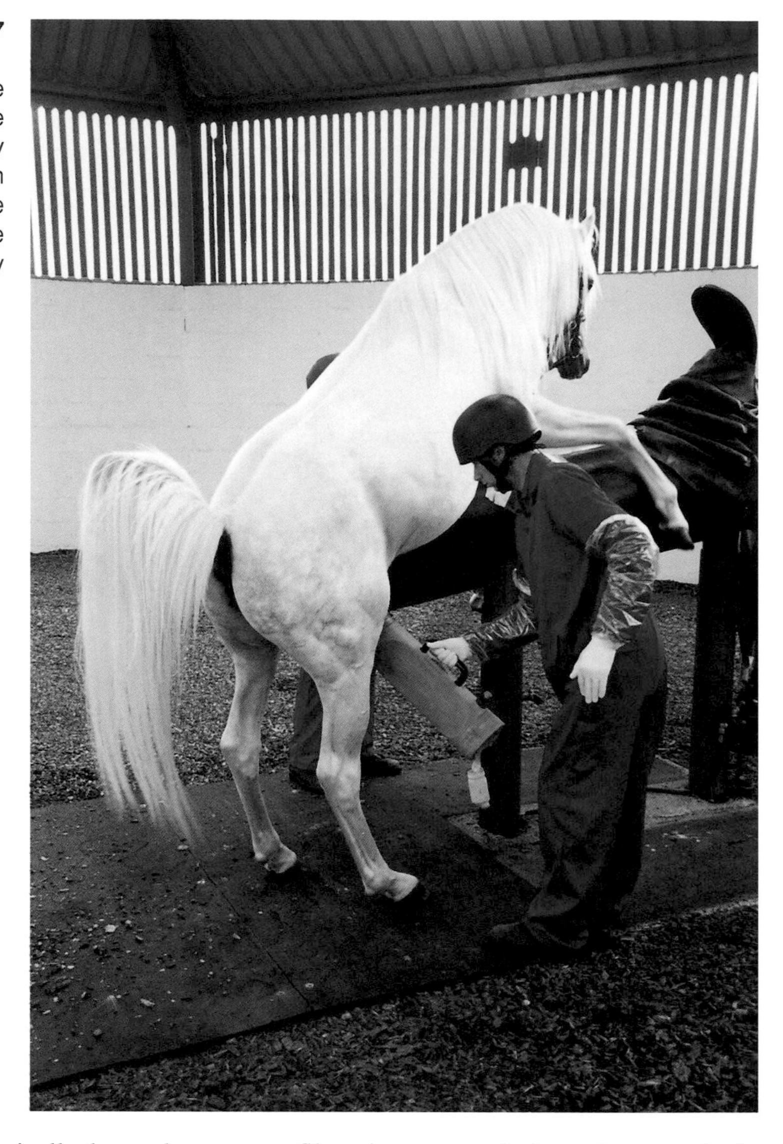

Figure 6.7

Care should be taken to remove the AV gently when the stallion dismounts. He should not be hurried in any way

Ejaculation typically lasts about ten seconds with the sperm being contained in the first three or four pulses. Some collection bottles have a filter system to reduce the amount of seminal plasma passing through with the sperm and holding the AV pointing slightly downwards during ejaculation can reduce the amount of plasma, which is more viscous in consistency, from passing into the collection bottle from the inner liner of the AV. If a filter is not used then the sample is generally filtered immediately once it is taken to the laboratory.

Insemination

The AV with the ejaculate should be taken to the laboratory area as soon as possible after collection (Figure 6.8). If

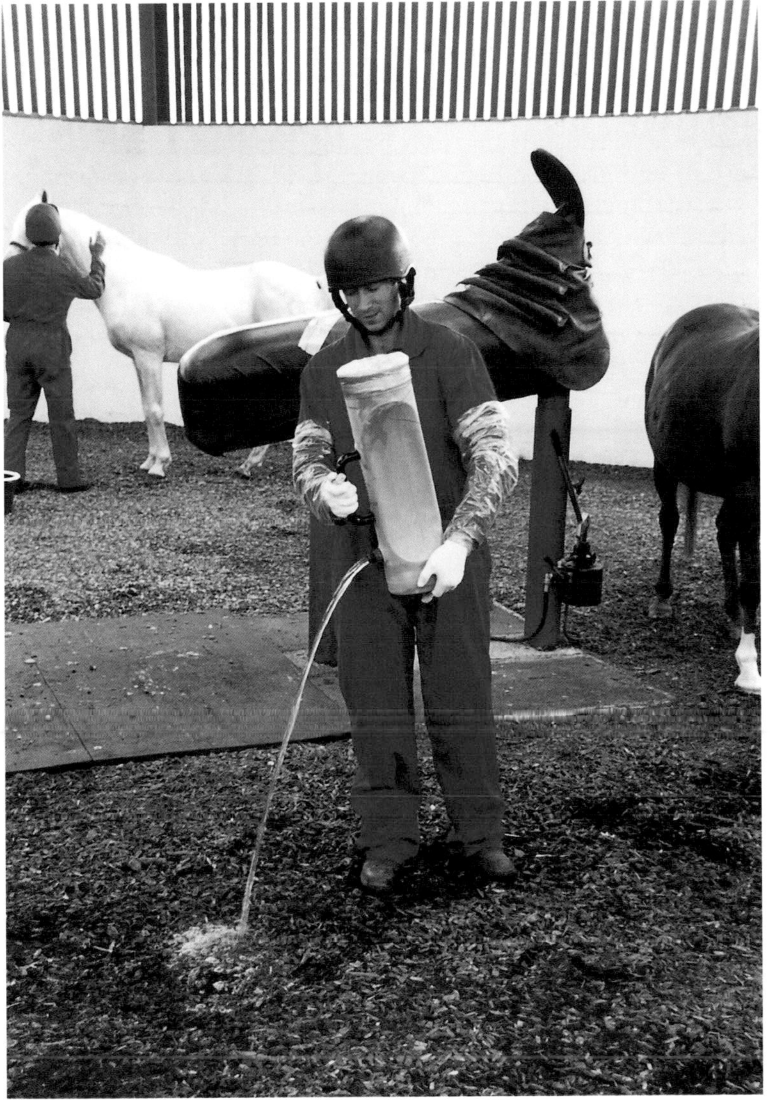

Figure 6.8

The collection bottle is taken immediately to the laboratory area for preparation and the warm water is removed from the AV

the sample is to be used immediately it can be stored in an incubator or warm water bath, but nearly all AI farms will incorporate it with a semen extender to optimise longevity whilst any preparations for insemination are made. The most common semen extenders are made from milk-based formulas and antibiotics can be added to the extender to reduce the number of bacteria present. This is of particular use with mares that suffer severe uterine inflammation following natural service and fail to conceive because of the inability to reduce the inflammation prior to the arrival of the conceptus in the uterus following successful fertilisation. If the sample is to be stored or transported prior to insemination, extender is always added and the sample chilled slowly to about 4–6°C. Specially designed containers called Equitainers can provide the correct environment for transportation of chilled semen. The temperature can be safely maintained in this container for up to 48 hours, sometimes longer.

If the semen is to be transported prior to insemination, it is essential that it is properly prepared and that communication between the mare owner and attending veterinary surgeon is maintained.

Mares are normally inseminated shortly before ovulation occurs – about 12–24 hours is the ideal range. This will obviously require the mare to be examined once she is in oestrus and during the next few days so that she can be correctly assessed for the optimum time for insemination. Transported semen is generally taken direct to the attending veterinary surgeon so that it can be correctly prepared prior to use. The success rates of using correctly prepared chilled semen are becoming as high as those using fresh semen and the preparation techniques are improving all the time. The use of frozen semen, however, has not yet shown such a high success rate and as much as 50 per cent of sperm is damaged during thawing. This is partly due to the individual variations between each stallion's sperm, as some do not respond well to storage of any form, as well as variations between each mare's fertility. However, as previously mentioned, techniques for AI are developing and improving all the time and high levels of fertility with frozen semen may soon become commonplace. To date, frozen semen from over 200 stallions is available in Europe and this number is increasing each year.

The speed at which the sperm are cooled and the temperature used for storage have a marked effect on the survival rate of the sperm following storage. A storage temperature for chilled sperm of 4–6°C is considered preferable if a relatively slow cooling rate has been possible. Research has shown that the critical damage range for sperm cooled too rapidly is between 20–25°C. Sperm can be cooled rapidly from normal body temperature – that is, about 37°C to 20°C, but the optimum cooling rate to reduce from 20°C is noted to be -0.05°C/minute to -0.1°C /minute to reduce the risk of any damaging effects of the cooling process.

Freezing sperm (cyropreservation) can be compared with hibernation. The function of the sperm cell is reduced to an absolute survival minimum without taking away the ability to fertilise an ovum. The freezing and thawing process exerts extraordinary stresses on the sperm cell – first there is the initial exposure caused by the cooling, then ice crystal damage and dehydration of the cells caused by the formation of crystals. To survive all this, the sperm have to be prepared with extreme care and even then, as mentioned earlier, the current success rate for frozen semen is only just over 50 per cent. Prior to freezing the sperm must be separated completely from the seminal plasma; usually this is done by the use of a centrifuge. Another more complicated method used by expert collectors is to use an open-ended AV and collect only the sperm-rich fraction of the ejaculate which is normally ejected in the first few spurts. This obviously requires a bit of practice! The sample is usually diluted with extender before separation with the centrifuge to aid in reducing shock to the sperm by cold and centrifugal forces. The sperm are then examined to calculate the number of straws that can be filled with a set number of sperm and placed into an appropriate freezing extender, which normally contains an energy and protein source, a protectant (glycerol) and electrolytes as well as antibiotics.

Today, there are several different packaging methods used for freezing sperm. The most common method is 0.5 ml or 5 ml sealed straws. Studfarms that regularly use straws for all insemination purposes quite often have a mechanical unit that automatically fills the straws – the most advanced farms have computerised equipment to assist with the whole procedure.

In general lay terms the actual freezing procedure begins once the straws are filled. They will then be immersed into the first freezing liquid which is liquid nitrogen vapour. This will cool the straws to -160°C at a set rate. The time the straws are held in the vapour will depend on the packaging and does vary. Once the straws are ready to be removed from the nitrogen vapour, they will be immersed immediately into liquid nitrogen, which will reduce the straw temperature further to -196°C. Once the straws have reached this temperature they are ready for storage. From current research, there appears to be no time limitation for storage of frozen sperm in liquid nitrogen. This is a very generalised outline of the freezing process and there are wide variations between individual laboratories, packaging systems and, most importantly, between each stallion used as to the actual times and temperatures required for optimum success. Thawing of the straws is normally carried out by putting the straws into water of a defined temperature for a set period of time – again there are wide variations between ideal temperatures and immersion times.

The most accurate way to establish a baseline for managing each stallion is to carry out trials prior to the start of breeding. These trials mean that each stallion's semen can be assessed and optimum preparation, shipping methods and amount of semen required for each insemination can be established. Sub-fertile stallions' sperm tends to have immediate lower motility rates and this may preclude their sperm from being transported for any distance to mares. For management purposes, trial samples are routinely examined and the motility rates of each stallion's sperm are checked every 10–15 minutes after warming. The ideal rate would be that at least 500 million actively motile sperm remain within the sample after 24 hours of cooling (common insemination rates for fresh semen are usually in the region of 250–500 million motile sperm). Sub-fertile horses should be assessed daily and the timing for insemination may need fine tuning to be successful. Some studfarms will inseminate a mare every other day until she ovulates, others will artificially manipulate a mare's cycle to coincide with a stallion's collection routine so that the timing for insemination with fresh semen is improved. Insemination of a mare with a sub-fertile stallion's semen can be carried out each day, or twice a day until ovulation occurs to achieve normal fertility rates.

Mares are prepared for insemination using minimal contamination procedures. The equipment used for insemination should be sterile and non-toxic. Most veterinary surgeons carrying out this technique use specialised equipment that has no spermicidal effects. Some rubber products, such as the rubber bungs used in syringes are reported to have spermicidal properties, a factor that is obviously not ideal! There are also reported variations between some stallions' semen as to its resilience with certain insemination techniques.

If the sample to be inseminated has been stored then it should be prepared carefully, with veterinary guidance if necessary, once the mare has been prepared. This reduces the length of time the sperm may be exposed to further stresses before insemination. Some veterinary surgeons will prepare a small sample from one of the straws sent to assess the quality of the sperm after storage. It is also common for some farms to inseminate the mare on two consecutive days; however, these repeat inseminations are not strictly necessary and may, in some cases, be detrimental. The pregnancy rates of repeat inseminated mares in research herds indicates similar rates to those receiving only a single insemination. Repeat inseminations may also expose compromised mares to a higher risk of uterine inflammation following each insemination resulting in a reduced success rate. If any cooled sperm is to be stored for a later insemination it should be kept refrigerated as the transport containers do not maintain optimum storage temperatures once opened.

The mare to be inseminated is brought into the stocks and will normally have her tail covered to prevent any contamination. The covered tail is then generally held or tied out of the way. The mare's vulva is thoroughly cleaned to remove all faecal material and rinsed well.

The semen is held in an insemination syringe connected to the insemination pipette. The pipette is inserted into the mare's vagina with a gloved hand. Again, it is essential that any lubricants used are non-spermicidal. The pipette is inserted through the cervix and the contents of the syringe put directly into the uterus. The semen is normally deposited slowly to reduce the risk of any damage being caused by the process. Once the insemination is complete, the pipette is normally drawn back into the hand and removed slowly to avoid any air being drawn into the genital tract.

It is common practice for each ejaculate to be split into several amounts. There is some variation between each stallion as to how many times each ejaculate can be split without compromising fertility and careful evaluation will need to be carried out to establish a sensible split amount for each individual stallion. Obviously, a stallion whose fertility is already compromised to any degree should be assessed extremely carefully before this practice is used, especially as there are environmental factors that may also contribute to reduced success rates even with fertile horses. Consultations with the farm's veterinary surgeon are vitally important to establish the best policy for splitting ejaculates for each of the stallions used for AI. Careful routine monitoring of each stallion's sperm throughout the breeding season is of particular importance so that the early changes in the average number of motile sperm present can be assessed.

Embryo Transfer

Embryo transfer is a technique that is used to transfer an embryo from one mare to another. As with artificial insemination, it is prohibited for use in Thoroughbred horses, but is becoming almost commonplace in its use with other breeds.

In simple terms, the mare is mated, or inseminated, in the normal way and the fertilised ovum is flushed from her uterus and placed into a recipient mare's uterus. The implantation procedure can be carried out either surgically or non-surgically, but has a higher success rate under surgical conditions. It is a highly-specialised technique and is generally only practiced by experienced veterinary surgeons.

The main objective of embryo transfer is to allow a mare to breed perhaps three or four foals a year using surrogate mares to carry each to term. Other reasons for its use are to allow a high-level competition mare to be bred without having to stop her training or competing for any length of time, or alternatively to allow a foal to be produced from a mare who is physically unable to carry a foal to term herself – perhaps due to injury or some other similar factor. Correctly prepared, each fertilised egg can be transported safely – even shipped overseas if necessary and implanted in a surrogate mare many thousands of miles away.

There are obviously sensitive implications, as with any method of artificial reproduction, and careful consideration should be given to the reasons for using a technique such as embryo transfer. The main reasons for and against are similar to those detailed with artificial insemination and, in many ways, this technique requires even stricter levels of registration, especially if a number of foals are to be bred from the donor mare each season.

To be successful, the two mares – the donor mare and the recipient mare – must have their oestrous cycles synchronised so that each is at exactly the same stage when transfer of the embryo is performed. This can be managed by artificially manipulating each mare's normal cycle, or by having a large number of recipient mares available; however, the most practical solution is to artificially synchronise the two individuals. Obviously, the reproductive health of both individuals is important; for example, elderly mares have a lower conception rate, as do those compromised by varying degrees of sub-fertility – such mares may prove to be unsuitable for such a procedure. Recipient mares are normally chosen for their ability as broodmares – as with foster mares, the heavier breeds are considered to be well suited to the role and some studfarms who use embryo transfer on a regular basis do keep mares purely for recipient purposes.

In simple layman's terms, the embryo is normally flushed from the donor mare's uterus at about seven days from mating. This is about the stage when the fertilised ovum arrives in the uterus from the fallopian tube and is the optimum stage of embryo development. Transfer of older or younger embryos has indicated lower success rates, but it is noted that less than seven-day embryos survive transport by freezing to a higher degree than those of greater than seven days. This is carried out under minimum contamination procedures by inserting a catheter into the mare's uterus and introducing a quantity of sterile saline fluid. The fluid is then drained back out of the uterus into suitable collection receptacles, usually through a filter. This procedure is carried out at least twice if necessary at each attempt to recover the embryo. Once the embryo is safely collected, it will be examined under a microscope to check its development and suitability for transfer. If collection and transfer are to occur immediately after each other, then the embryo can be normally maintained at room temperature. However, as mentioned earlier, it is now possible for embryos to be stored and shipped to a mare at a different location prior to transfer. The preparation of the embryos for transfer is very specialised and should only be carried out under the guidance of the attending veterinary surgeon immediately after collection.

There have been significant improvements in the pregnancy success rates with embryo transfer over the last decade and this will, no doubt, only continue to improve as more efficient and sophisticated techniques become available. The storage of embryos by freezing for future use is relatively well known in human medicine and is a technique that is also used with equines to allow embryos to be transported. Chilled storage and shipment of embryos using the Equitainer system has also been successful. To date, chilling embryos rather than freezing produces a higher pregnancy success rate but this is changing; and it will also become possible for semen from influential stallions to be stored for use long after their death. Further research indicates that such limitations are likely to be short lived and artificial conception procedures will become more widely available and routine.

Work on the equine genome should provide us with knowledge of an individual's propensity for unsoundness, problems in athletic performance, as well as the reasons for sub-fertility in mares and stallions. This information could be used to reduce the percentage of horses that 'break down' in training with conditions ranging from degenerative joint disease to tendon injury and from muscular to respiratory problems, by eliminating these individuals from the breeding stock. At the same time, the introduction of non-Thoroughbred stock without these deleterious genes could be used to produce a hybrid vigour in what otherwise may be a self-perpetuating decrease in the breeding quality of Thoroughbreds as far as health and soundness are concerned.

Scientific advances currently being developed and envisaged for the future will challenge both management and veterinarians together with those responsible for breeds in ways as yet undreamed of and not experienced in the last century.

CHAPTER SEVEN

Sub-fertility in Breeding Horses

Sub-fertility is a term used to describe a wide range of problems. Infertility is a term that is often used to describe the same problems, but more correctly describes a complete inability to breed. A mare that has been successfully pregnant before and then fails to conceive at another time is not, strictly speaking, infertile. The same applies to a stallion that has been fertile in the past. The main issue with sub-fertility is the cost in time and labour involved to maintain a reasonable level of productivity and/or conception. On a commercial studfarm, no matter what type of horse is being bred, or the stud fee involved, reproductive efficiency is of prime importance.

To discuss the factors that predispose the mare and stallion to periods of sub-fertility, whether temporary or permanent, it is perhaps correct to discuss each sex in turn. The overall reproductive health of the mare is particularly important in determining the health of the resulting offspring. Also, the relatively complex nature of the mare's reproductive system compared to that of the stallion, predisposes her to a higher level of stresses. In the past, little consideration was given to the effect that management techniques can have on the fertility of both mare and stallion. In fact, it is only relatively recently that consideration has been given to the reproductive status of the stallion in any great detail.

Infertility and Sub-fertility

The term 'infertility' is one that should, strictly speaking, be reserved for mares and stallions which are unable to breed; 'sub-fertility' implies a level of achievement in establishing conception which is reduced below the average normal level. Infertility is, therefore, an absolute situation whereas sub-fertility is more a subjective evaluation.

Infertility

The conditions affecting mares and stallions which prevent them from achieving conception when mated with a fertile stallion or mare, respectively, are fortunately comparatively rare. In mares, they are mostly associated with congenital abnormalities affecting parts of the genital tract or genital organs. These structural abnormalities are usually caused by abnormalities in chromosome composition or numbers (for example, the XX sex chromosomes being replaced in the individual by XO, XY, XXX or a combination of these variations).

The chromosomal abnormalities are not necessarily present in all tissues but in those affecting the organs concerned. Hermaphrodites and agnesis (lack of gonads) are terms used in connection with these conditions.

In the mare, the XXX and XO combinations are the most common and are associated with small or non-functional ovaries. Structural defects, such as an absence of cervix, or small inactive testes in the male, may be due to congenital problems not based on chromosomal abnormalities. Some of these may, however, have a genetic origin or be the result of failure in development of the individual while a fetus.

It is more difficult to diagnose the cause of infertile stallions; most are probably due to genetic or inherited features resulting in asperma (no sperm) or defects which prevent the sperm from possessing normal fertilising capacity.

Sub-fertility

The problem of sub-fertility is much more widespread and diverse than that of infertility.

In the first place, when labelling a mare or stallion as being sub-fertile, we have to be careful not to label an individual as sub-fertile purely on the basis of not conforming to our gold standard of normality. The latter may be based on an arbitrary definition skewed in part to our expectations within objectives set by commercial rather than biological requirements.

For example, we may expect a mare to breed a foal every year or, perhaps, five foals out of every six years. The individual that breeds a foal every other year or one that delivers only three or four out of six years may be described as sub-fertile but the reasons may well be related to management and a need to achieve conception in the winter and early spring, rather than the summer, being the main cause of the individual's failure.

We should, therefore, use the term sub-fertile only when there is definite veterinary evidence of abnormality, a point which we shall return to later in this chapter.

The same reservations apply to stallions where 90–100 per cent conception rates are the aim. If the stallion achieves only 60 per cent, the term sub-fertility may be applied. There is probably more reason to accept this in stallions than in mares, providing the stallion has had the same chance of achieving a 90 per cent rate as the individual with which it is compared. The number of mares mated and their own quality of breeding performance has to be taken into account in these comparisons.

The reason for sub-fertility in stallions, as with infertility, is probably the result of genetic make-up and the presence of, as yet undetermined, inheritance of genes that limit either libido or sperm output from the testes, or introduce some deleterious composition of components of the semen that reduces the capacity of sperm to fertilise the egg or to survive long enough in the mare's genital tract to do so. Let us now examine the various components in the pathway to sub-fertility.

Management

Many individual mares fail to conceive because they are mated too soon and the period between deposition of spermatozoa in the genital tract and the release of the egg (ovulation) allows the spermatozoa to die or lose their capacity to fertilise the egg. The period differs both with the stallion and the mare. One individual stallion may deposit sperm which are capable of fertilising the egg many days (up to seven, on record) following ejaculation into the mare; while in others the sperm appear to survive for only 24 hours or less.

The need for mating 12–24 hours prior to ovulation is therefore greater with some stallions than with others; and this may also apply to the mare because there is a variation in the 'hostility' of the conditions of the genital tract. Sperm and semen are foreign material and the sperm have to overcome the adverse conditions of the mare's genital tract. Where endometritis or infection is present the mare herself may determine the length of the period in which the sperm survive.

An even more important consideration is to achieve mating before rather than after ovulation. In the latter event, the egg itself becomes refractory to fertilisation within hours of being shed. After 24 hours there is little chance of conception occurring.

The synchronisation of mating with ovulation is one of the main justifications for the veterinary gynaecological examinations described in Chapter Four. Other decisions of management which are crucial for high levels of fertility include an accurate teasing programme and the appropriate use of veterinary assistance with its helpful gynaecological examinations of the cervix and ovaries.

Ensuring that a stallion actually ejaculates at the time of mating is another way in which management contributes to fertility percentages. There may be difficulty in certain individual stallions in determining whether or not ejaculation has occurred at any given mating (see Chapter Five).

Normal Variations in the Sexual Functions of the Mare and Stallion

We must accept that it is not natural for every mare to produce a foal each year. There are a number of reasons behind this statement. Firstly, mares have a relatively long pregnancy combined with only seasonal breeding activity, normally late April to August. Opportunities for annual conception are consequently limited and, in many individuals, the uterus needs time to recover after the pregnancy. In circumstances of the arbitrarily selected breeding season for Thoroughbreds, the possibilities of successful conception may be reduced to, at best, two or three heat periods. This may be described as the other side of the coin of management; that is, if a mare is missed at one heat period this may reduce by a third the number of oestrous periods in which conception could be achieved in that individual in that year.

Of course, the use of drugs, such as prostaglandin, can nowadays increase the chances by increasing the number of oestrous periods in which a mare may be mated. For further descriptions of the use of prostaglandin and other drugs in relation to management, see Chapter Two.

Under natural conditions, the peak period for ovulation occurs in April to September when each oestrous cycle is naturally active. Outside the natural breeding season mares are in a state of anoestrus, reflecting the inactive state of the pituitary in producing the hormones FSH and LH that control the sexual activities of the mare.

A mare cannot conceive when the pituitary is inactive and producing minimal levels of these hormones. Of course, we are now able to control this to a certain extent by artificially employing increased light in winter as well as by keeping mares in warm surroundings with high levels of nutrition. In this respect, we are simulating conditions of spring whereby there is a corresponding increase in the activity of the pituitary in the late winter and early spring months, thereby providing more opportunities for conception through the induction of oestrous periods and ovulation (Figure 7.1).

Another normal quirk of nature which may reduce the chances of a mare conceiving is the so-called lactational anoestrus that individuals may suffer when they are suckling their foals. The hormone prolactin, which is associated with milk production, may also reduce the activity of the ovaries through its action on the pituitary. This is one reason that some mares may suffer what is known as being every other year breeders.

The quality and quantity of a stallion's semen may vary with the season of the year. It has been shown that a parallel change occurs in hormonal status as between winter, spring and summer. However, this factor does not seem to affect fertility of the stallion under natural breeding conditions, only where the semen is required for artificial insemination and, in consequence, is split so that several mares can be inseminated in one ejaculate. In these situations, the quality of the semen is all important as to whether the stallion used for AI can achieve high levels of fertility (see Chapter Six).

Sub-fertility and Pathology or Disease

As is the case with all conditions and diseases, the important objective of the clinician is to establish a diagnosis of cause. It is from this basis that treatment and preventive measures may be put into operation (Figure 7.2).

Diagnosis, in the case of sub-fertility, should follow well-established procedures described below.

First, it must be emphasised that many symptoms (clinical signs) may have an interrelated effect and that sub-fertility may therefore be the result of one feature compounded by others. For example, poor conformation of the perineum, as described below, may lead to the taking in of air into the vagina and from there it may enter the uterus, especially during heat when the cervix is relaxed. The individual thus affected suffers from the combined effects of poor vulval conformation, an irritant and bacteria entering the genital tract as a result and the setting up of inflammation and infection within the uterus.

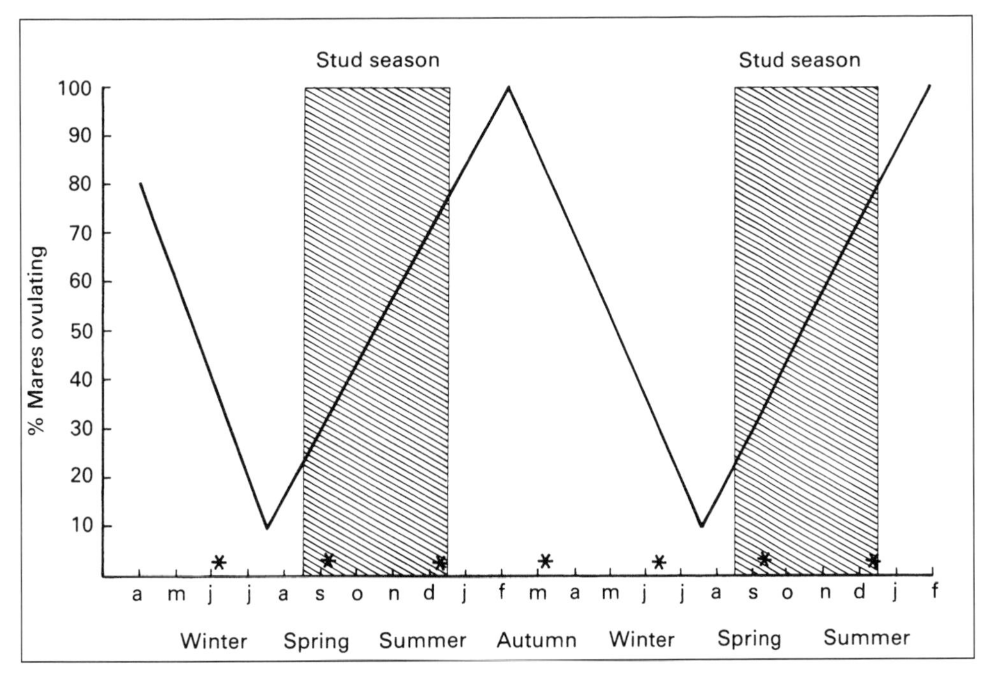

Figure 7.1

Data collected by Dr Virginia Osborne of Sydney University (1950s) show the percentage of mares ovulating during different months. Asterisks mark the solstices

Figure 7.2

Genital tract of a mare, illustrating the position of a cervical swab as it penetrates the cervix to collect material from the posterior part of the uterus

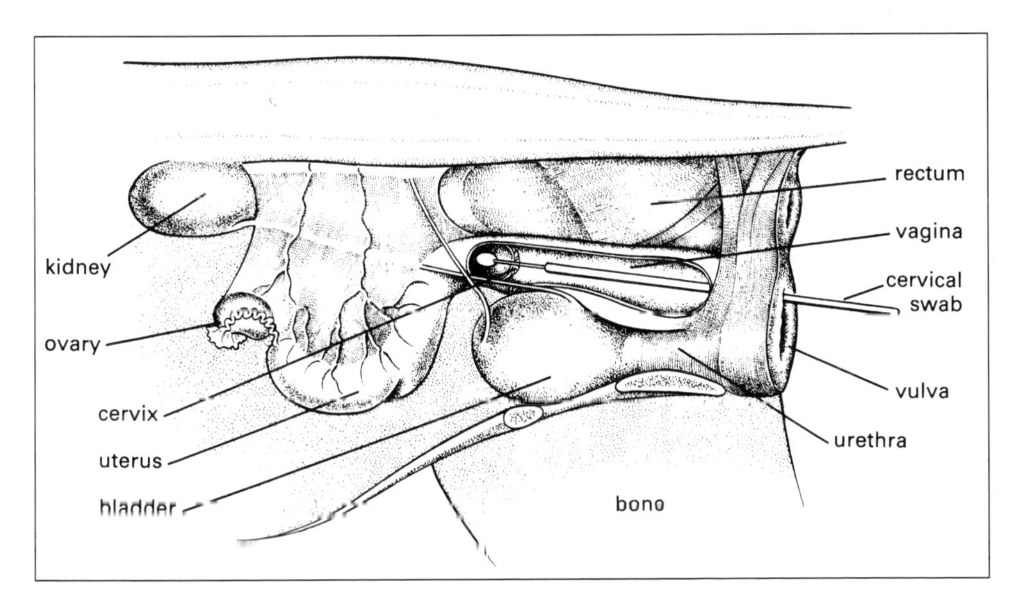

Oestrogen, the hormone of the heat period, also plays a role in what the clinician may describe as endometritis (inflammation of the uterine lining) and infection, while the colloquial description is that of a 'dirty' mare; that is, one exhibiting a discharge from the genital tract.

Conformation of the perineum

Normally, the genital tract is guarded against the entry of air and bacteria into the uterus by three valves formed by:

1. The vulva and its relationship with the pelvic brim.
2. The arrangement of the fold that divides the anterior from the posterior vagina.
3. The cervix.

Good conformation entails that the vulval orifice lies below the brim of the pelvis, at least to the greater extent of its length (see Figure 7.3).

The floor of the vagina runs horizontally to the fold described above and then, still horizontally, to the cervix.

The abnormal situation which makes the entry of infection into the genital tract more likely is when the vulval aperture lies largely above the brim of the pelvis (see Figure 7.4) and this may become accentuated by the retraction of the anus and upper commissure of the vulva becoming pulled in an anterior direction so that the vulval lips become sloping and, eventually, horizontal.

Another problem, often experienced in mares that have foaled recently and in older mares, is for the floor of the vagina to slope downwards so that urine and/or uterine fluid pools on the vaginal floor.

The cervix becomes naturally relaxed during oestrus which tends to breach the integrity of the third valve

Figure 7.3

Diagram to show the arrangement of the mare's anus (a), vulva (b), and the floor of the pelvis (c). It also shows: (left) good conformation, with the majority of the vulva below the level of the pelvic floor; (centre) poor conformation; leading to a situation where (right) the upper part of the vulva is tending to sink forward, allowing air into the tract

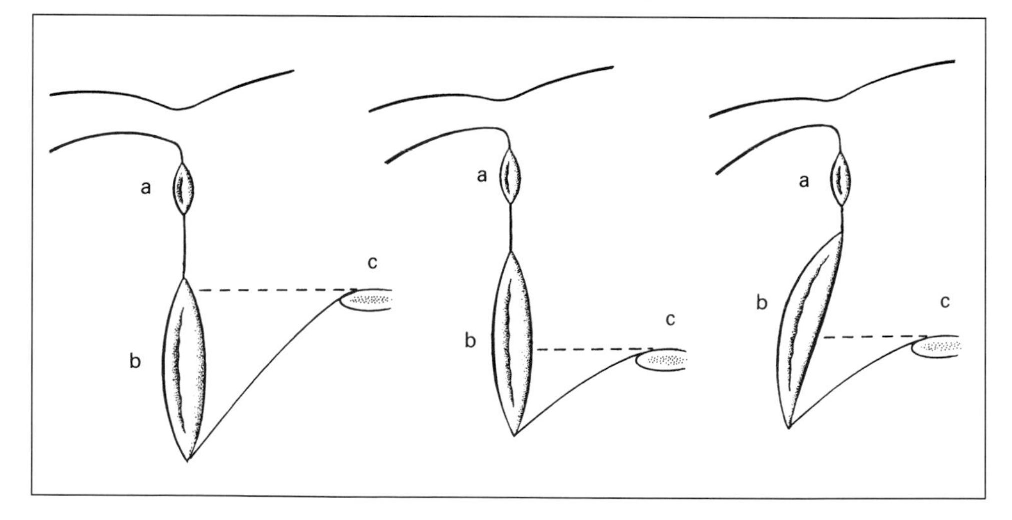

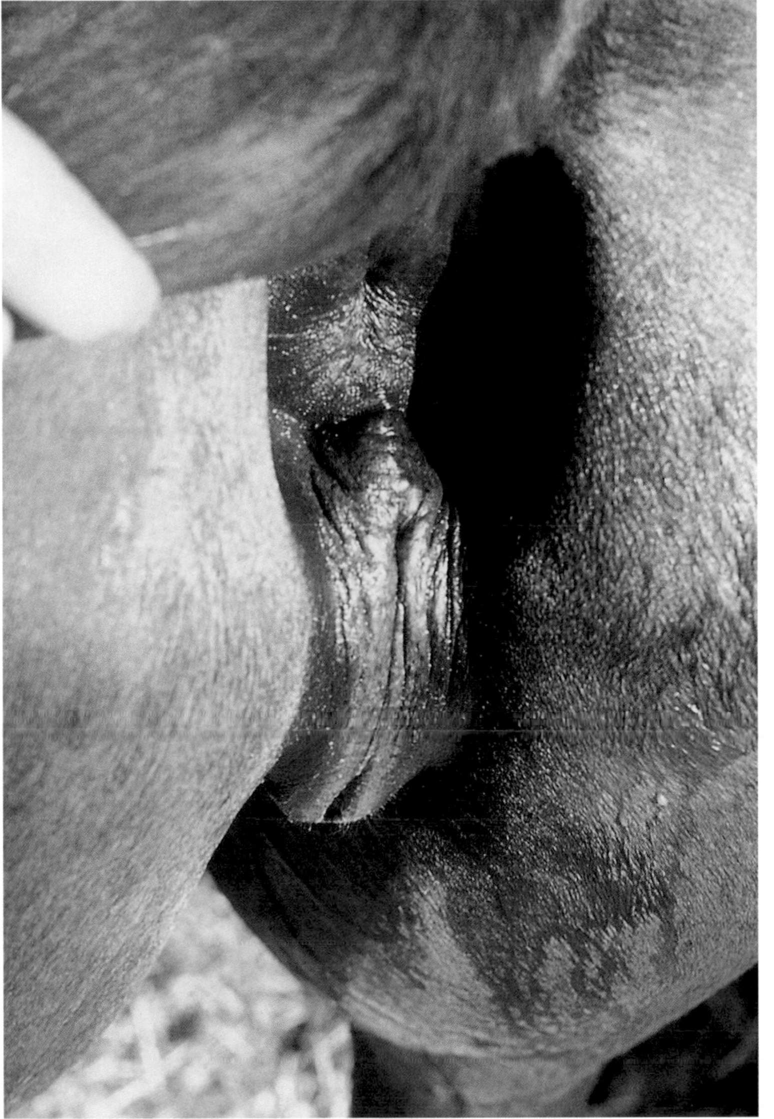

Figure 7.4

A mare with poor vulval conformation. The vulva has become sloping, with a sunken anus predisposing the mare to genital inflammation

guarding entry to the uterus. Also, the cervix may become damaged at foaling, resulting in adhesions or other defects which accentuate the lack of patency of the cervical barrier.

All of these conditions may be treated by the clinician employing surgery of the vulval lips, administration of hormones, such as oxytocin, and antibiotics to counter infection. Surgery consists of one of two operations. The most commonly employed is the Caslick operation, designed to restore the integrity of the valve at the perineum by closing the upper commissures of the vulva (see Figures 7.5–7.7) to an extent which brings them together to the level of the brim of the pelvis. First introduced in 1937 by Caslick in the USA, this operation

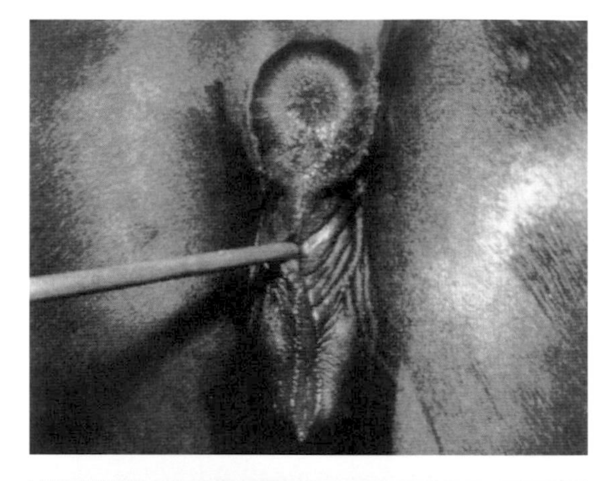

Figure 7.5

A well-formed vulva, showing good conformation

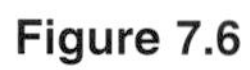

Figure 7.6

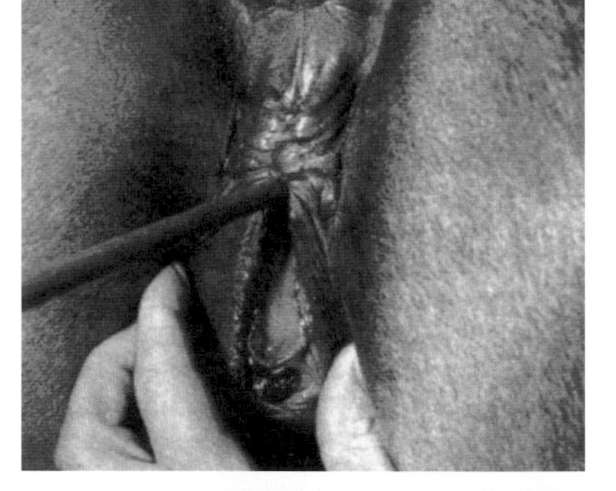

A Caslick operation has been performed on this vulva

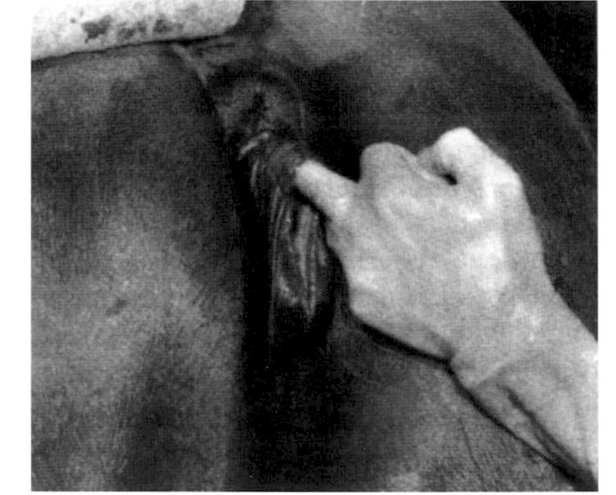

Figure 7.7

The effect of the Caslick operation showing a reduction of the vulvar opening by joining the lips surgically has been described as the single most important contribution to the problem of sub-fertility that has yet been discovered. Many mares, over the years, have been enabled to breed successfully because of this relatively simple operation.

The other surgical procedure of more recent times (1982), which has received the name of the Pouret operation after the distinguished French veterinarian who first introduced it, is designed to separate the tissues supporting the anus and rectum from those of the roof of the vagina, thereby releasing the vagina to move in a backward direction and the vulva to fall below the level of the brim of the pelvis. This operation is successful but is required only in severe cases of malformation of the perineum; and, sometimes, the effects may be reversed, over time, as the tissues contract and the vulva is again drawn backwards and upwards.

Infection and endometritis

Endometritis is the inflammation of the lining of the uterus, namely the endometrium.

It occurs in an acute form in which poly-morpho-nuclear leucocytes (PMN) invade the mucosal lining and is frequently associated with infective agents, particularly bacteria and, sometimes, fungus. It has also been suggested that herpes viruses may play a part in causing endometritis.

The chronic form is characterised by accumulations of fibrous material in a generalised form or associated with the glands. The technical details of these differences are not appropriate to this text, but the reader should understand that chronic changes are more associated with a degenerative process occurring with age and repeated pregnancies, whereas the acute form is largely of a temporary nature depending on the elimination of the factors causing endometritis – for example, infection, air contamination.

To understand acute endometritis it is necessary to consider the immune status of the uterine lining. During oestrus the glands secrete mucus and the lining becomes suffused with blood as the blood vessels dilate under the influence of oestrogen. The secretions thus produced have microbe killing capacity and form part of the immune barrier to the entry of infection into the uterine lining and beyond.

The same type of barrier is found on all mucosal surfaces of the body, whether these be in the airways, the throat or eyes. When this barrier is disturbed or weakened, infective agents overcome the resistance and establish themselves on the lining membranes. In the uterus, the bacteria most commonly associated with endometritis are *Streptococci* and *E. coli*. However, a whole range of bacteria may be recovered in any particular case and, often, there may be more than one type of bacteria involved.

It is important to emphasise that, in most cases, the presence of bacteria and, therefore, infection, is secondary to other happenings, such as the entry of air into the uterus, discussed above.

The late John Hughes, the distinguished Californian reproductive clinical scientist, showed in 1988 that the introduction of *Streptococci* into the genital tract of the normal mare was eliminated quite quickly by the natural defence mechanism of the uterine lining. Bacteria are, therefore, more a symptom than a cause of infection in the mare's uterus. It is only when the defensive mechanisms are faulty or overcome by excessive challenge that infection occurs.

The only exception to this are the three venereal pathogens, *Klebsiella*, Contagious Equine Metritis (CEM) and *Pseudomonas aeroginosa*. These bacteria may be transmitted from mare to mare by the stallion and set up infection in the recipient mare. For this reason they are named venereal; that is, organisms transmitted at coitus. It is these organisms, therefore, which are most importantly identified by the system of cervical swabbing performed routinely.

Even with these bacteria, we have to note that there are strains which are more infective (that is, capable of setting up infection) than others. *Klebsiella* capsular types 1 and 5 are the most infective, whereas type 7 is common but does not appear to have the same degree of infectivity. CEM may lie dormant in a mare without causing endometritis but, on the whole, is the most important equine venereal organism because in most cases it appears to be highly infective. *Pseudomonas* is easily imparted onto the stallion's penis where it becomes a long-term inhabitant unless eliminated by treatment. It may be transferred from the penis to a mare, but a susceptible mare is more likely to become infected than one that is less or not susceptible.

Having introduced these terms let us now consider their implication in relation to endometritis and infection.

The susceptible mare

This term has been used increasingly in recent years to describe individuals who are diagnosed as suffering from endometritis which, when cleared by treatment and/or sexual rest, recurs following mating. The description of becoming re-infected is often used because of the close association between endometritis and infective agents. The re-infection often follows mating and, therefore, the term susceptibility to coital challenge is a phrase often used.

At mating the stallion's penis and ejaculate are introduced into the mare's genital tract resulting in the inevitable challenge of bacteria and foreign protein. This challenge is normally dealt with by the immune status of the tract together with secretions containing anti-bacterial and anti-inflammatory compounds that ensure minimal to no reaction on the part of the genital tract to challenge.

In susceptible mares, the challenge evokes both an exaggerated inflammatory response and, within that response, the conditions in which bacteria flourish. An example is *Pseudomonas* acting as a venereal agent that poses a challenge to older and susceptible mares.

Pregnancy and birth

The fetus and its membranes that occupy the uterus for eleven months are, perhaps, the most significant challenge to the health of the genital tract. Although, of course, a natural process of occupation of the uterus and subsequent passage through the birth canal (cervix and vagina), the fetus is, nonetheless, a foreign body composed of genetic material that is different, even if related to, its dam.

There is, therefore, a potential immunological stimulus to which the maternal system might respond if it were not for mechanisms that normally provide protection. These mechanisms are not fully understood but involve localised suppression of inflammatory responses that would be evoked by the body under other circumstances. In addition, the size of the fetus and its membranes containing the amniotic and allantoic fluids entails a very substantial stretching effect on the uterus, with a similar stretching of the cervix, vagina and vulva during the passage of the fetal foal during birth.

The whole genital tract is exposed, therefore, to a process from which it has to recover each year after pregnancy has terminated. This recovery entails expulsion of all the remnants and fluids of the pregnancy and the return of the uterus to its non-pregnant size. Although this recovery usually takes place, even by the time the foal heat occurs, some individuals require a longer period; possibly one or several heat periods. In exceptional circumstances and in older mares recovery may not take place until the following year or, in very exceptional circumstances, more than one year.

The recovery process is enhanced by the prevention of air being taken into the genital tract after foaling; especially if the air in the environment is dusty and liable therefore to lead to dust particles entering the uterus. This occurs particularly as mares rise to their feet after foaling when the tissues of the vagina, vulva and cervix are stretched to their maximum following birth. If the conformation of the perineum has required a Caslick operation to have been performed, reconstitution by resuturing should be carried out as soon as possible after foaling and the afterbirth has been expelled.

If portions of the placenta are left in the uterus and/or the placenta is abnormally thickened or diseased, recovery of the uterus after foaling may be further delayed.

Recovery of the genital tract is assisted by the natural process of recurring heat periods because the oestrogen produced at this time helps to mobilise the defences of the uterus against infection. It may even be that nature intended the foaling heat to cleanse the uterus rather than allow a new pregnancy.

There is a close relationship between the effect of birth and pregnancy and subsequent breeding results. Conception in maiden mares is in the region of 90 per cent but the rate becomes progressively lower in foaling mares and repeated pregnancies may lead to gradual deterioration of the mare's genital tract with chronic and acute endometritis developing.

Veterinary treatment following foaling consists of administration of oxytocin (the hormone which causes the uterus to contract and expel fluid); and washing out of the uterus with normal saline and/or antibiotic solutions (Figure 7.8) may be used to assist recovery.

Hormonal imbalance

In the past, claims have been made that hormonal imbalance is the cause of sub-fertility. However, the measurement of hormone levels in the blood fails to reflect the receptor status of the tissues to that hormone and, without that knowledge, the concept of imbalance in levels of oestrogen, progesterone or the pituitary hormones FSH and LH is not really meaningful. Further, changing levels of sex hormones are the background to the oestrous cycle and pregnancy so that the term hormonal imbalance is something of a misnomer.

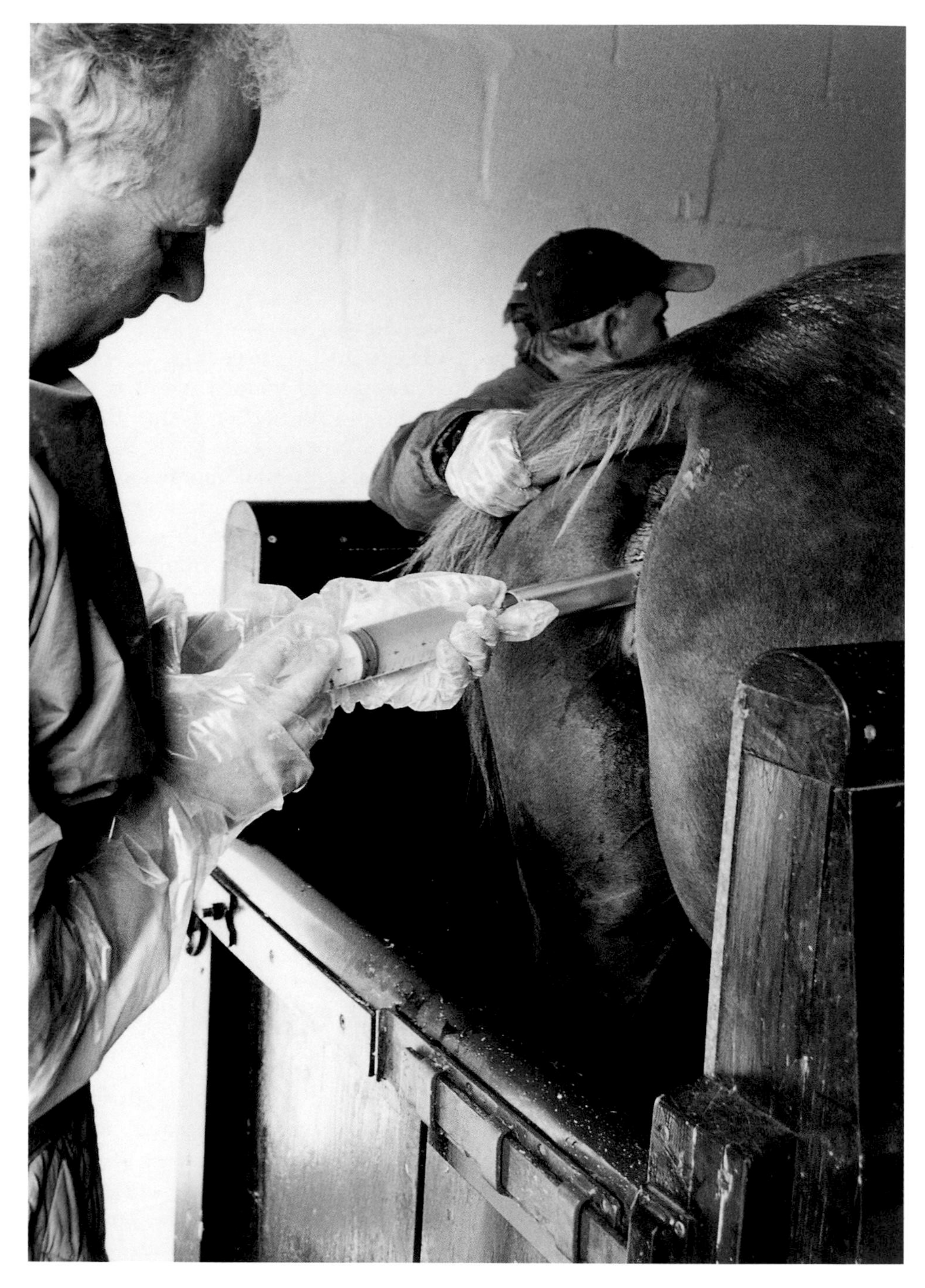

Figure 7.8

Washing out of the uterus with an antibiotic solution

The exception is when there is a pathology which causes a substantial and measurable hormonal imbalance, the most notable of which is the granulosa cell tumour of the ovary or when the uterine lining degenerates into the condition known as pyometra and the uterus fills with pus.

Ovarian tumours

Tumours occasionally form in an ovary from the granulosa cells which line the follicles.

The ovary becomes enlarged and honeycombed with cyst-like spaces containing bloodstained fluid (Figure 7.9).

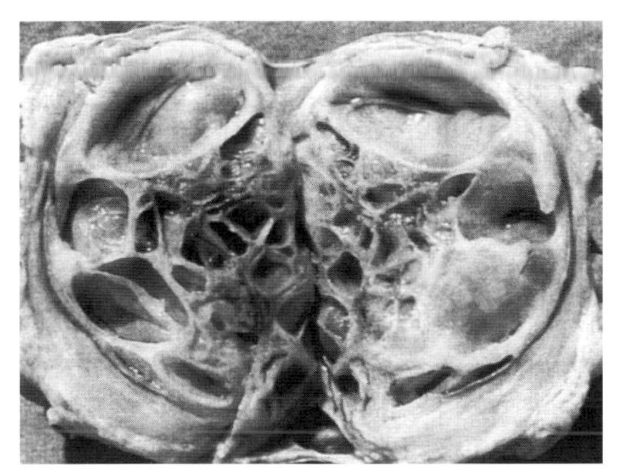

Figure 7.9

Section of granulosa cell tumour showing the cystic spaces which are fluid-filled in life

The mare cannot breed unless the affected ovary is removed but, once this is performed, fertility is usually restored and the mare can function adequately with one ovary.

Granulosa cell tumours may produce large quantities of testosterone which cause the mare to become aggressive. Other forms seem only to prevent the formation of yellow bodies and, therefore, an absence of progesterone. These individuals suffer prolonged low-grade oestrus.

Managing Sub-fertility in the Mare

Inability to conceive, repeated uterine infections and/or inability to carry a pregnancy through to term are the main visible factors of sub-fertility in the mare; however, there may be several underlying causes. From a management point of view, it is important to establish the main causal factors as soon as possible to avoid substantial veterinary expense, delays in breeding and consequently financial costs and losses to the owner.

It is important for every breeder to understand the causes of sub-fertility so that irreversible damage is not done to the mare's reproductive tract by slow action. Today it is common for mares, particularly on larger studfarms, to be examined thoroughly prior to mating, for swabs to be taken and detailed preparations made prior to breeding. Due to this practice, slight changes can be picked up quickly.

However, on smaller studfarms where regular veterinary attendance may be prohibitive due to cost, such problems may go unnoticed for some time. Some of the factors that cause sub-fertility in mares are easily put right – careful and thorough management practices will help in almost all cases.

Controlled breeding, such as in-hand breeding, can affect a mare's breeding potential. The enforced breeding season, such as that for Thoroughbreds (15 February to 15 July), can dramatically affect a mare. In the wild state she would not begin to cycle properly until spring and continue to cycle into summer; with the Thoroughbred's set breeding season, some mares are only just coming to the peak in their reproductive activity when the season is over. Over many centuries, the evolutionary process has ensured that foals are born at the optimum time of year for survival – when the weather is warm and the grazing at its most nutritious.

Selection of stock for breeding, on the basis of performance and conformation, may also predispose the individual to reduced fertility. When horses are selected on this basis alone little thought is given to reproductive potential and many only manage some level of fertility with veterinary intervention. For example, in the wild, a sub-fertile mare would still be mated but would fail to produce offspring regularly and therefore any inherent problems would not extensively be passed on to future generations.

Today, the many techniques used on a regular basis by studfarms ensure that sub-fertile mares get in foal each year. Twins are also common, particularly with Thoroughbreds. Before the use of ultrasound, twins were almost impossible to detect until birth; however, today it is possible to detect twins as early as 16 days from mating. A commonly used veterinary technique is to squeeze one of the twins leaving the remaining twin to continue its development to term. Therefore, it is possible that a large percentage of Thoroughbreds were twins at conception and this predisposes production of twin pregnancies when they themselves are bred.

Nutritional status is a factor that is often overlooked. However, on a more general basis, it is sensible to consider the influence of domestication on the modern horse.

It is common knowledge that the horse's natural method of feeding is generally seriously compromised by modern management techniques and this can predispose digestive problems such as colic and laminitis. Reproductive status can also be compromised by nutrition. Underfeeding can delay the onset of puberty and it can, in the long term, cause permanent damage. Underfeeding in adults can delay the onset of oestrus and result in a lack of follicular development as well as altering the normal reproductive behaviour. Some nutritionally compromised horses will remain in deep anoestrus.

A compromised nutritional status can develop from lack of correct feeding, a poorly balanced diet, a systemic illness, tooth disease or overgrowth and, perhaps most importantly of all, parasite infestation.

Another common factor in reduced conception rates is the failure to detect oestrus in the mare. This is more common on smaller studfarms where veterinary examinations are kept to a minimum.

There may be several reason why this may occur:

- Poor understanding by the stud manager of the oestrous cycle.
- The erratic behaviour of mares during the transitional period from anoestrus to oestrus.
- Inadequate teasing records.
- Inadequate teasing techniques. Some small studfarms do not have a teaser, or stallion with which to tease their mares regularly and may be forced to rely on veterinary assistance alone. This can work if the stud staff fully understand the mare's likely status and are able to give as much information as possible to the veterinary surgeon before the mare is examined.
- Maiden mares that are afraid or nervous of the teaser stallion.

Breeding during the foal heat – the first oestrus period after foaling – is still a controversial practice. Some research has indicated that breeding on this heat can result in a higher rate of uterine infection and subsequent absorption of the pregnancy at an early stage. However, some mares do conceive successfully on this heat.

Normally, foal heat matings depend on a careful assessment of the mare for suitability. Her uterus will be examined by rectal palpation and ultrasonography to check for the stage of involution after foaling (Figure 7.10). This means whether the uterus has adequately returned to its normal non-pregnant size and consistency. Some young mares display a good level of rapid involution after foaling, but older mares may take some time to return to normal. If the mare has had a difficult foaling it is wise to leave her to run a full cycle before mating is considered. Swabs are also taken from through the cervix to obtain a sample of the uterine cells, which will indicate if inflammation and infection are present. Again, a mare showing signs of inflammation or infection should not be mated on this heat. A common compromise for many breeders is the use of the hormone prostaglandin to shorten the mare's normal cycle. This is generally given a week or longer after the end of the foal heat and should result in the mare returning into oestrus.

Older mares who have bred successfully for many years may display reduced fertility as they age. The uterine lining of the mare is not renewed as in humans and any damage that it suffers over the years from matings and pregnancies will result in permanent scarring. This scarring will eventually prevent the proper implantation of a conceptus and the mare will continually fail to become pregnant. The changes in her uterus may make her prone to post-coital infections that she is unable to clear in time for the arrival of the fertilised ovum (Figure 7.11). She may suffer from reduced muscle tone and the muscular seal of the vulva may be incomplete, causing her to take air into the vagina and, consequently, cause a chronic, low-grade, uterine infection. Older mares may undergo cyclic changes and may develop erratic oestrous patterns and changes in ovulation.

In conclusion, careful preparation of the mare prior to the breeding season and before mating can assist in reducing the level of sub-fertility. Understanding each mare as an individual, even if she is only on the stud for a matter of days, is

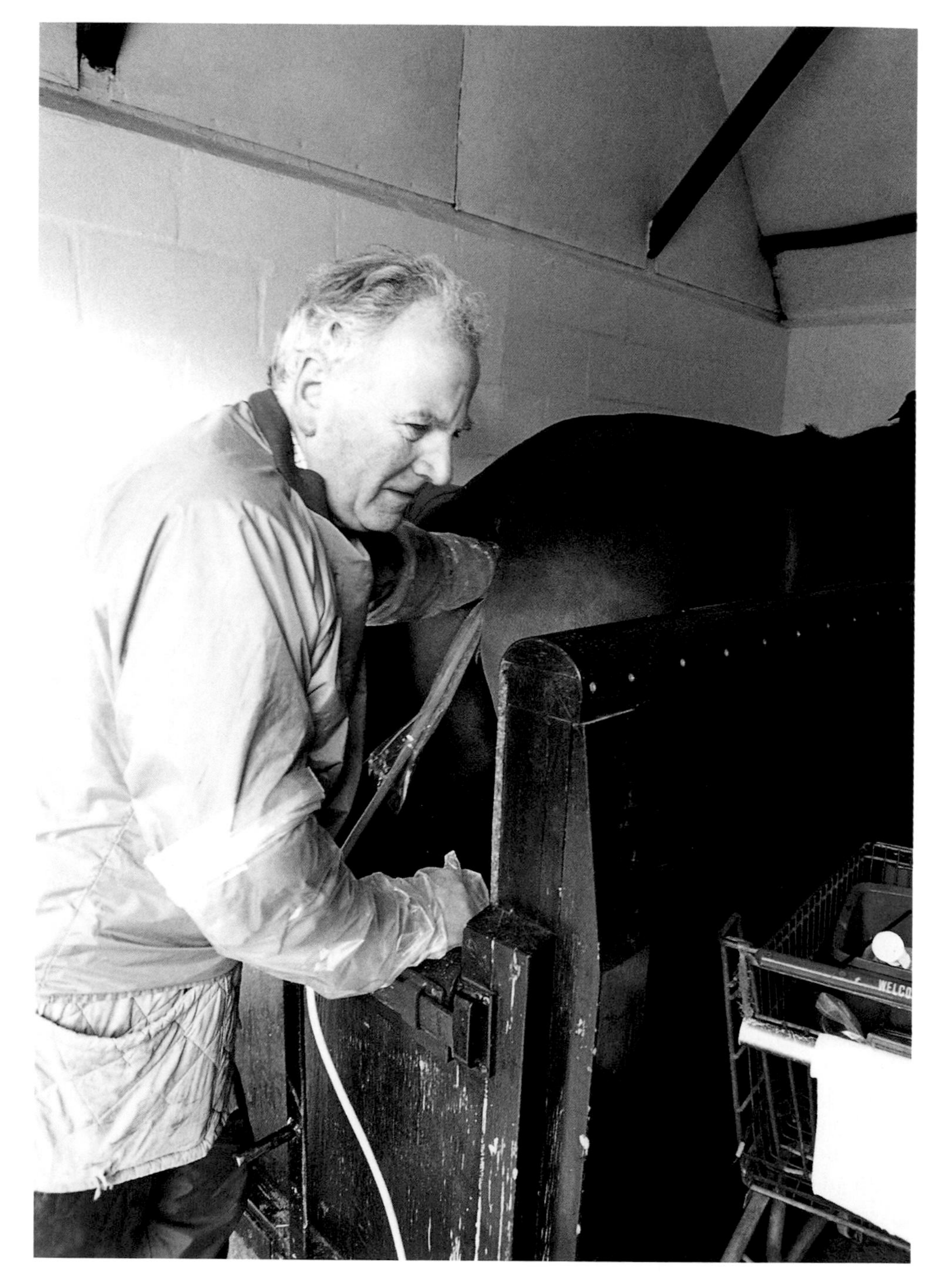

Figure 7.10

Examination of the mare's uterus, post-foaling. Using ultrasonography enables the veterinary surgeon to assess the level of recovery of her uterus following pregnancy

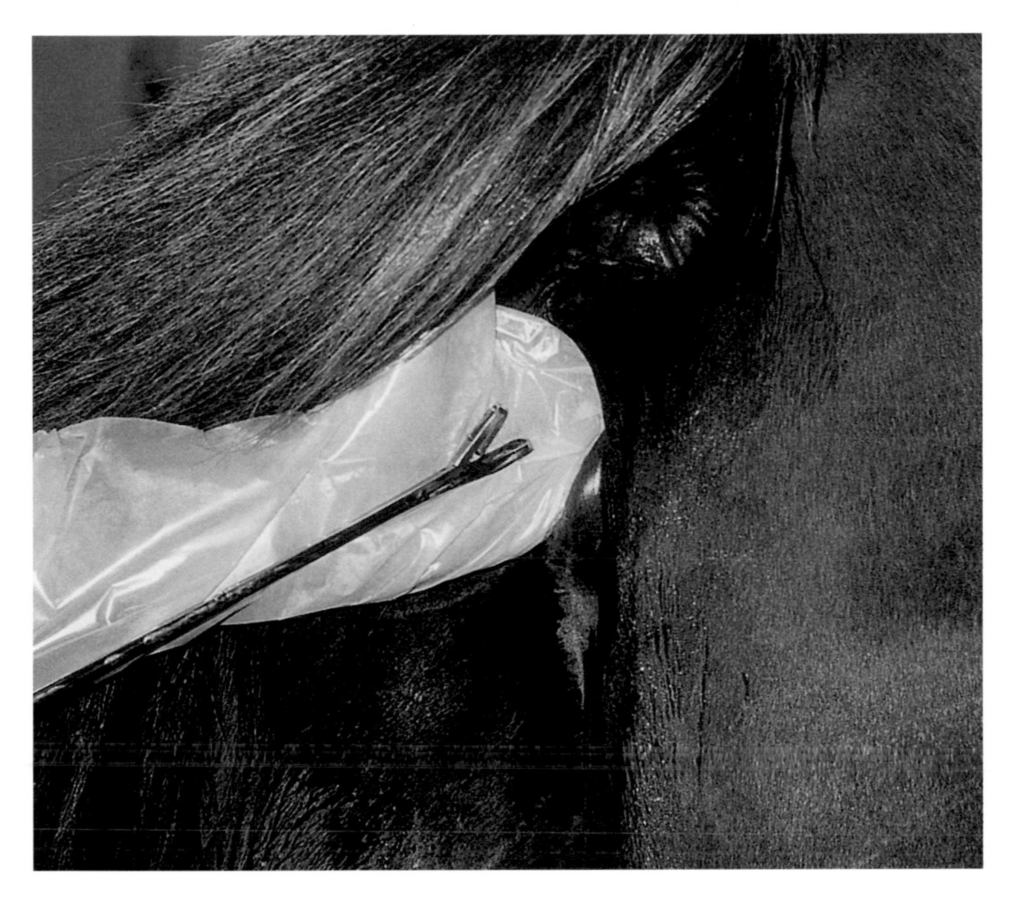

Figure 7.11

A uterine biopsy may be carried out to assess the condition of the endometrium in a sub-fertile mare. This procedure is commonly carried out in the late summer/autumn to allow time for treatment and recovery

of particular importance. A good stud manager will be able to assess each mare shortly after her arrival and, by using her previous breeding history, her age and condition, decide on the best management plan for her.

Today the availability of quality equine veterinary surgeons to most studfarms has enabled previously difficult mares to successfully conceive much earlier in the breeding season and to carry a healthy pregnancy to term.

However, nature nearly always has the last word when it is time for a mare to stop breeding.

Sub-fertility in Stallions

As with mares, the term sub-fertility is a matter of degree. In stallions, complete infertility or sterility is a comparatively rare phenomenon but conception rates vary from horse to horse. It is sometimes said, therefore, that one horse is more fertile than another.

As with individual mares and groups of mares, allowance must be made for deficiencies in management and, in addition, for the breeding states of mares presented to the horse. A horse with a high proportion of problem mares, such as those suffering from sub-fertility, foaling late in the breeding season or consisting of a high proportion of older mares, may have rates of conception which are lower than the average.

The fairest and most appropriate method of comparison and of assessment of any given stallion is to use means introduced by underwriters when a stallion is insured against sub-fertility. This system appraises the ratio of matings per oestrous cycle of mares presented to those conceiving.

Reasons for sub-fertility in stallions

Lack of libido – that is, a horse showing no interest in its mares, failing to mount, failing to maintain an erection or failing to ejaculate – are links in the chain of sexual drive which may be lacking in any particular individual.

Lack of sexual drive may be due to insufficient LH produced by the pituitary and/or testosterone by the testes. Because sexual drive is based on testosterone, it is this hormone which plays a decisive role.

Painful lesions of the back, hind limbs or genital regions may prevent the horse exhibiting the normal sequence of sexual behaviour and prevent completion of the ejaculatory process. Failure of stud management to recognise ejaculation may also contribute to the stallion's ability to achieve conception in a high proportion of his mares.

Ejaculation is usually evaluated by observing tail flag or feeling the urethral pulse. The latter method is probably the more reliable, but in some cases, seminal plasma may be ejaculated without sperm and the horse is led away from his mare in the erroneous assumption that successful mating has taken place.

If ejaculation is occurring, then the semen quality is the all-important measure. The number of live normal sperm per unit volume (Nl) of the sample is multiplied by the total gel-free volume. This allows the ejaculate to be evaluated in terms of total number of normal live and active sperm.

It has been estimated that the minimum number is 300,000,000 for a mating to be successful. However, this can only be a rule of thumb assessment because numbers may vary considerably according to any given stallion.

Most stallions ejaculate far in excess of this gold standard number. But there are occasions when the stallion produces well in excess of the minimal number but is still sub-fertile. Often the reasons for this are unknown. However, there is evidence in other species, such as the bull, that the seminal fluid produced by the accessory glands may have some fertility reducing content; and when the sperm is separated by artificial means from the seminal fluid normal conception is achieved. This procedure would not, of course, be allowed in Thoroughbreds.

Infection of the horse's urethra or accessory sexual glands with bacteria such as *Klebsiella* is comparatively rare but, if infection is established, this would interfere with fertility. Blood in the semen is another element which may cause sub-fertility.

Managing Sub-fertility in the Stallion

Reproductive efficiency in the stallion is vital. On a commercial studfarm, a stallion may have a book of 80 mares (some studfarms allow as many as 200 mares per stallion, but the average would perhaps be nearer to 65). The aim of the stud manager is that each mare will only need to mated on one heat period to conceive. Although this is the ideal, the reality is that at least 25 per cent of the mares will require mating on more than one heat period before they conceive, a further, say 5 per cent, of the original 25 per cent will need mating on three or more heat periods before conception. For a stallion who already has a large book of mares, this may mean he is mating upwards of 120 times during, in many cases, a relatively short breeding season. It is therefore necessary for him to mate normally every day, for the majority twice a day, throughout the peak of the season. Some stallions with very large books of mares, those in the region of 120 per season, may need to mate as many as four times a day throughout the peak. On a commercial studfarm, it is easy for the number of covers required of a stallion to escalate, resulting in the potential for serious economic loss, especially if he was already struggling to maintain a basic level of reproductive efficiency.

As with the mare, stallions are rarely selected for fertility alone and in many breeds this fact alone has contributed to very low conception rates; perhaps as low as 50 per cent with some breeds. Artificial management of most domesticated stallions can affect them to a greater degree than it does to a mare. Stallions tend to be kept relatively isolated from the other horses and this can play a large part in the stallion's general attitude and ability when mating with his mares (see Chapter Five). Some stallions are particularly susceptible to management stresses.

The use of drugs in young horses, for example steroids to improve muscle, libido and growth rates, is not common today. Such drugs, if used with breeding stallions, produce almost the opposite effect, causing a loss of libido and fertility, sometimes permanently. The effects of any drug vary between horses and it is important to monitor each individual's reaction so that an adverse reaction can be avoided during the breeding season. This is an important factor that should not be overlooked even with commonly used medication such as 'bute'.

The nutritional status of the stallion is of prime importance to maintain high levels of sperm production. Although the stallion requires an optimum balanced diet, it is important that he should not be allowed to become overweight as this may make it difficult for him physically to mate with his mares and, in the long term, may shorten his life at stud. Obesity is known to decrease libido and fat deposits around the scrotum will increase sperm temperature causing degeneration of the sperm producing cells.

Over-use of a stallion throughout the breeding season will nearly always cause reduced fertility. Each stallion varies and by keeping careful records it is possible to clearly track any drop in the reproductive efficiency of the stallion during each season. By looking back through the records, it may be possible to link this to a previously busy period; perhaps he was mating more than once a day every day for two weeks. The real key is understanding how many times each stallion can be bred without reducing the number or quality of the sperm in each ejaculate. Some research indicates that the sperm reserves are depleted by 80 per cent after mating once a day every day for one week. When this occurs the stallion can only ejaculate those sperm which have reached maturity that day. If bred every day the total sperm produced does not change, but the concentration per ejaculate will be reduced.

Although there will be times when it is impossible to reduce the demands on the stallion, it is important to remember that there may be a temporary period of reduced fertility as a result.

If the stallion is unwell, or in pain, it will directly affect his ability in the covering barn. Any stallion that is unwell should be relieved of his covering duties until he has recovered.

CHAPTER EIGHT

Life Before Birth

Pregnancy is the popular term for gestation, the period of growth and development of the new individual conceived at the time of fertilisation of the egg. The period of gestation in the mare is, on average, 340 days for Thoroughbreds and 335 days for ponies.

The emphasis on a new individual is important because this illustrates the autonomy and genetic difference between the mare and her fetal foal. This difference has led to the description 'the fetus is equivalent to a foreign body and acts as a parasite, gaining nourishment and sustenance from the mare without contributing to the well-being of the host'.

The new individual starts as a single cell and develops into the foal that we see for the first time at birth. Then, it contains all the tissues and essential structural and functional elements for independent existence and further development to the horse of our pleasure and usage, reaching sexual and musculo-skeletal maturity by about age four years. However, it is during the period of gestation that the most rapid developments have to be achieved if the foal is to survive and be normal.

In this chapter, let us look at the various elements, peculiarities and special relationships of the foal in its life before birth.

Conception

The egg consists of a single cell about the size of a grain of sand. The spermatazoa are even smaller and many millions are contained in each ejaculate of a stallion. After coitus the spermatazoa travel rapidly up both horns of the uterus and into each of the fallopian tubes. In these tubes they await the descent of the egg after it has been expelled from the ovary (ovulation).

The egg is fertilised by the entry of one spermatozoon and subsequently is resistant to the entry of any other male cell; it cannot be fertilised a second time. The union of the egg cell (ovum) and the sperm cell (spermatozoon) 'activates' the egg and the inherited material (chromosomes and genes) combine to form a single cell.

This single cell then divides repeatedly, so that at first two cells, then four, then eight, then 16 are formed. At this early stage the term 'embryo' is often used instead of fetus. The term 'blastocyst' is also used to describe the hollow ball of cells which enters the uterus from the fallopian tube.

The fertilised egg takes five days to travel down the fallopian tube and enter the uterus. This has an important practical significance, because the uterus may be treated with antibiotics or flushed out in the treatment or prevention of endometritis in sub-fertile mares during this period without risk of disturbing the embryo. Conversely, if for any reason we need to prevent pregnancy continuing (for example, in the event of a mismating), successful flushing cannot be achieved until at least five days after ovulation, but, it must be emphasised, not from the time of mating.

Development and Growth

In the uterus the cells continue to multiply but at the same time certain cells become differentiated into organs, blood, muscle, skin, etc. By about day 20 an outline of the foal has appeared in miniature. From day 20 onwards the organs and tissues that have been formed start to grow.

Of course not all the tissues will be fully formed in the first 20 days (for example, hair does not appear until about the seventh month). The organs will not necessarily mature until a much later stage; the lungs, for instance, grow as an organ from an early stage of pregnancy but cannot function normally until about day 300 after conception. For this reason a foal born in a very premature state cannot survive.

Just as the young need body-building substances, so the fetus depends on an adequate diet to meet its demands for growth. In addition, it must receive the vital gas oxygen and dispose of waste products (carbon dioxide, ammonia, etc.) which are potentially poisonous if allowed to accumulate in the body. These processes, which in the outside world are carried out by the lungs, kidneys and digestive tract, are performed for the fetus by the placenta, an organ developed especially for the purpose.

In recent years, studies of human fetal development and newborn status indicate that the development of the microstructure within most organs is completed by the end of pregnancy. Thus, the human infant is born with a total number of terminal air ducts in the lungs and glomeruli (filtering units) in the kidneys; the human individual develops no more in numbers and although size of organs increases for some years, the density (number per gram) of the glomeruli and terminal bronchioles remains the same. If we lose these microstructures for reasons of disease or injury we cannot grow replacements. This is in contrast to an organ such as the liver, which can regenerate if the need arises.

We will consider later the effects of intrauterine growth retardation (IUGR) and its potential consequences for the individual in later life.

The development of microstructure during pregnancy has been shown to be similar in animals, including the horse, to that present in human development.

When the embryo reaches the uterus on the fifth day, the cells continue to divide, arranging themselves around the central cavity of the blastocyst. Then begin the two major processes of differentiation and growth which continue until birth. The ability of cells to differentiate into specialised layers and tissues leads to organ formation, while growth is necessary to achieve the size required for independent survival.

The two processes of differentiation and growth are continuous although they occur at differing rates; differentiation is most intense during the first 40 days, growth the most obvious between 150 and 300 days.

At the time of fertilisation of the egg, the new individual is the size of a grain of sand, by nine days its diameter is about 2 mm, at three weeks it is 50 mm. The changes in weight, length and character during pregnancy are significant (see Figure 8.1).

Nourishment of the Fetus

In the early stages of development the fetus is nourished from fluids which surround it first in the fallopian tube, and then in the uterus. Once inside the uterus, it develops special outgrowths from its body containing numerous blood vessels. This is known as the yolk sac placenta.

Between days 20 and 40 the yolk sac placenta decreases in size and importance, the role of the exchange between mother and fetus being taken over by the true placenta which is connected to the fetus through the umbilical cord.

The yolk sac placenta is a pouch containing many blood vessels which grows from the gut of the embryo. The pouch is bathed in uterine fluid and capable of extracting the necessary nutrients for the early development of the fetus.

The true placenta develops as a very fine membrane filled with fluid and undergoes progressive development, becoming increasingly substantial. By day 50–60 the membrane develops the fine velvet-like surface that we see when the afterbirth is expelled at foaling.

The true placenta is unique to the horse compared to other mammalian species because it covers the whole of the uterine surface from about day 100 of pregnancy onwards. All other mammalian species restrict their placenta to discrete areas of contact with the uterine wall. In women, the placenta is

Figure 8.1

The length and weight of a fetus in relation to stage of pregnancy

Days from conception	Approximate length from head to tail	Approximate weight
56	10 cm	9 g
112	28 cm	70 g
224	56 cm	9 kg
280	84 cm	19 kg
340 (full term)	97 cm	45 kg

disc-shaped, in the pig, band-like and, in sheep and cow, it is attached by button-like structures.

In passing, it is worthy of note that the diffuse attachment of the mare's placenta means that there is no extra area for the presence of a second placenta so that, in the case of twins, each placenta competes with the other for attachment to the uterine wall. The restriction in area of attachment means that both twins are disadvantaged and the pregnancy results in abortion or undersized and undernourished foals should they go to full-term.

The equine central attachment to the uterine lining of the mare has six cell layers between the fetal and maternal bloodstreams. Three of these layers are part of the placenta and three part of the uterus.

These layers are:

1. The wall of the fetal blood vessel.
2. A layer of supporting (connective) tissue.
3. The epithelial (outer) layer of the placenta.
4. The epithelial (outer) layer of the uterus.
5. The supporting connective tissue layer.
6. The fine capillary wall of the maternal blood vessel.

In terms of nourishment and exchange of nutrients and waste material in the fetal and maternal bloodstreams, respectively, the pathway between the two bloodstreams is known as the diffusion pathway along which travel the molecules of nourishment and life support, such as oxygen. Those of waste material, such as carbon dioxide and tissue waste, take the opposite route (Figure 8.2).

If we compare the arrangement with other species, the number of cell layers in many species is reduced, usually by the placenta eroding the maternal layers, and in some cases, losing some of

Figure 8.2

The close relationship between the blood vessels in the placenta and the wall of the uterus

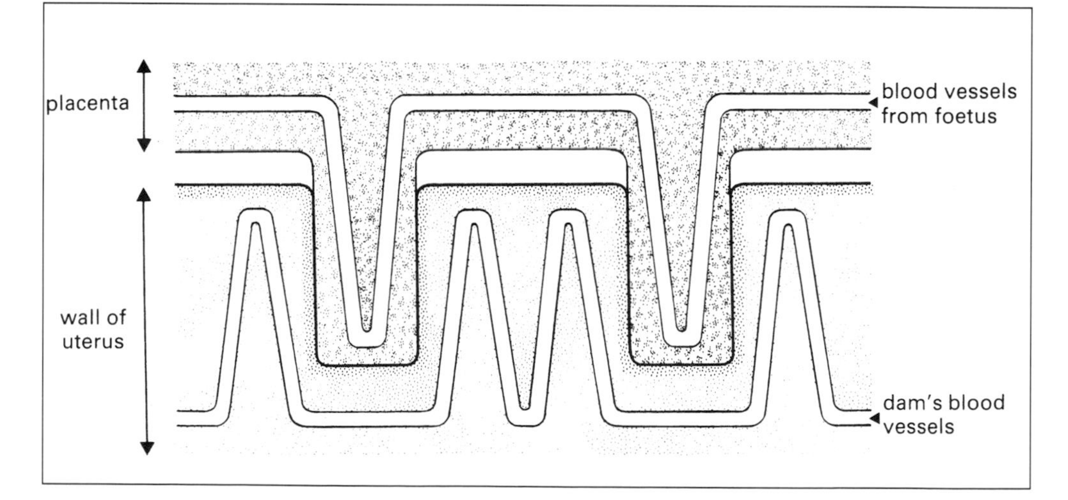

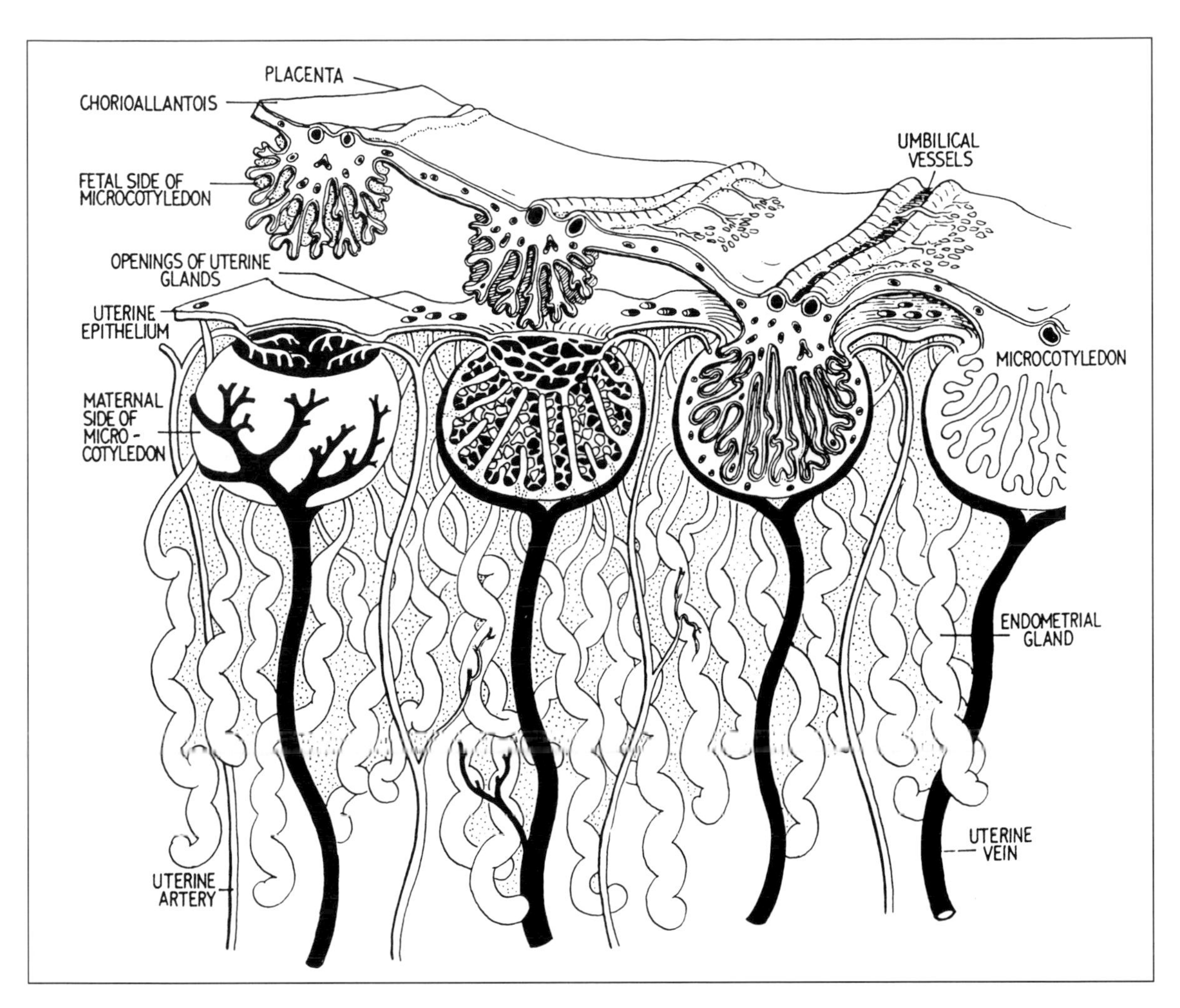

Figure 8.3

The mature equine placenta, showing the structure of the microcotyledons, of which four are shown: the two on the left are 'unbuttoned' from their position in the uterine wall

its own. The equine placenta does not erode the uterine tissue and, therefore, when it peels away after birth, it does not usually cause much, if any, bleeding.

There is an intricate relationship between the fetal and maternal sides, commonly called the utero-placental junction (Figure 8.3). Cotyledons (buttons of the sheep and cow which can readily be seen with the naked eye) are not present in the equine placenta although there is a corresponding arrangement in the form of microcotyledons that is, microscopic buttons. There are many millions which cover the entire surface of the placental membrane and fit into opposite receiving 'buttonholes' on the maternal side.

Each micro-cotyledon is composed of an outer capsule with arterial blood vessels entering at the top. These divide into capillaries through which the blood passes back into veins. Veins form one large vein draining away from the lower part of the capsule.

On the placental side arteries also carry blood driven by the fetal heart into capillaries. The two systems fit together like the clasping of hands. Veins convey the blood back into the umbilical cord and thence it passes to the fetal foal's heart.

The direction of flow in the placental and maternal blood vessels is in opposite directions and this makes the exchange between the bloodstreams more efficient based, as it is, on the principle of simple diffusion in which gases and substances pass from areas of high to those of low concentration. Oxygen in the maternal bloodstream is relatively plentiful compared with that within the fetal bloodstream, which takes up the oxygen and carries it via the fetal heart to the tissues of the fetus. Carbon dioxide and other waste material enters the heart through the veins of the fetus and is then driven by the pumping heart into the arteries which carry it through the cord to the placenta.

Thus, the umbilical vein contains blood which is high in oxygen and nutrients whereas the arteries entering the placenta are high in carbon dioxide and waste material; the reverse quality is true in the bloodstream in the independent individual where the arteries carry blood rich in oxygen.

The placenta itself is an organ of considerable substance, at birth weighing something in the order of 5–10 kg. It is an organ which, like any other, requires oxygen and nutrients for its health. The pathways involved in diffusion between the fetal and maternal bloodstream and that involved in maintaining the placenta are illustrated in Figure 8.3. The placenta is also a source of hormones, such as corticotrophin releasing factor (CRF) that causes the release of ACTH from the pituitary, as well as ACTH, progesterone and progesterone-like substances.

The placenta is thus actually engaged in the maintenance of pregnancy as well as in the development and maturation of the fetus itself. It probably plays a major role in mediating the end of pregnancy at the time of foaling. The placental glands are active in producing substances which overcome the natural reaction of the uterus to reject the presence of foreign material.

Umbilical Cord

The umbilical cord runs from the fetal foal's navel to the placenta and is composed of two arteries that arise from the aorta where it divides into two vessels (iliac arteries), thus carrying blood directly from the heart into the placental membrane.

The two arteries enter the membrane at a point where the two horns of the placenta meet. One artery supplies blood to the body and non-pregnant horn of the placenta and the other supplies the pregnant horn and body. Both arteries divide into smaller and smaller branches until entering the micro-cotyledons as capillaries.

As described above, the blood in the micro-cotyledons leaves in veins that collect to an increasing size until eventually adjoining to form the one umbilical vein that passes in the cord to the fetal foal's navel (umbilicus) where it passes forward to the liver discharging its blood into this organ. In other mammals, part of the venous bloodstream is diverted through the ductus venosus, a channel which bypasses the liver and goes directly into the vena cava (the major vein of the body leading to the heart). There is no ductus venosus in the horse and the entire blood flow from the placenta passes through the liver.

The consequences of this in terms of blood pressure and its flow has not yet been determined by scientists, but this quirk of nature may well have some bearing on failure of pregnancy (abortion) in certain circumstances. A quite common finding at post mortem of aborted fetuses is engorgement of the liver indicating that a failure in the circulation has been associated with the demise and expulsion of the fetus.

The average length of a cord is about 70 cm but some cords are much longer (up to 110 cm). A cord is naturally twisted but not in an acute sense as this would obviously interfere with blood flow. Due to its length the cord may lie in coils and, sometimes, becomes entangled with the foal's hind legs.

The cord also contains the urachus which is a duct (tube) leading directly from the fetal foal's bladder to the allantois. Urine passes from the bladder through this duct into the allantoic cavity contributing to the formation of allantoic fluid.

Fetal Membranes

The placenta is part of the fetal membrane, the outer surface of which is attached to the uterus and has already been described. The inner surface is the allantois which is an outgrowth of the urinary system which fuses with the chorion, the surface attached to the uterus (see Figure 8.4).

The fetal foal itself is surrounded by a fine membrane, the amnion. This has the property of protecting the foal from the allantoic fluid, contact with which would be harmful. It also has a smooth surface and maintains the amniotic fluid with its protective and nourishing basis for the foal. The membrane and fluid help to lubricate and facilitate the foal's movement in utero as well as contributing to a smooth passage through the birth canal at foaling.

Amniotic fluid is clear, straw-coloured, slightly sticky fluid containing cells rubbed off the foal's skin. It is formed partly by the blood vessels of the amniotic membrane and partly from secretions produced by the foal. It has a physiological composition that is similar to internal fluids that bathe the cells of the body and is, therefore, ideally suited to come in contact with the airways of the fetal head and neck, eyes, ears and skin. It is frequently swallowed by the fetus and this probably assists in the development of the gut both in terms of lubrication and as a means of distending the stomach as it develops.

In the first third of pregnancy the volume of amniotic fluid is in the region of 600 ml, but by the end of pregnancy the volume is some seven or eight times greater.

Allantoic fluid consists of a yellowish-brown fluid which accumulates in increasing quantities during pregnancy. Around day 40 of pregnancy there is about 60 ml; by day 60 about 1200 ml and at the end of pregnancy 8 litres.

The fluid is formed by the placenta and urine passing via the urachus. It is, therefore, a receptacle for unwanted salts and compounds which are not eliminated through the placental/uterine connection. At birth, the fluid

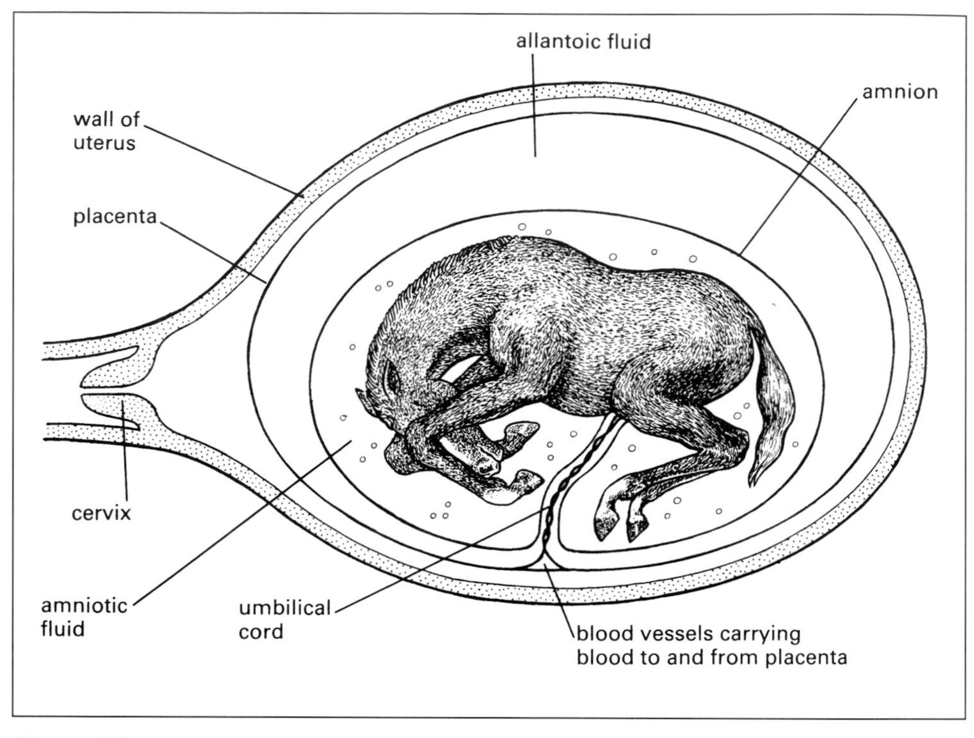

Figure 8.4

The relationship between the amnion, the placenta and the wall of the uterus

escapes when the placenta ruptures and forms the 'breaking of the water'. This fluid contains many cells rubbed off from the placenta and amnion and the hippomane.

The hippomane is a soft, flat, roughly oval-shaped body measuring about 14 cm x 1.5 cm. It is usually brown- or cream-coloured but, sometimes, white. It contains high concentrations of various salts such as calcium, sodium, phosphorus, potassium and magnesium. There is usually only one hippomane but occasionally smaller ones develop and, sometimes, it breaks up into several fragments.

The hippomane appears to form in a similar manner to crystals, cells providing a nucleus around which salts and other substances attach themselves. The term hippomane comes from the Greek word meaning 'horse madness'.

Pregnancy Diagnosis

The diagnosis of pregnancy plays a very important part in stud management during the mating season. Once a mare has been mated by a stallion it is necessary to diagnose whether or not she is pregnant or should be mated at a subsequent oestrus.

Since echography was introduced as a means of diagnosing pregnancy it has been possible for veterinarians to perform a diagnosis at around 16 days following a previous mating. Before the advent of echography it was possible only to make a positive diagnosis at about day 40 from mating employing rectal palpation. This meant that many mares that were not pregnant were missed because they did not show signs of oestrus at the day 15–20 post-mating period.

The use of echography is described in Chapter Four. The rectal examination including echography is usually performed routinely on day 16 from mating. It must be emphasised that 16 days from mating may be only 14 days or less from ovulation. It is important, therefore, for sufficient care to be taken when diagnosing a negative result. Further, the fetal sac may be mobile at this time and although the presence of a fetus may be established with a 95 per cent certainty, the risk of a 5 per cent inaccurate diagnosis at this time makes it reasonable to repeat the examination two or three days later. The same care applies to missing a second fetus, that is, a twin, at an early stage of examination.

As far as pregnancy is concerned, a vaginal examination may help to establish a negative result when the cervix is found to be moist and relaxed. In addition, blood progesterone measurements may be used to establish a negative diagnosis because concentrations of less than 4 ng/ml suggest that a mare is not pregnant; and those below 1 ng/ml indicate that the mare is in oestrus.

As pregnancy proceeds, ultrasonography becomes more accurate to a 100 per cent level by day 40. From day 45 to day 120 the eCG hormone test may be performed. The MIP (mare immunological pregnancy) test is employed by laboratories to measure the blood levels of this hormone. This is a highly accurate test with regard to establishing the presence of endometrial cup production of the hormone eCG, but there is about a 5 per cent inaccuracy related to those mares who have formed cups but the fetus has died. In these cases, the pregnancy test is positive but the mare is not in foal.

Large quantities of oestrogen-like hormone are produced by the fetus and pass into the mare's bloodstream to be filtered through the kidneys into the urine. A further pregnancy test, which is reliable from about day 100 of pregnancy onwards, involves laboratory tests for this hormone (Cuboni test). This is a reliable diagnosis but has the disadvantage that early detection of a fetus is not possible and urine collection may be a tedious process in some individuals.

Progestogen concentrations in a mare's bloodstream may be measured during the last half of pregnancy and are usually in the region of 6 ng/ml, depending on the particular antibody used in the test in different laboratories. However, each laboratory has its own reference values and, in some, the normal values may be higher. However, the value of 6–10 ng/ml is well established and higher values may indicate either that the mare is near to foaling or that there is some pathology of the placenta.

Maintenance of Pregnancy

We have already described the fetal foal as a foreign body or parasite within the uterus of its dam. As it grows, the uterus accommodates this increase by re-modelling of the uterine wall which consists of the lining on the inside, circular and longitudinally running muscle layers in the middle, interspersed by connective tissue and, on the outside, the peritoneum. Re-modelling involves all of these elements in a quite substantial increase of length and area. Following birth, these all return to their non-pregnant state thus completing the cycle of events from conception; the entry of the relatively minute blastocyst into the uterus, its enormous increase in size together with fluids and membranes and then back to the non-pregnant state of the barren mare.

Further, in the early days of pregnancy the uterus is quite active in propelling the conceptus around the surface of the two horns and body. Up to day 15 from ovulation, the conceptus is mobile and propelled by muscular contractions of the uterine wall so that it comes in contact with the whole uterine surface. It is thought that this movement prevents the release of prostaglandin thereby maintaining the yellow body formed when the egg was shed and fertilised. It is essential for continuance of pregnancy that the hormone progesterone continues to be produced by the yellow body beyond its usual oestrous cycle length of 16 days.

Progesterone is the hormone of pregnancy because it helps to keep the uterus quiescent – that is, avoiding major contractions which would expel the fetus as, indeed, occurs at the time of foaling. Other hormones involved in maintaining pregnancy, facilitating re-modelling of the uterine wall to accommodate the increasing uterine content and in the development of the

Figure 8.5

The various changes and hormonal events which occur during pregnancy

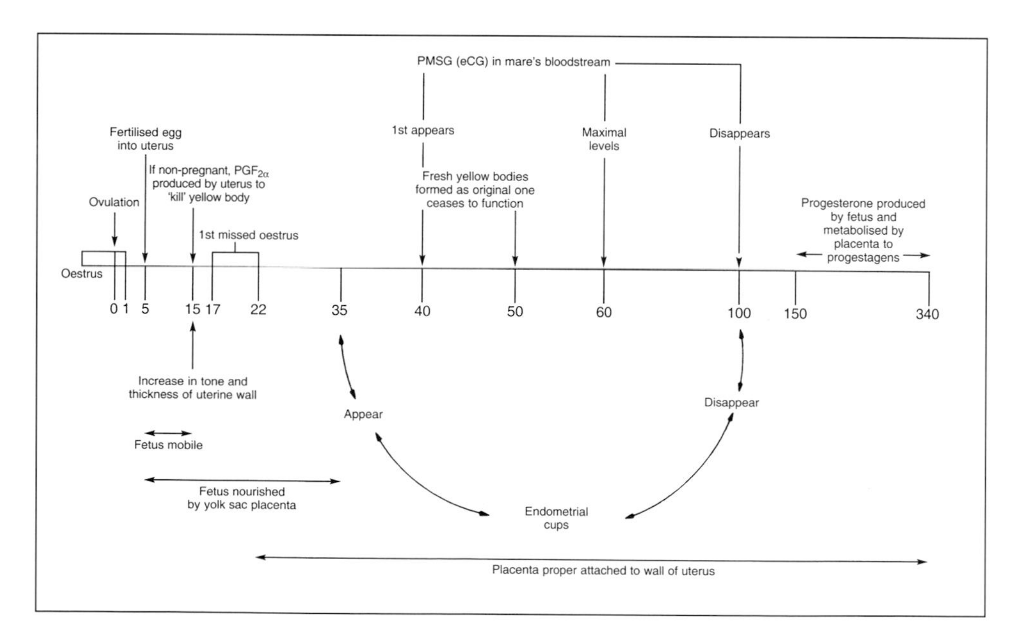

fetus, both of differentiation and growth, include the hormones oestrogen, growth hormones, prostaglandins (PGE not PGF 2alpha) and prolactin.

Hormones control the state of the uterine lining, the amount of blood flowing to the uterine cotyledons, activity of the uterine glands, sensitivity of uterine muscle to stimuli and the degree to which the uterus can expand to accommodate the developing foal while maintaining the cervix in a tightly closed condition.

On the fetal side, hormones control blood flow to the placenta, the development of the placenta itself and fetal growth and development to full size and maturity.

The interrelationship and sequential activity of various hormones is illustrated in Figure 8.5. The yellow body formed at the time of conception has its life extended due to the presence of the conceptus in the uterus. From day 17 onwards other follicles increase in size and, at about day 35, the hormone eCG is produced by the endometrial cups that develop in the lining of the uterus adjacent to the placenta. These consist of a string of saucer-like areas in the uterine surface and consist of cells that have invaded uterine mucosa (lining) from the placenta. These cells produce the hormone eCG (equine chorionic gonadotrophin) composed of follicle stimulating hormone and luteinising hormone in large quantities.

The cups continue to function until around day 90 to day 120 of pregnancy. The cells are recognised and eventually rejected by the mare's immune system. The effect of eCG is to cause the ovaries to produce more follicles which ovulate, thereby taking over the role of progesterone production from the orig inal yellow body.

By about day 120, when the endometrial cups cease to function, the ovaries cease to produce progesterone and become inactive for the rest of pregnancy, only producing follicles at the time of birth leading up to the foal heat.

The source of progesterone in the last two-thirds of pregnancy is from the fetus and placenta. The fetal adrenal gland produces pregnenalone which is converted by the placenta into progesterone and then metabolised; that is, changed in form by enzymes to what are known as progestagens. Progestagens are compounds which have a progesterone-like structure and function. Progesterone itself is not found in the maternal bloodstream during the last two-thirds of pregnancy but higher concentrations of progestagens are present.

Care of the Mare during Pregnancy

During pregnancy, the main management responsibility should be to protect the mare's future reproductive ability as well as allowing every advantage to the developing fetus. It is of particular importance to understand the changes that are occurring within the mare's reproductive system during pregnancy so that a suitable programme of care can be established.

Foaling problems are minimised by keeping the mare in good condition throughout pregnancy, as well as optimising the mare's recovery post-foaling. This factor is particularly important on commercial public studfarms where the aim is to breed from the mare each year and where it may be difficult to provide individual care for each mare. Good husbandry as well as management techniques will all help to ensure optimum well-being for both the mare and the foal during pregnancy, foaling and after birth.

Housing

Pregnant mares are normally kept separately from other groups of mares as they are probably the adult group most susceptible to infection risks. It is not necessary for a normal fit pregnant mare to have special stabling during the early months and, in fact, many studfarms do not move the pregnant mares to foaling boxes until within a few days of giving birth. The decision as to when to move a mare to a foaling box will be taken depending on the facilities available on each individual establishment. Some studfarms have sufficient space in their specialist foaling units to allow the mares to be moved two to three weeks before they are due. This is perhaps the ideal on larger studfarms as it allows the mare a chance to become accustomed to her new environment. However, mares due to foal during the summer months, or in warmer climates, may not be moved to specialised stabling at all and may indeed intentionally be left to foal outside in small foaling paddocks.

The normal considerations for stabling are of prime importance with the pregnant mare. Although healthy adult horses can withstand a wide range of temperatures, a consistent temperature within any stabling is important. Draughts will have a chilling effect on any stabled horse and these should be avoided without compromising ventilation. The effect of stable design and ventilation on the respiratory health of stabled horses is well documented and stabling for all breeding horses requires particular attention. As pregnant mares increase in size and width, they are more prone to injury from narrow doorways; sliding doors are commonly seen on larger studfarms for this very reason. The walkways between stabling should also be designed to be non-slip and wide enough for pregnant mares to be safely led and turned around in.

Exercise

During the early months of pregnancy, the broodmare does not have very different needs to those of a non-pregnant mare. Some mares may continue to race and compete during the first trimester of pregnancy – correctly managed, this level of work will not affect the developing fetus if the mare remains fit and healthy. By the second trimester of her pregnancy, her workload should be reduced accordingly. Some level of moderate exercise is important for the mare, regardless of how close to foaling she is. Self-exercise by being turned out in a paddock is ideal but if the mare has to be box-rested for any particular reason then walking in-hand each day is essential. Throughout pregnancy, the fetus is dependent on the circulating blood from the mare for all its nutritional needs; exercise will increase the flow of blood to all the organs, especially the placenta, enriching the fetus with nutrients and oxygen.

During pregnancy, it is important to keep pregnant mares as settled as possible. Normally, the mares will be put into small groups with similar foaling dates – this also assists with reintegrating a mare back with her companions after foaling. Sometimes it is not possible to avoid introducing a new individual to an established herd, but this should be done in as quiet a manner as possible – perhaps turning the new mare out later in the morning when the established group has already had chance to let off steam. Abortion has been associated with stress – whether it is psychological or physical.

Once the mares are close to term, they will probably become more sedentary and their appetites reduce due to the sheer size of the foal inside them. Oedema and stiffness of the lower limbs is very common in the later stages of pregnancy and exercise will help to ease the discomfort that this may cause. Some mares may also develop abdominal oedema towards the end of their pregnancies as their milk production is increased in preparation for birth. Normally this oedema will develop from the udder following the line of the main veins supplying blood to the area and it does reduce with exercise.

Any excessive abdominal oedema in pregnant mares should be assessed as soon as possible by a veterinary surgeon. Extreme abdominal oedema may indicate a serious condition where the abdominal muscles and the pre-pubic tendon, which supports the uterus, become damaged or ruptured. The incidence of rupture of the supporting structures for the uterus is rare. Reported cases of complete rupture appear to be more common in the heavier breeds, particularly in older mares who may also have poor muscle tone due to age or lack of exercise. A mare with this type of injury will require very careful management and specialised veterinary assistance during foaling. Although it is known for some affected mares to carry subsequent pregnancies to term, it is unlikely that such a mare would be retained for breeding purposes.

Other rare and serious complications such as torsion of the uterus are also recorded in the later stages of pregnancy, when the sheer size of the growing foal causes high levels of physical stress on the mare. This condition is most commonly discovered during surgical treatment for colic but may also be one of the causes of uterine haemorrhage. Uterine haemorrhage is always very serious and more often than not fatal, but if identified early, some mares can be treated successfully.

Nutrition

During the early stages of pregnancy, there is no need to change or increase a pregnant mare's diet unless she is in poor condition. Her nutritional demands will not increase until the last trimester of pregnancy and will not peak until after the foal is born and she is lactating. However, it is important to maintain pregnant mares in good condition throughout the whole of pregnancy. As mentioned earlier, good body condition will allow the mare to recover more quickly post-foaling and provide the foal with the optimum environment during pregnancy. It has to be noted, however, that many mares will go on to produce relatively strong foals even though they themselves are severely nutritionally compromised. Nature has a wonderful way of providing in these circumstances, but allowing this situation to continue past the short-term will ultimately result in a mare who fails to get in foal, or fails to carry a pregnancy to term. Some breeds are more resilient than others; some of the native breeds can cope with high levels of nutritional stress before their pregnancies are affected, whereas the Thoroughbred may not be able to maintain a viable pregnancy if a poor nutritional environment persists.

Conversely, some mares are overfed from the minute they are confirmed as being in foal. The old theory of feeding for two should be discarded. Allowing mares to become overweight will exacerbate the problems of later pregnancy, such as limb oedema and stiffness, and may also affect the mare's recovery post-foaling, as well as putting stress on her vital organs which are already working at peak levels to provide for the pregnancy.

Parasite control

Parasite control is a vital part of horse management, regardless of the status of the horse (see Chapter Fifteen). A mare with a heavy worm infestation will be compromised in many ways.

During pregnancy, the mare is physically challenged to produce healthy offspring – her digestive and circulatory systems are all working at peak capacity. A worm burden will compromise nutritional levels and causes stress on the circulatory system with migrating parasites causing minor haemorrhages and aneurysms which result in the pregnancy being compromised as well as putting the mare at an increased risk of colic or further complications. Mares with infestations will also put their newborn offspring at risk. For example, infection with *Strongyloides westeri* (small roundworm) in the foal is directly transmitted through sucking; the parasite is adept at transferring itself to its newborn host through the milk the mare produces. Most adult horses have some degree of resistance to this parasite; however, a foal has no such resistance and its immature gut can be seriously and permanently damaged by a worm burden at this stage. Foals that become infested will remain compromised for the rest of their lives due to intestinal ulceration.

Routine care

As the pregnancy progresses, increasing and changing bodyweight may predispose mares to foot and limb problems. Routine farrier attention is very important at this time to keep hooves well trimmed and supported. Most broodmares have their shoes removed when they are at stud and this is preferred unless the mare has a particular problem, although for obvious safety reasons hind shoes should be removed. Regardless of whether shod or not, the pregnant mare requires the same frequency of farrier attention as any competing horse. Mares who have a pre-existing or old injury may also suffer more discomfort as their pregnancy progresses and these mares should be continually assessed to avoid the risk of exacerbating original problems or causing secondary injuries.

Routine vaccinations

Most public studfarms have a set vaccination requirement for all visiting mares and this will include routine protection against conditions such as influenza and tetanus, as well as more specialised requirements for vaccination against equine herpesvirus (EHV) for all pregnant mares. The use of vaccination against other conditions, such as rotavirus, is becoming increasingly common.

The infection risk to breeding horses on public studfarms is particularly high. This is mainly due to the changing population of mares arriving for the breeding season. Each studfarm may have a different policy regarding vaccination and, surprisingly, there are still some horses who remain totally unvaccinated for the whole of their lives. The cost of vaccinating a horse is small when it is compared to the very real cost in terms of avoidable loss of life and/or veterinary fees in the event of a disease outbreak.

The standard requirement for mares visiting a public studfarm would be an up to date annual vaccination for influenza and tetanus. Some breeders also like to give the mare a booster tetanus vaccination when she is about one month from foaling. All visiting pregnant mares will also be required to be vaccinated for EHV if they are to give birth at stud. This vaccination is usually given in the fifth, seventh and ninth months of pregnancy – at least two of these vaccinations must have been given for protection to be considered adequate. Insisting on correct vaccination for all visiting mares, particularly for foaling mares, is an essential part of any stud management policy.

All of the commonly used vaccinations for EHV, such as Duvaxyn EHV 1,4, are recorded as completely safe at any stage of the mare's pregnancy – this is because most vaccinations currently used as routine contain the inactivated or killed virus.

CHAPTER NINE

Abortion

Abortion is the term used for expulsion of the fetal foal from the mare in a non-viable state; that is, when it has no chance of survival. This is usually taken as being less than 300 days of pregnancy. After 300 days, there is a chance that the foal will be capable of survival given moderate assistance. The term premature is used for delivery between day 300 and day 320 of pregnancy, whereas the term dysmature is used for foals that are born in a premature-like condition (see Chapter Thirteen) but during the full-term period of between day 320 and day 360 of pregnancy. Stillbirth describes a full-term foal which is born dead from about day 320 onwards.

Of course, all these different terms are defined arbitrarily and used frequently in different senses. For example, a foal born dead at any stage, even during the full-term period, may be described as an abortion or a stillbirth. A dysmature foal may be described as premature. There are also exceptions as, for example, a foal born at day 280 of pregnancy but surviving (see Chapter Thirteen). This is biologically a premature foal but one which has been switched on and is ready for birth (see Chapter Eleven).

The emphasis in this chapter is on the conditions which cause fetal ill-health and death, thereby causing the mare to expel the fetus in a non-viable condition or dead. Abortion may be regarded as the fatal and extreme outcome of a uterine condition which, in a less acute form, may mean premature delivery and the possibility of survival of the foal delivered as a result of ill-health. In addition, the fetus may be healthy but some process or stimulus on the maternal side causes the mare to expel the fetus in a non-viable state. Let us, therefore, examine what is known of the various states of ill-health and maternally triggered evacuation of the uterine contents.

Placental Ill-health

The placenta is an organ of supreme importance to fetal health (see Chapter Eight). It is responsible for the exchange of nutrients and waste products between the fetus and the mare. Any damage or lack of function puts fetal health at risk.

Twins used to be the major cause of abortion in Thoroughbreds because of the lack of room in the uterus for attachment of two placentae (Figure 9.1). The competition between the two placentae damaged both. Twins are therefore a good example of the outcome of placental damage, twins being either aborted, born prematurely, in a dysmature state, or surviving full-term but undersized and disadvantaged. We will return to this point when discussing intrauterine growth retardation (see Chapter Thirteen).

The placenta may be damaged by one or a combination of the following:

- Restriction of blood supply to the placenta itself. This may result from a restriction of entry of nourishment and oxygen into the placental tissues so that they become damaged. This often happens in an area of the body or cervical pole region of the placenta, involving a progressively larger area over time. We recognise these areas at birth when delivery of the placenta reveals surfaces thickened and/or denuded of chorionic villae, often with a sticky, sometimes copious exudate. This is largely the result of the uterine glands producing excess secretions in an area where attachment to the uterine surface is lost. These areas of damage may be caused by restriction in blood supply to the placenta as a result of insufficient development of blood vessels or some interference in the circulation at any point along the vessels supplying the area. This interference may stem from thrombi or emboli forming in the vessel or from circulatory deficiencies of blood pressure or cardiac output from the fetal heart. There is insufficient evidence available to substantiate the problem arising in individuals, but it must be remembered that the fetal circulation from the fetal cardiac ventricles to the return of blood in the veins back to the heart is in the order of 200 cm, depending on the length of the cord which may vary from 80–120 cm and, in addition, the blood has to pass through the liver.
- The placenta also gains nourishment from the uterine surface itself and there may be a restriction in certain areas due to chronic changes in the mare's uterus. This is particularly likely in older mares, but much depends on the health of the maternal uterine lining at the time of

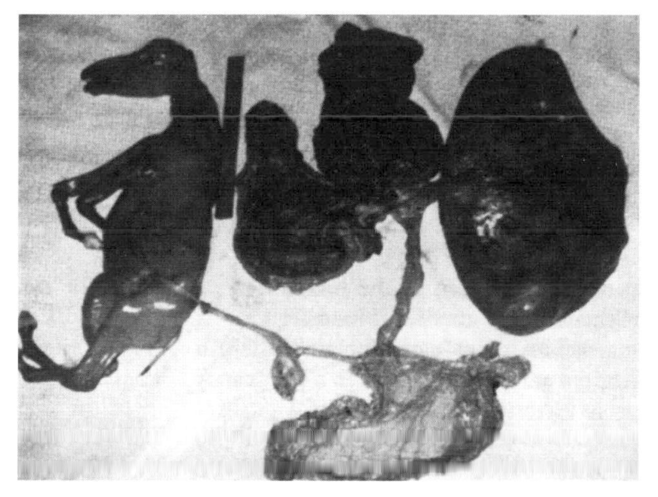

Figure 9.1

When twins are aborted one has usually been dead for some time and has started to degenerate, the other may be well preserved. Here, twin fetuses are shown, aged about seven months. A ruler has been laid against the one on the left which died some time before abortion. The fetus on the right is still enclosed in the placenta and was living at the time of abortion

conception and any residual damage that may be present following a previous pregnancy. The umbilical cord is 80–120 cm long and there is always the risk that the fetal limbs, or, even, body may impinge on the cord at some point. This may produce sufficient interference in blood supply to cause damage to the placenta of a hypoxic (lack of oxygen) or ischaemic (lack of blood supply) nature, leading to placental damage.
- Any infectious agent capable of multiplying within body tissues may be involved in placental damage. The most common bacteria are *Streptococcus, E. coli* and *Staphylococci*; those also found most commonly in association with endometritis.
- In addition, fungal elements may be involved in placentitis, as damage to the placenta is often termed, especially when damage occurs at the cervical pole (Figure 9.2).

It must be emphasised here that infection of the placenta and resulting placentitis may be primary or secondary in origin. Primary infection occurs as a result of resident infection in the uterus at the time of mating or when the cervix becomes relaxed and infection gains access from the vagina. Secondary infection would be that arising when the tissue of the placenta becomes damaged by circulatory causes (as described above) and infection gains entry because of damage already present.

Equine herpesvirus type 1 may infect the mare and the virus pass across the utero-placental junction causing infection and death of the fetus. The virus is carried across in leucocytes that have

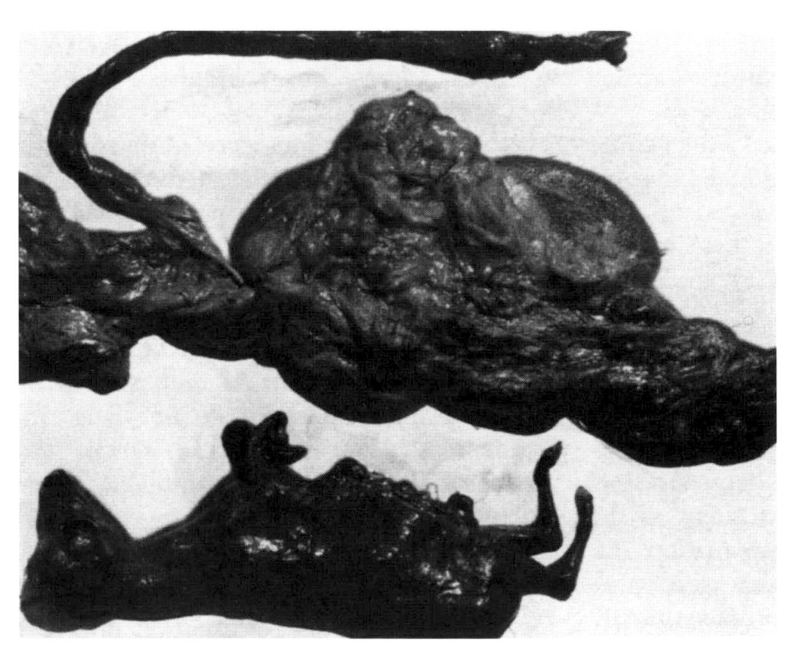

Figure 9.2

A fetus with its membranes aborted on the 120th day of pregnancy. It is approximately 18 cm long. The normal size at this stage would be approximately 20 cm; it is under size for its gestational age, probably as a result of the infection which caused the abortion become infected and gain entrance to the fetal circulation from the mare. The virus may also cause vasculitis (inflammation of the lining cells of the arteries) resulting in abortion before the virus actually passes into the fetus itself, and the abortion occurs because of the effect of the virus on the mare's uterine quiescence so that the fetus is expelled precipitously.

The typical situation, as described in research done in the 1940s and 1950s, is for a mare to abort without warning in the seventh to ninth month of pregnancy. The fetus is expelled with its membranes and may be found fresh with no external evidence from the placenta or fetus except, possibly, a jaundiced appearance of the hooves.

However, in recent years with the advent of laboratory capacity for identifying viruses, it has been shown that infection may be present in fetuses aborted much earlier in pregnancy than seven months and even be present in foals born at full-term and showing evidence of illness. The picture of EHV-1 abortion is therefore nowadays known to be much wider than the typical seven- to nine-month period abortion described by Messrs Dimmock and Edwards in the USA in the 1930s.

Further, abortions caused by EHV-1 may be associated with abortions in which the fetus is not expelled fresh but in a degenerate state; and also where the afterbirth is retained rather than expelled with the fetus.

In practice, therefore, we cannot assume that any abortion or any foal dying in the first three or four days after birth is free from EHV-1 infection unless laboratory tests are performed. This emphasises the need for all such cases to go to post mortem examination. EHV-1 infection is essentially an infection of the mare's respiratory system, but it is highly infectious and knowledge of its presence is essential if epidemic outbreaks of the disease are to be prevented and contained.

In the laboratory, diagnosis is made partly on the gross appearance of the aborted fetus but mainly on culture of the liver, lung and spleen of the fetus for potential growth of virus by which a diagnosis can be made positively. There are, nowadays, also tests based on immunological properties by which the virus may be identified in tissue on laboratory examination.

The subject of EHV-1 infection is addressed in the advice contained in the Horserace Betting Levy Board Code of Practice (see Chapter Ten).

Equine arteritis virus is another cause of abortion as a result of its effect on the small arteries of the mare; that is, vasculitis. It also causes fever and general malaise which may add to its capacity to trigger abortion in an affected pregnant individual. Diagnosis is made upon laboratory examination and the recovery of the arteritis virus.

Hormonal and Immunological Problems

Many people believe that a failure of progesterone production on the part of the mare is a cause of abortion in the early stages of pregnancy. On the basis of this assumption, many mares are placed onto varying doses of progesterone or a synthetic progesterone, allyl trenbolone (Regumate).

There is no firm evidence as to whether or not this is effective and studies reporting the relationship of maternal progesterone concentrations in individuals that lose their pregnancies under 100 days gestation suggest that the progesterone levels decrease after and not before loss or death of the conceptus.

The other hormones which have an influence on the uterus are oestrogen, cortisone, prostaglandin and oxytocin. In general, all of these hormones are associated more with the act of expulsion of the fetus than with its maintenance because they are involved in stimulating uterine contractions. However, this statement is too simplistic and it must be emphasised that each of the hormones also plays a part in the development of the fetus and are essential for the continuation of pregnancy; the balance and interaction between each hormone being the determining factor.

It is reasonable to suppose that abortion may be brought about, in some cases, by failure in the control hormonal balances but, in our present state of knowledge, we can only guess at the reasons why these failures occur or what hormone levels are involved.

There are many gaps in our basic knowledge of this particular field of biology and the horse owner together with his or her veterinarian are faced with a certain number of inexplicable happenings as far as mares who have aborted are concerned.

The same applies to immunological deficiencies or excesses involved in the relationship between the fetus and its placenta with the maternal immune response to what is, essentially a foreign body. Little is known as to how the immune response of the mare is mediated into an acceptance of the fetus through pregnancy, as is normally the case.

There is undoubtedly a genetic element that may make some individual matings fail because the host reacts unfavourably to the presence of fetal tissue within the uterus. Some matings may result in an incompatibility between the host mare and her 'fetal parasite'.

Errors of Development and Implantation

In other species, we know that abortions may be the direct consequence of defective genetic or chromosomal material in the newly-formed individual. It is reasonable to argue that the abortion or loss of pregnancy, where a fetus has malformations, is one way in which nature controls the genetic health of the species. In other words, serious abnormalities are not allowed to live and reproduce themselves. Not all deformities are limited by abortion, as some foals are born with cleft palate, parrot jaw and other defects.

Failure of the placenta to become attached (implanted to the uterus) is often put forward as a reason for abortion in the first 30 days of pregnancy. Even by day 35 the fetus is lying free in the uterus and its membranes are not firmly attached to the uterine wall. The fetus may be particularly vulnerable at this stage.

Any disturbance of the intricate mechanisms maintaining pregnancy may pose a threat to the safety of the fetus. We cannot hope to explain many of the non-infective causes of abortion nor to take measures to prevent them. A common reason put forward for abortion is the length of the umbilical cord; usually this is in the region of 70 cm length. The longer the cord the more stress this may place upon the circulation from the fetus through the placenta and its return to the fetal heart, and there may be a greater risk of the cord being entangled in fetal limbs or compressed by the fetal body. Compromise of the fetal circulation has been discussed above.

Influence of Management

To what extent can management be responsible for whether or not a mare aborts? This is largely a theoretical consideration because it is extremely difficult to relate cause and effect in any particular individual.

If pregnant mares are subjected to abnormal stresses, such as being transported by air or road, put through the sales ring, handled roughly or excited by unusual events (for example, low-flying aircraft, or hounds in the vicinity of their paddock), we might expect an abortion in many cases. However, based on the small number of studies carried out, there is no conclusive evidence that any of these factors actually cause abortion, any more than surgical procedures or the suffering of severe pain from conditions such as laminitis or colic.

On the other hand, there are individual cases where a correlation between such happenings and abortion is evident. It may be that the key to this conundrum is that some mares are more sensitive to losing their pregnancies than others; they are, in effect, individuals looking for a reason to abort. Fortunately, these individuals are few compared to the many who seem to be able to maintain their pregnancy despite quite horrific events taking place in their vicinity and causing them extreme degrees of stress. This subject requires further study before we can hope to identify such individuals and take measures to avoid their aborting.

The older a mare, the more likely she is to abort and, therefore, vigorous culling of these mares and those with bad breeding records might make a significant contribution to the problem of abortion.

Nutrition is unlikely to cause abortion unless levels of energy intake fall below certain minimum requirements of quality or quantity, which is rarely the case. However, recent work has shown that low levels of nutrition can affect the development of the fetus and we shall return to this subject later (see Chapter Thirteen) when considering the subject of intrauterine growth retardation.

CHAPTER TEN

The Codes of Practice for Studfarms

One of the most important management factors for studfarms is maintaining the health and productivity of all animals that are resident on the farm. An outbreak of disease can cause the loss of valuable, perhaps irreplaceable, breeding animals as well as massive financial loss. The outbreak of foot and mouth disease in the UK in 2001 has demonstrated the effect of a significant disease outbreak to the whole population. Horses cannot contract foot and mouth but they can act as mechanical carriers, spreading the virus from one place to another on their feet. Although the significant equine infectious diseases are unlikely to have such a wide-reaching impact outside of the horse industry, the control measures that become necessary in the event of any infectious disease outbreak can be just as wide-reaching and damaging to nearly all horse owners. Most studfarms rely on the bulk of their annual income being earned during the breeding season by providing facilities to board and foal mares, as well as the sale of nominations to the stud's stallions. The outbreak of serious infection on any studfarm will, in most cases, result in the farm being closed for several weeks, sometimes months. All movements of horses to and from the stud will also be stopped – this will not only result in visiting mares being essentially 'locked in' to the farm, but will also mean that mares booked to the stallion who have yet to arrive will probably go elsewhere.

Additionally, there is the reputation of the studfarm to be considered and this factor alone can sometimes work against reducing infection risk. No stud wants to be thought of as being involved with an infection outbreak – people remember such occurrences long after they have forgotten the number of champions that the stud may have produced in the past. Sadly, it is not uncommon for some less responsible studfarms to cover up a case or cases of serious infection and continue to trade as normal. Obviously, the long-term risk to horse population by such practices is very serious indeed.

Today, broodmares may be sent many thousands of miles each year to visit stallions at stud – to the other end of the country or even to the other side of the world. The sheer volume of movements of horses throughout the year means that very strict controls have to be put in place to avoid the outbreak of disease. In mainland Europe, conditions such as contagious equine metritis and equine viral arteritis are endemic, but, due to control procedures, cases in England are now relatively rare. It may be that some of the conditions that require controls are not life threatening in the majority of cases, but some of the infections do kill or cause permanent damage, and all have the potential to cause serious implications to the national horse population.

These diseases do not discriminate between horse type or purpose, the quality of the studfarm or the horse owner. The main concern for studfarms is not just the physical, emotional and financial damage that an outbreak can cause, but also the fact that these conditions are extremely contagious. Infection can mean that horses become carriers for life, some organisms may remain in the stabling, fencing or land for many, many years – being almost impossible to eradicate. This all sounds very dramatic and it is easy to become blasé about the risks, particularly when reported cases have not occurred for many years; however, in 1996 outbreaks of CEM were recorded in England for the first time since the late 1970s and each year there are reported cases of equine viral arteritis and equine herpesvirus-1. All studfarms, regardless of whether the horses are bred naturally or by artificial methods, should develop a policy for control of disease and follow the guidelines for reducing the risks to their horses – this policy should be firmly adhered to without any exceptions.

Due to the seriousness of infection risk to breeding horses, an annually reviewed code is published by the Horserace Betting Levy Board called the Codes of Practice. It is aimed at the control and prevention of venereal diseases in horses – all breeding horses, not just Thoroughbreds. The main diseases covered are contagious equine metritis (CEM), equine viral arteritis (EVA) and equine herpesvirus-1 (EHV-1); however, in recent years strangles has also been included. Strangles is not a reproductive disease, but it can have similar implications on the affected studfarm to any of the venereal diseases.

The main aim of the Code is to advise as to common practices to reduce the risk and spread of venereal disease within the horse population. Precautions are equally important when using artificial insemination or embryo transfer and so an additional Code of Practice is published by the British Veterinary Association for these breeding methods.

The Codes of Practice are only recommendations and there is no compulsion to adhere to their guidelines. However, as mentioned earlier, due to the increase in travelling horses all over the world and to the increase of walking-in mares to stud, the Codes are vital to the well-being of all horses.

On Thoroughbred studfarms particularly, the practice of walking-in mares is becoming increasingly common. The term 'walking-in' is used to describe the situation when mares are brought to the stallion studfarm just for the act of mating and then taken back to their home or boarding stud. This practice is very common in areas where stallion studfarms are concentrated, such as Newmarket in the UK. Many stallion studfarms in these areas have a policy of not taking in boarding outside mares, to reduce risks such as infection outbreak for the resident broodmare band as well as reducing risks for the walking-in mares. These mares should be treated in the same way as if they were permanently resident at the stallion stud.

To understand how these diseases can be prevented, it is important to understand what causes these diseases, how they are spread, the signs of each condition and action to be taken in the event of any outbreak. An outbreak of some disease, such as CEM or EVA, may result in affected horses becoming carriers or shedders. The future for carriers/shedders in these circumstances is very grave.

Contagious Equine Metritis

In the UK, contagious equine metritis (CEM) is a notifiable venereal disease by law. This requirement is set out in detail under the Infectious Diseases of Horses Order 1987, meaning that a case has to be reported immediately even if it has not been confirmed but only suspected. All reports should be made to the Department of the Environment, Food and Rural Affairs (DEFRA), formerly known as MAFF.

The organism that causes CEM is *Taylorella equigenitalis*. It was first identified in Newmarket in the 1970s and it caused widespread infection, as the bacterium was not recognised prior to this time.

The bacteria are carried on the external genitalia of the stallion and are transmitted at mating to the mare, or via the seminal fluids with artificial insemination. Stallions act as carriers for the disease and do not show any outward signs of infection. Rarely, stallions may suffer internal infection and pus may contaminate the semen. The acutely infected mare will normally show signs of genital inflammation and discharge as well as reduced fertility. Affected mares may return to oestrus at any time, usually at shortened intervals and will fail to conceive until the infection is cleared. The discharge is clearly seen around the vulva and tail, with matting of the tail also being common. Chronically affected mares may have a deep-seated infection that shows limited external signs. Mares may also be carriers, like the stallion showing no external signs of disease but remaining very infectious. Colt foals born to affected mares may themselves be carriers, transmitting the disease several years later when they are at stud.

Diagnosis of infection is made by taking swabs (Figures 10.1–10.3) from the affected mare (cervix and clitoris) and stallion (urethra, urethral fossa and sheath). In mares, the organism has been isolated from the cervix, urethra and clitoris. However, it commonly persists in the clitoral fossa and sinuses. In affected mares, it may be necessary for the clitoris to be removed surgically if infection cannot be controlled by any other method. There are restrictions on fillies and mares to be exported to the USA that require all female horses to undergo surgical removal of the clitoris.

A clitoral swab should be taken routinely each year and repeated if the mare is to be covered by another stallion after her original mating that year. Even pregnant mares can safely have a clitoral swab prior to foaling. Following the Codes of Practice, such swabs should be taken after 1 January each year. Swabs are also taken from the endometrium of the mare; this should be done prior to service during the time that the mare is in oestrus. Endometrial swabs (taken from the lining of the uterus during oestrus via the open cervix) are repeated, one each heat

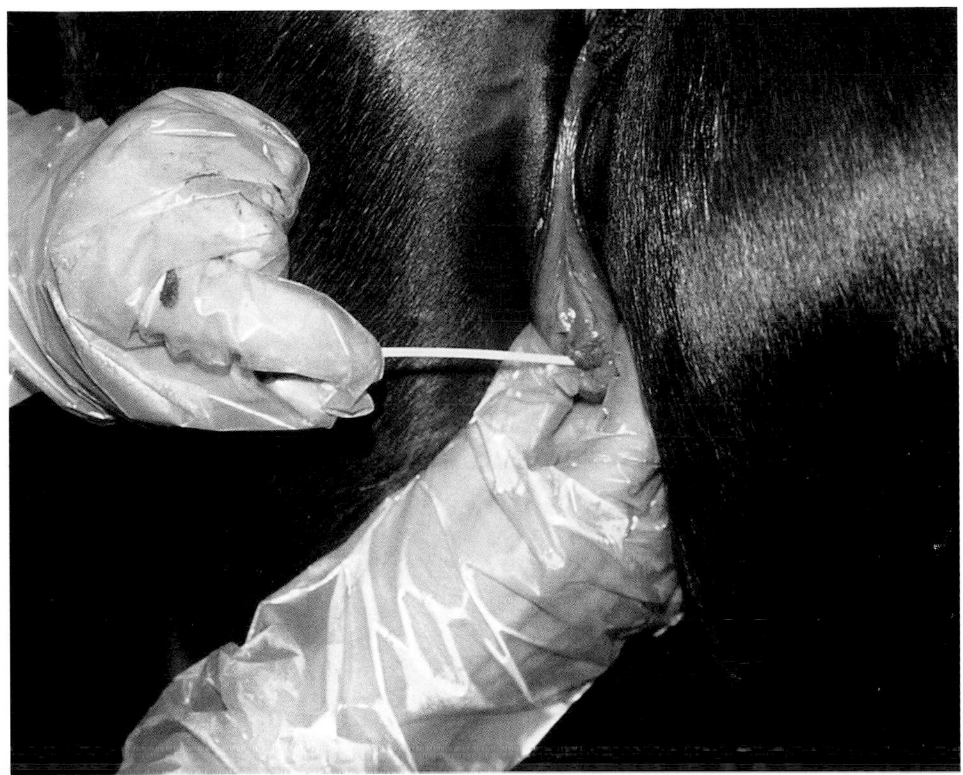

Figure 10.1

Clitoral swabs are taken from the clitoral fossa and sinuses

period that that mare is to be mated, regardless of the fact that she may return several times to the same stallion. This is of particular importance if the mare returns to heat unexpectedly after mating. In this case, it may be wise to repeat a complete set of swabs, especially if more than one mare returns to heat unexpectedly or any external signs of infection are suspected.

Under the Codes of Practice, mares are split into risk groups: high-risk and low-risk.

A high-risk mare may be defined as a mare from which CEM has been isolated within the last two years. She will be removed from the high-risk category once she has been mated after treating and had a foal, which has been swabbed negative for CEM. Foals born to high-risk mares should be swabbed under the guidelines of the veterinary surgeon, but the recommendation is normally three times at intervals of not less than seven days before they are three months old. High-risk mares may also be classified as such following mating by an affected stallion or teaser in the last breeding season. Due to variations in global policies for disease control, a mare may also be termed high-risk if she has been mated to a stallion outside the UK, Ireland, USA, France, Germany, Italy and Canada; or if she has not been bred, but has arrived from outside of these countries. A low-risk mare is one that does not fit into any of these categories.

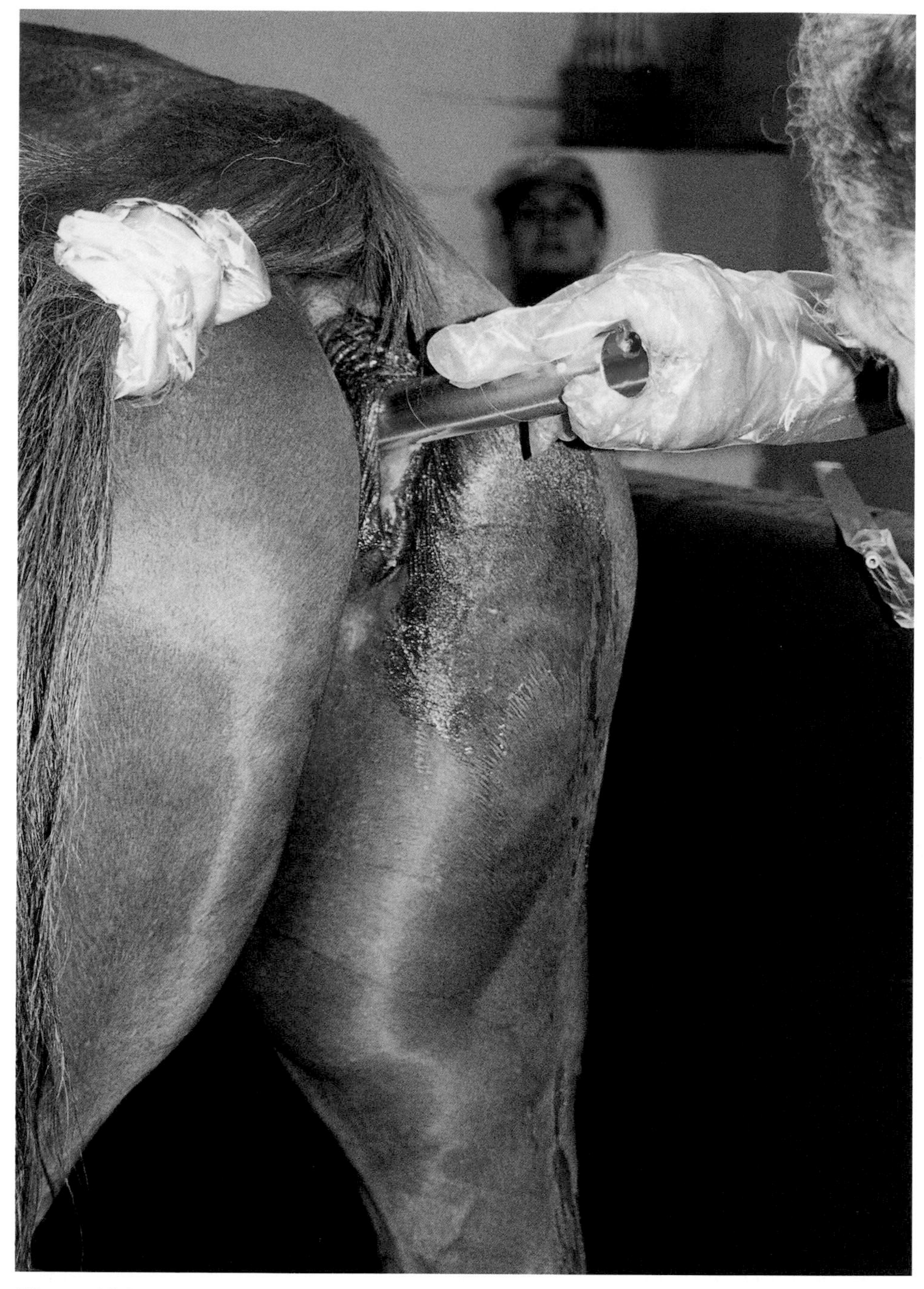

Figure 10.2

Cervical swabs are taken using a speculum to avoid the risk of contaminating the sample by touching any other part of the reproductive tract

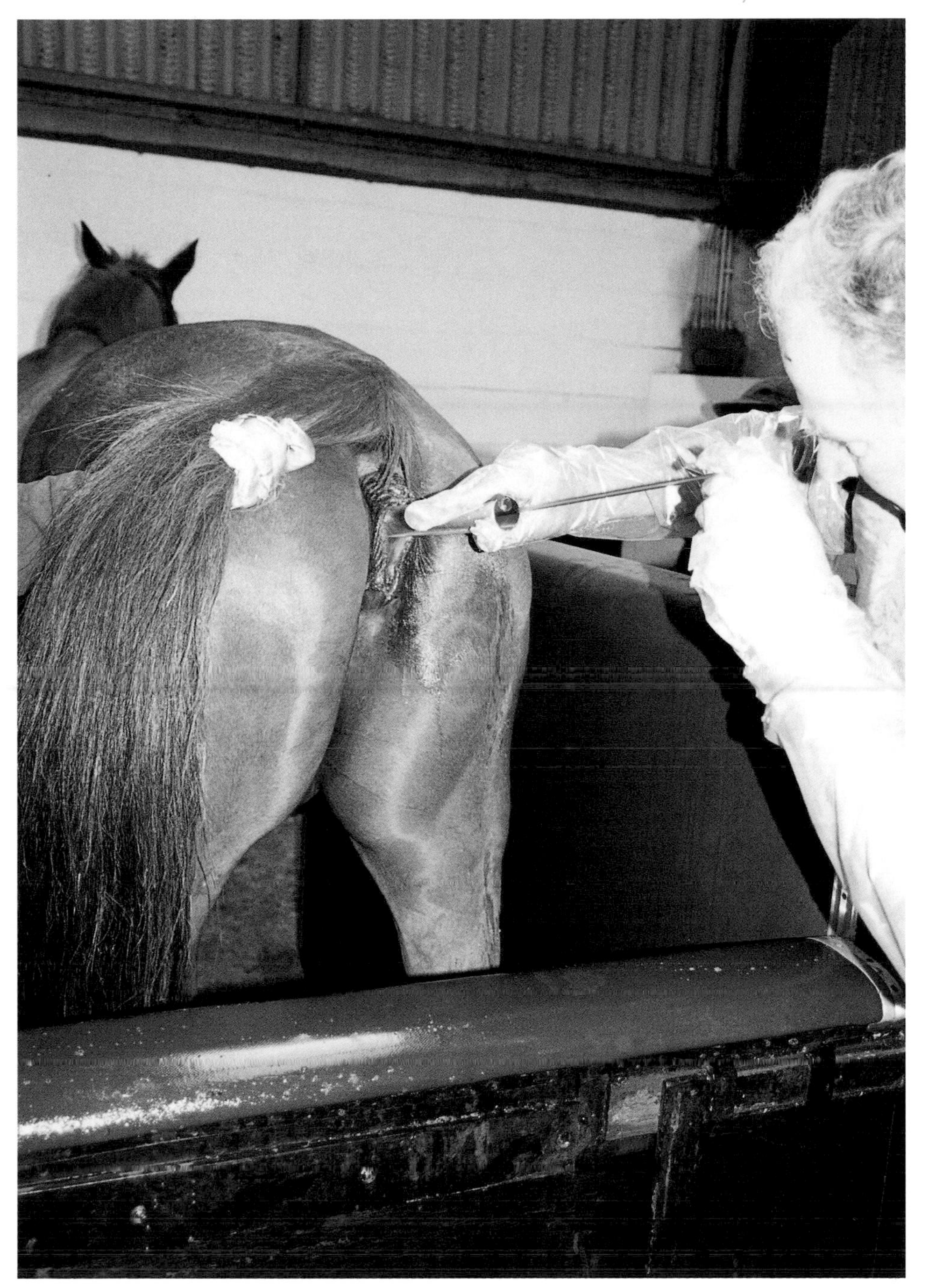

Figure 10.3

Cervical swabs can only be taken when the mare is in oestrus

High-risk mares should have a clitoral swab taken prior to arrival at stud, as well as another taken after arrival. An endometrial swab should be taken during oestrus and prior to mating. A subsequent endometrial swab should be taken on each subsequent oestrus period that the mare is to be mated. A low-risk mare should be swabbed before mating and have endometrial swabs taken during oestrus before mating and at each subsequent heat period as before.

Walking-in mares, particularly those who are termed high-risk, should only be accepted from boarding studs known to and approved by the stallion stud.

Stallions should also routinely be swabbed at the start of the breeding season. Swabs are taken from the urethra, urethral fossa and penile sheath and from the pre-ejaculatory fluids. Importantly, these swabs should also be repeated at the end of the breeding season.

Swabs should only be accepted when cultured by a recognised laboratory, registered specifically for CEM (see Figure 10.4). In the 1970s the organism was identifiable after two to three days of culture, but outbreaks in the 1990s have shown that identification may take up to four to six days. The bacterium has now been identified in two different strains and it is of concern to the laboratories that negative cultures may now take more than six days to be confirmed.

Most responsible studfarms also insist on the last five years' breeding history of the mare being detailed by the owner and forms are produced for Thoroughbreds by the Thoroughbred Breeders' Association for this purpose (Figure 10.5).

It should also be noted that indirect infection of horses may also occur due to poor stud hygiene. Infection can be passed via contaminated water or utensils, as well as on the hands of the staff that handle the tail area of the mare or the penis of the stallion or teaser. Normally, disposable gloves are routinely used when handling or examining any mare, stallion or teaser and each stallion will normally have his own utensils.

The use of teaser stallions on many studfarms is a factor that may have contributed to the more recent outbreak. As detailed above, infection can be passed indirectly and the teaser stallion is a potential risk, especially if he is used for 'bouncing' mares when genital-to-genital contact may be possible. The teaser's handlers may also pass the infection if they touch the teaser's penis without gloves and then handle the mare.

It is most important to remember that horses can be infected with CEM regardless of whether or not they have been used for breeding previously. Only stringent adherence to the Codes of Practice and a high level of stud hygiene will avoid lack of identification of affected horses and uncontrolled transmission of the infection.

Klebsiella pneumoniae and *Pseudomonas aeruginosa*

Both the *Klebsiella* and *Pseudomonas* infections are spread in a similar fashion to CEM. *Klebsiella* is the most dangerous as it can become established in the reproductive tract of a healthy young horse, whereas *Pseudomonas*

LABORATORY CERTIFICATE
(CERTIFICAT LABORATOIRE)
(FOR USE IN THE UK DURING THE 2000 SEASON)

For use only by Approved Laboratories* December 1999 to November 2000.
(Laboratoires agréés en 1999/2000)

Swabs contained in transport medium and labelled as collected from the stallion/teaser/mare named:
(Nom du cheval)

....

Passport number (where available): *(Numéro SIRE/carnet signalétique)* ....

from the following sites: *(Prélèvements effectués)* ....

....

were submitted by *(Nom du vétérinaire ayant effectué les prélèvements)* ....

for bacteriological examination on (date[s]) *(Faitle)*..

I *(Je)* ....

of (Laboratory) *(Nom du laboratoire agréé)* ....

certify that the above swabs were examined under specific conditions of microaerophilic and aerobic culture with the following results *(Le/la sousigné/e atteste que les prélèvements mis en culture sous conditions d'aérobie et de microanaérobie ont livré les résultats suivants):*

Taylorella equigenitalis (CEMO) **WAS/WAS NOT** ** isolated
(Métrite contagieuse des Equidés) *positif/négatif*

Pseudomonas aeruginosa **WAS/WAS NOT** ** isolated
(Pseudomonas aeruginosa) *positif/négatif*

Klebsiella pneumoniae **WAS/WAS NOT** ** isolated
(Klebsiella pneumoniae) *positif/négatif*

Where *K. pneumoniae was* isolated, capsule type(s) identified were ....
Type(s) capsulaire(s)

NAME AND QUALIFICATIONS *(Responsable du laboratoire agréé)* (PLEASE PRINT)..

SIGNATURE...DATE..

LABORATORY NAME AND ADDRESS *(Nom et adresse du laboratoire agréé)* ....

....

....

....

*An Approved Laboratory is one whose name is published in the Veterinary Record by the Horserace Betting Levy Board in December 1999.

**Delete as appropriate. Where post-coitus swabs were examined for the CEMO only, delete the lines which are not applicable.

†In the event of a positive *Klebsiella pneumoniae* isolate, capsule typing should be performed and the results detailed to aid the determination of potential venereal pathogenicity.

Figure 10.4

Example of the laboratory certificate provided to confirm that swabs have been cultured under correct conditions. It also confirms whether any significant bacteria were isolated

CONTAGIOUS EQUINE METRITIS AND OTHER EQUINE BACTERIAL VENEREAL DISEASES (2001 SEASON)

MARE CERTIFICATE

Certificate to be completed by mare owner and lodged with the prospective stallion stud farm owner before the mare is sent to the stallion stud farm.

Name of mare ....

Passport number (where available) ....

Name and address of owner ....

....

....

1998 stud visited ....

mated with ....result ....

1999 stud visited ....

mated with ....result ....

2000 stud visited ....

mated with ....result ....

Additional information including the results of positive bacteriological examinations for CEMO, *Klebsiella pneumoniae* and *Pseudomonas aeruginosa* at any time:

....

....

NAME (PLEASE PRINT) ....

SIGNATURE..

DATE ....

NOTICE:
The Thoroughbred Breeders' Association (TBA) strongly recommends that breeders consider insuring their mare against being locked-in when she visits a boarding stud or stallion stud in the UK or Ireland for the purposes of being covered. The TBA Insurance Scheme will cover the daily keep charges and veterinary treatment directly associated with the eradication of the disease at a premium of £25 per mare. Please contact the TBA on 01638 661321 for further details.

Figure 10.5

Example of a CEM form provided annually to record a mare's breeding history over five years tends, in many but not all cases, to become prominent in susceptible animals.

The same policies as for CEM should be maintained to avoid the risk of infection from horse to horse. Swabs taken for CEM can also be used to check for both *Klebsiella* and *Pseudomonas*; the accepted endometrial swab certificate allows indication of infection for all three organisms to be detailed.

Infected animals should be isolated and not used for breeding until the infection has been cleared. This includes stopping the use of an infected stallion for artificial insemination.

There are different types of *Klebsiella*, some of which would not be considered pathogenic; for example, capsule type 7 which is quite common. However, three types, called capsule types 1, 2 and 5, are known to be significant and can be sexually transmitted. If *Klebsiella* is identified, the veterinary surgeon will perform tests to determine which capsule type is present – this must be performed by a specialist laboratory.

Pseudomonas aeruginosa is recognised in several different strains, not all of which are associated with true venereal disease. It is difficult to differentiate between the strains and so, normally, any identified isolate will be treated as harmful unless proved otherwise. If the infection is isolated from the stallion's penis, it can be extremely difficult to eradicate completely.

Equine Viral Arteritis

EVA is a contagious viral disease. It occurs globally and is endemic as close as mainland Europe. As with CEM, cases of EVA are seen most regularly in the UK in the non-Thoroughbred population. In 2001 in Germany and France, there were recorded cases of EVA infection in the Thoroughbred population. This outbreak caused significant additional control measures and testing to be carried out during the 2001 Thoroughbred breeding season. Many studfarms, particularly those in the central areas for Thoroughbred breeding, such as Newmarket in England and around County Kildare in Ireland, requested additional testing of all mares arriving from outside of the country – essentially treating all mares as high-risk. Not only does this additional testing result in a further financial burden to the breeder, but due to the specific timing of testing required, some mares will unable to be mated early in the season, a factor that is of particular importance to those breeding Thoroughbreds. This virus is particularly significant as not only does it cause abortion and pregnancy failure but it may also be fatal.

Horse become infected with EVA by:

- Sexual transmission during mating.
- Insemination with infected semen.
- Contact with aborted fetuses and fluids.
- Droplet transmission from coughing and sneezing.

Stallions are a particular source of the infection. The virus is prolific in the infected stallion's sex glands and he may shed the virus in his semen. Although he may appear to have recovered from the acute illness and his fertility is not affected, he may continue to shed the virus for months, years or even for life. Although the stallion commonly infects mares by mating or insemination with infected semen, the infected mare will then infect other mares by droplet transmission. As is common with viruses, EVA is resistant to climate changes and can easily survive being chilled or frozen in semen. The carrier state is not, yet, known in mares.

The signs of infection do vary. Another factor that makes EVA so significant is that some horses are obviously ill, while others show no external signs at all, so infection is difficult to diagnose. The signs of infection include fever, lethargy, depression, swelling of the lower limbs, conjunctivitis, swelling around the eye socket and eyelid, nasal discharge, 'nettle rash' and swelling of the sheath and mammary glands. Pregnant mares may abort.

Normally, affected animals are identified from serological tests on blood samples but nasal pharyngeal swabs are also useful. If an infected mare has aborted, the virus can be isolated from the fetus and membranes, so it is essential that these are sent to the laboratory for examination.

As mentioned above, EVA is commonly found in the non-Thoroughbred population. Perhaps this is due to a more relaxed attitude towards screening for infection amongst other breed types, whether the horses are used for breeding or not. Competition horses that travel extensively may come into contact with a much larger number of horses from all backgrounds. The possibilities for transfer of disease in such situations are vast. This is one of the many reasons why racehorses and competition horses of all disciplines should be kept separately from breeding horses.

Prevention of EVA infection is essential in any breeding operation and particularly so with EVA, as affected horses may exhibit no signs of infection. Studfarms generally have a policy of testing and isolation to help minimise the risk of an infected horse being allowed contact with the rest of the breeding stock. This normally involves compulsory blood testing of all horses on a similar basis to that of CEM swabbing. That is, every horse coming onto the studfarm must have had a blood sample taken to check for EVA after 1 January of that year. Imported horses should be sampled prior to leaving their original country, sampled again on arrival to this country and another sample taken at least 14 days after arrival. In the meantime, they must be kept in isolation from all other horses. For AI and embryo transfer, the status of the stallion only in the case of AI and the mare and stallion in the case of embryo transfer must be made available. It is essential that any prospective purchaser of either semen or embryo from overseas insists on this procedure.

A horse that has previously been infected with EVA will be termed seropositive. That is to say that any blood sample will indicate the presence of antibodies against the virus (high level and/or a rising level of antibodies in two blood samples taken at intervals of at least ten days). The horse may not present a risk to other breeding stock by being seropositive, but must be checked to be certain that it is not still infectious and, in the case of a male horse, that it is not a shedder. Some stallions are vaccinated against EVA and may, as a result, become seropositive on blood sampling. Prior to vaccination, a blood sample should be taken to prove that the horse was seronegative before vaccination. Horses that are proved not to be shedders but are seropositive should still tested every year – it may be required that the horse is sampled on more than one occasion to show that the level of antibodies in the blood has not changed; therefore, to indicate that the horse is now free from any infection. A stallion or teaser that is proven to be seropositive and a shedder will almost certainly have a very grave future.

If all horses that come onto the studfarm are tested, regardless of whether or not they are used for breeding, then this will dramatically reduce the risk of accidental infection. There have been cases where a foster mare has been brought onto a stud for an orphaned foal and the mare has then been found to be the source of infection. In a situation such as this, where time is of the essence in ensuring the best chances of a successful fostering, then the foster mare and orphan foal should be kept in isolation until such time as the mare's status is able to be known and test results available.

Foaling a mare that is infected with EVA should be carried out in isolation and, if a mare has aborted, the fetus and any available fluids and membranes should be sent to a recognised laboratory for examination.

There is a very high risk with competition horses, which travel internationally and may be used for exported frozen semen. At this time, it is not required for any horse or semen to be tested from any country inside the EU, only from outside. To reduce the spread of infection, it is ideal if horse owners and purchasers of semen have tests carried out even though they may not be required by law. Travelling of horses in enclosed spaces may also increase the risk of a horse becoming infected by respiratory transfer of the virus, so actual contact is not essential for infection to occur.

In the event of a case of EVA, a strict isolation procedure for all horses on the studfarm should be followed. As with CEM, EVA is notifiable and DEFRA should be informed immediately, although the farm's veterinary surgeon will almost certainly do this directly. All matings and movement of horses to and from the stud must be stopped immediately and owners of any horses that have left the stud must be notified. Any semen samples that have been sent out from the stud must also be stopped and the recipients notified.

The most sinister aspect of EVA infection is its ability to produce carriers in affected males. Although not all infected males become carriers, it is a common outcome. If a seropositive stallion is found, it is imperative to find out if he is shedding the virus in his semen. This is currently done by taking two ejaculates at intervals of seven days and then having them examined by the recommended laboratory. Test matings are also commonly carried out – obviously, these must be done with the horses in strict isolation. The usual procedure is to choose two seronegative mares, which are then blood sampled to confirm their status. The mares are then mated, usually twice a day for two consecutive days. The mares and suspected carrier stallion must remain in isolation for a further 28 days, when repeat blood samples are taken. If the mares remain seronegative then it is unlikely that the stallion is a carrier. If one or both of the mares become seropositive then the stallion is confirmed as a carrier and must not be used for any further mating or AI. A stallion that is found to be a carrier will have two possible futures – euthanasia or castration followed by another six weeks of isolation. The seropositive mares must remain in isolation until they are no longer infectious.

Vaccination against EVA is not a short cut to good practice and disease control. At present, the use of a vaccine called Artervac is most common with stallions at stud. Even in 2000, the vaccine was available only under licence and full clinical trials have yet to prove its efficiency.

Equine Herpesvirus Type 1

Equine herpesvirus-1 (EHV-1) is a common contagious virus, which causes respiratory disease, abortion and paralysis in horses.

All types of horses can be infected with EHV. Pregnant mares are particularly vulnerable and should be kept in isolation from all other types of horses. The disease commonly spreads via the respiratory route, but an aborted fetus and its fluids are also a source of infection; for this reason, any abortion should be treated as suspicious and sent to a laboratory for examination. Foals infected with the respiratory form can infect other pregnant mares and foals. The virus can remain in the stabling and paddocks for several weeks and indirect infection can therefore occur. In a similar fashion to EVA, mares and other horses infected with EHV-1 may become carriers. They may transmit infection without showing any indication of infection themselves. Carriers may show some signs of illness from time to time and the virus is always contagious at this time. Testing for EHV-1 must be done by a laboratory; blood testing is not appropriate for abortion, so aborted fetuses and membranes are most useful in diagnosis. For the respiratory and paralytic form, blood samples and throat swabs are taken.

Infected pregnant mares normally abort in late pregnancy at about 8–11 months, but can abort as early as four months. Once a mare becomes infected, she can abort at any time from a few weeks after infection to several months later. Long journeys and other stresses can increase the risk of infection.

If an infected foal is born alive, it is usually poor at birth, showing signs of weakness, jaundice and respiratory distress. They generally die within a few days. Infected foals are very contagious to all other horses.

EHV-1 causes mild respiratory disease in weaned foals and yearlings, normally in the autumn and winter. The signs are generally a mild fever, coughing and nasal discharge.

Controlling the spread of EHV-1 infection is vital. The disease itself is not notifiable but any horse suspected of being infected should be kept away from broodmares, especially those that are pregnant. If possible, mares should be foaled at home and sent to stud with a healthy foal at foot. If this is not practical, send the mare to stud at least a month prior to her foaling date. Newly-arrived pregnant mares should be kept in small groups – those from overseas, from sales or in late pregnancy should be kept in isolation from all others. Pregnant mares should be kept as far as possible from weaned foals, yearlings, racehorses and competition horses, and should not be travelled with these groups of horses.

Stud hygiene is most important in reducing the risk of EHV-1 infection. The virus is susceptible to disinfectant and heat. Stabling and horseboxes should be cleaned regularly as routine. If an adequate level of hygiene is not maintained, the virus can remain in the environment for several weeks. It is ideal if separate staff can attend to the pregnant mares entirely, but if not, the pregnant mares should be seen to before all others.

Vaccination against EHV-1 is commonplace and is required by most studs before they will accept a pregnant mare to board. In the UK, the most commonly used vaccine, for Thoroughbreds, is Duvaxyn EHV 1,4.

If an abortion occurs, the strict guidelines as detailed in the Codes of Practice is essential. The most important factor with any outbreak is to ensure that all owners of mares who may have been in contact are notified so that they can take adequate precautions at their premises.

Strangles

Strangles is a bacterial infection caused by the bacterium *Streptococcus equi*. The signs are high temperature, coughing, nasal discharge and swollen lymph nodes that normally produce abscesses. The disease can be fatal if allowed to spread to other parts of the body. Normally the discharging abscesses are all that is seen and some horses are carriers without displaying any signs of illness at all.

From first exposure, incubation takes about one week. The bacteria are spread from the discharging abscesses and will contaminate any surfaces that the horse touches. Once the discharging stops, the risk of cross infection reduces. However, shedding of the bacteria can be intermittent and convalescing horses should be kept isolated until nasopharyngeal swabs have proved negative. The swabs need to taken at intervals of between five and seven days over a two-week period. Normally, three negative swabs will indicate that the horse is free from infection. Sadly, some horses that produce negative swabs following infection remain carriers. The only way to be certain of these individuals is to have swabs taken from the guttural pouch, sinuses and trachea.

Isolation Procedures

Most studfarms have some facility for isolation. Facilities for complete isolation should be considered essential for farms that regularly board horses from overseas, or from sales.

Essentially, an isolation yard should be sited away from the main breeding and foaling areas of the studfarm. The structure of the stabling should be such that complete disinfection and cleaning can be ensured. The yard should be at least 100 m from any other horses and no contact, either directly or indirectly with horses, should be possible. Ideally, the yard should be totally self-contained with its own feed and forage stores. The staff that attend to the horses in isolation should be separate from those who attend to the other horses if at all possible. If this is not practical then the isolation horses should be done after the healthy horses each day and the staff must maintain extremely high levels of hygiene. Footbaths, overalls and protective footwear should be kept for the isolation yard only. The yard should have its own stable tools, tack and grooming equipment – ideally made of materials that can be cleaned completely and easily.

Keeping horses in such high levels of

isolation is labour intensive and time consuming. However, it is the only way to reduce further risk of infection and any time spent properly in isolation reduces the long-term time and labour implications that would occur if any outbreak affected the whole stud.

Transporting horses may increase the risk of infection of some diseases. When transported, horses may become stressed and more susceptible to infection. If the transport used is not cleaned thoroughly and routinely with the correct disinfectants, viruses and some bacteria can remain in the environment for some considerable time.

Associations such as the Thoroughbred Breeders' Association can advise on insurance policies to protect against losses should a healthy mare be forced to remain on an infected studfarm. This use of this type of insurance assists with the financial costs or losses incurred by a mare owner should an outbreak occur on a studfarm that she is visiting and is commonly called 'lock-in' insurance.

Copies of The Codes of Practice are published by The Horserace Betting Levy Board each year and can be obtained direct from:

The Horserace Betting Levy Board
52 Grosvenor Gardens
London SW1W 0AU

Or, via their website at:

http://www.hblb.org.uk

Or, alternatively, from:

The Thoroughbred Breeders' Association
Stansted House, The Avenue,
Newmarket, Suffolk
CB8 9AA

CHAPTER ELEVEN

Foaling

The birth of a foal marks the end of pregnancy (gestation). It is a natural event which brings to a close the period of formation and development of the new individual within the maternal uterus. Normally, it is a beautifully coordinated and controlled event in which the fetal foal passes through the mare's birth canal and begins its life of independent status. In this chapter, let us therefore consider how this transition occurs and the biological events surrounding it.

Events Leading Up to Birth

Foaling is an act in which two individuals participate, mare and foal. A biological collaboration occurs throughout the process. Firstly, foaling does not occur until both mare and foal are ready for the event. This entails that the fetal foal is fully mature, which means a state in which it is fully capable of adapting to existence outside of the uterus (see Chapter Twelve). As far as the mare is concerned, preparations for birth must include a fully developed mammary gland containing colostrum of high immunoglobulin (IgG) content.

To achieve this coordination there is what might be described as a biological duet between mare and fetal foal resulting in the eventual triggering of the act of birth when both individuals are ready for the event. Although much of the duet is unknown in detail, there are landmarks which are clearly discernable and which may be summarised as follows:

- Foaling occurs at full term; that is, between day 320 and day 360 of pregnancy. The actual timing varies with the individual and this may be due to genetic factors on the fetal and/or maternal side. Individual mares often foal less than the mean length of pregnancy which is 340 days for Thoroughbreds and 335 days for smaller breeds; other individuals may consistently carry their foals for much longer than the average.
- Mammary development increases from about six weeks prior to the time of foaling. It may increase for a period and then experience a plateau of development before increasing again within a week or so of foaling. There are quite wide variations in

this respect. Some mares experience an increase in mammary size for longer or shorter periods; and mares foaling for the first time may develop their mammary size more rapidly and closer to foaling than mares that have had several foals previously.

- Within the mammary glands, pre-colostral secretions develop within a week or so of the mare giving birth. Availability for sampling of these secretions varies with the individuals; and the occasion of their being available for an examination depends both on the individual and the experience of previous foalings. However, the actual electrolyte content of the secretions provides a fairly accurate guide to the nearness of the intending event. Calcium and potassium content increases and sodium content decreases leading up to birth. The values may be taken, in practice, as indicators of whether or not a mare is likely to foal. As already indicated, IgG concentrations increase close to delivery and are essential in the process of passive transfer of immunity to the newborn foal.
- Leading up to foaling, the fetus and placenta produce increasing amounts of progestagens (progesterone-like compounds but not progesterone) and decreasing amounts of oestrogen. Oestrogens are produced by the fetal gonads and these increase rapidly in size in mid-gestation, then decreasing to only a small size at birth. Oestrogen concentrations in the mare's bloodstream rise and decline in association with these changes. However, it is the progestagens which show the most striking changes close to birth. From about 21 days prior to delivery, substantial amounts of certain progestagens increase and can be measured in the mare's bloodstream. Less readily identifiable in practice are the increases in prostaglandin and cortisol (cortisone) occurring in the fetus as the fetal foal becomes ready for birth. These changes occur in the fetus and are not reflected so much by levels in the mare's bloodstream. It is these two hormones which play the most significant role in events which trigger the onset of birth. Together with the action of oxytocin, released from the pituitary gland of the mare, a combination of effects occurs that produces the contraction of the uterine muscle responsible for the onset of foaling and expulsion of the fetal foal through the birth canal.
- The placental pole becomes progressively thinner during this period until at birth it is normally so thin that it ruptures readily at the end of first stage labour.

Physical and Physiological Events of Foaling

Let us begin by outlining the situation within the uterus in the days and hours immediately before foaling. The fetus lies in the uterus with the cervix closed and the lining of the birth canal in a sticky and contracted state. The birth canal is composed of the cervix, vagina and vulval lips surrounded by the bony hoop formed by the bones of the pelvis (Figures 11.1 and 11.2). It is through this hoop that the foal must pass during the birth process.

To achieve this passage the foal must

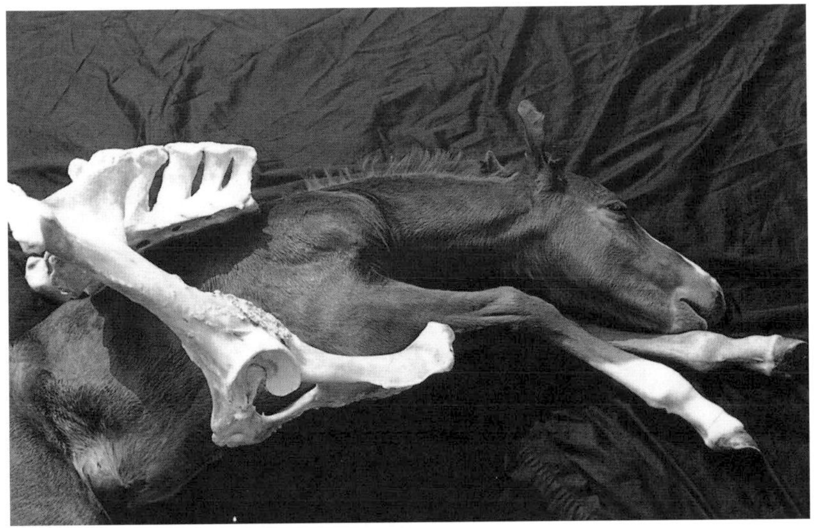

Figure 11.1

Normal posture, presentation and position of the foal passing through the 'hoop' formed by the bones of the pelvis

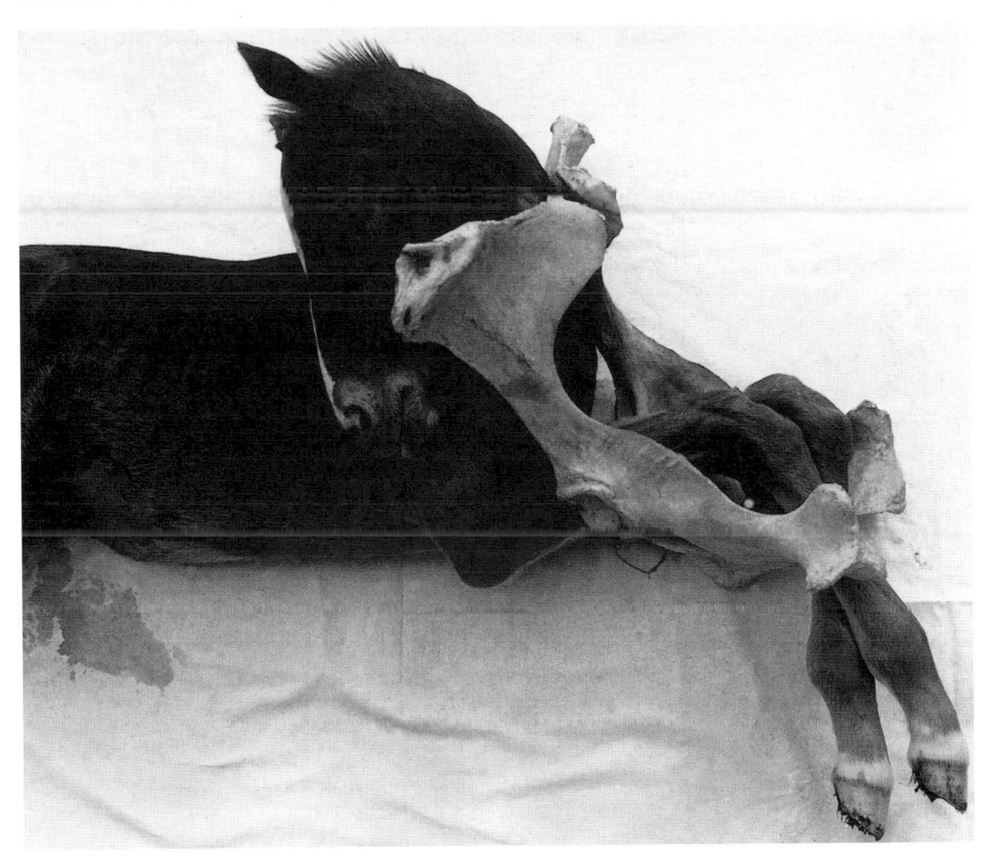

Figure 11.2

Abnormal posture of the foal with the head, neck and forelegs obstructing the passage through the pelvic outlet

come to lie in the most propitious manner, namely, with its forelimbs, head and neck extended and its body lying at an angle between the vertical and horizontal in order to be accommodated by the greatest diameter available within the pelvic hoop. It is as if the foal is leaping through the hoop.

On the maternal side, the cervix and the tissue forming a scaffolding around the vagina (that is, connective tissue) has to relax in order to accommodate the passage of the fetal foal. Even the ligaments of the pelvic attachment to the spine become more pliable, allowing some relaxation of the pelvic hoop. In addition, the lining of the vagina becomes lubricated by mucus and the vulval lips relax, again to accommodate the large cross-sectional area of the fetal foal.

As the uterine muscles contract under the influence of oxytocin, pressure within the uterus is transmitted through the fetal fluids. The foal becomes active and starts to turn from lying on its side or back towards a more ventral position and, importantly, extending its forelegs and head.

While these events are occurring the mare is showing signs of pain and sweating, forming part of first stage labour.

The cervix is dilating at this stage, due to the pressure brought to bear by the contracting uterus on the fetal fluids which cause the cervical pole of the placenta to bulge through the opening cervix. The placenta ruptures at its thinnest point at the placental pole allowing the escape of allantoic fluid. This marks the onset of second stage labour (see below). The fluid serves to lubricate the birth canal and the amnion forms a slippery covering thereby reducing friction between the foal and the walls of the vagina as birth proceeds. The amniotic fluid adds to the lubrication (Figure 11.3).

The forces of birth are those of pushing not pulling. The uterine contractions are considerable and become supplemented by the voluntary contractions of the mare's abdominal muscles as second stage proceeds. These voluntary efforts consist of fixing the diaphragm and compression of the abdominal contents by the circular and longitudinal muscles of the abdomen. In effect, the mare strains to push the foal through the birth canal.

Foaling as Viewed by the Onlooker

It is customary to describe birth in three stages.

First stage

The signs most noticeable in first stage are those of sweating, restlessness and dripping milk from the mammae (Figures 11.4 and 11.5).

These signs are caused by the release of the hormone oxytocin which causes contraction of the uterine muscle. Release is episodic and, therefore, the external signs tend to follow periods of decreasing intervals leading up to second stage.

The uterine contractions are not only rhythmical but spread in waves passing from the horns along the body of the uterus towards the cervix. Each contraction gives rise to a degree of pain which has its behavioural consequences which vary with the individual.

A similar individual response is

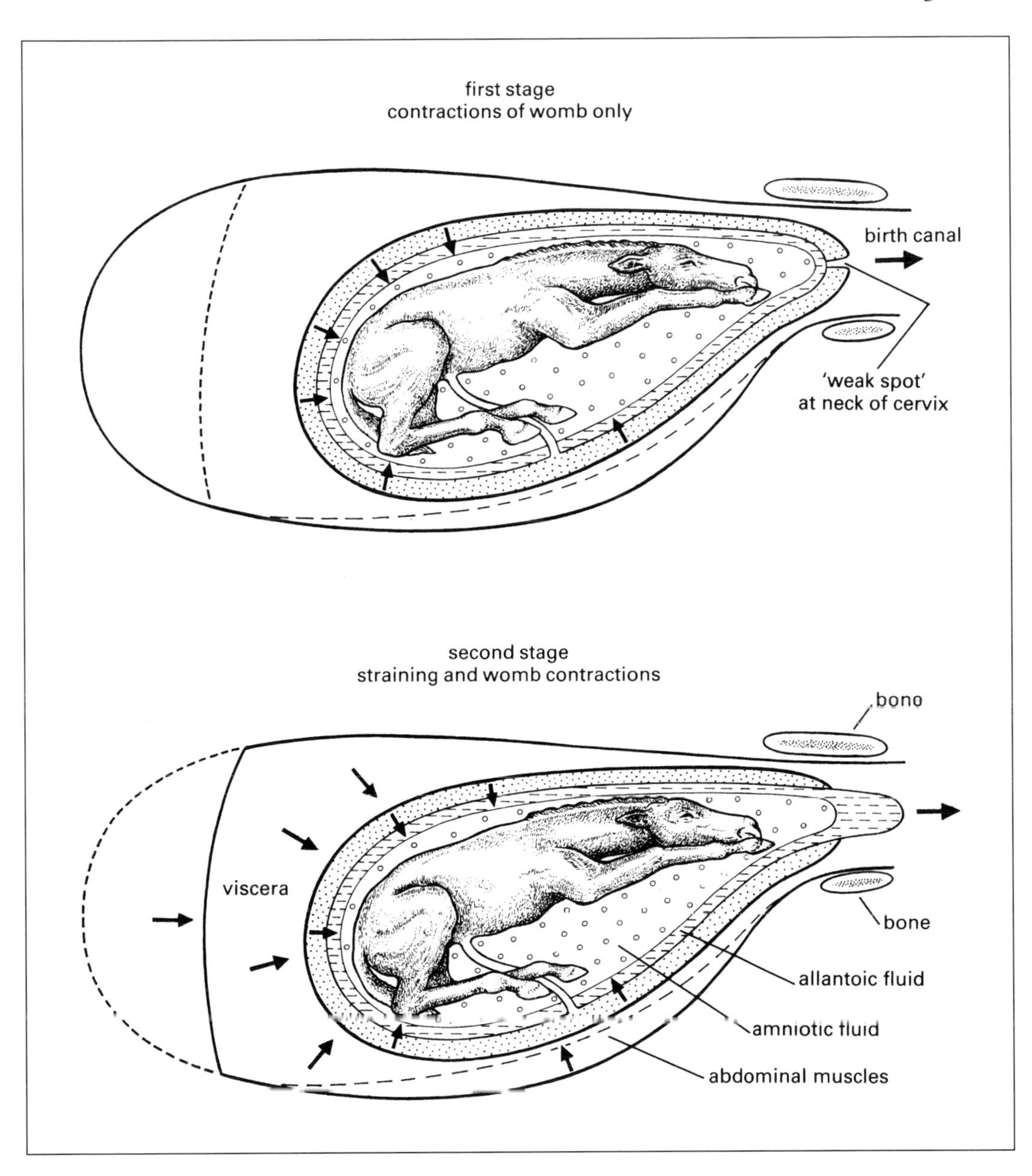

Figure 11.3

The forces of birth push the foal from its position in the uterus through the birth canal, which is bounded by the bony hoop formed by the pelvis. In first stage labour the muscles of the wall of the uterus contract and exert pressure (small arrows) on the contents, eventually causing the placenta to rupture at a weak spot close to the cervix which at this time is dilating. In second stage labour, the contractions of the uterus are supplemented by those of the abdominal muscles (large arrows), and the diaphragm is fixed at the position of inspiration (breathing in)

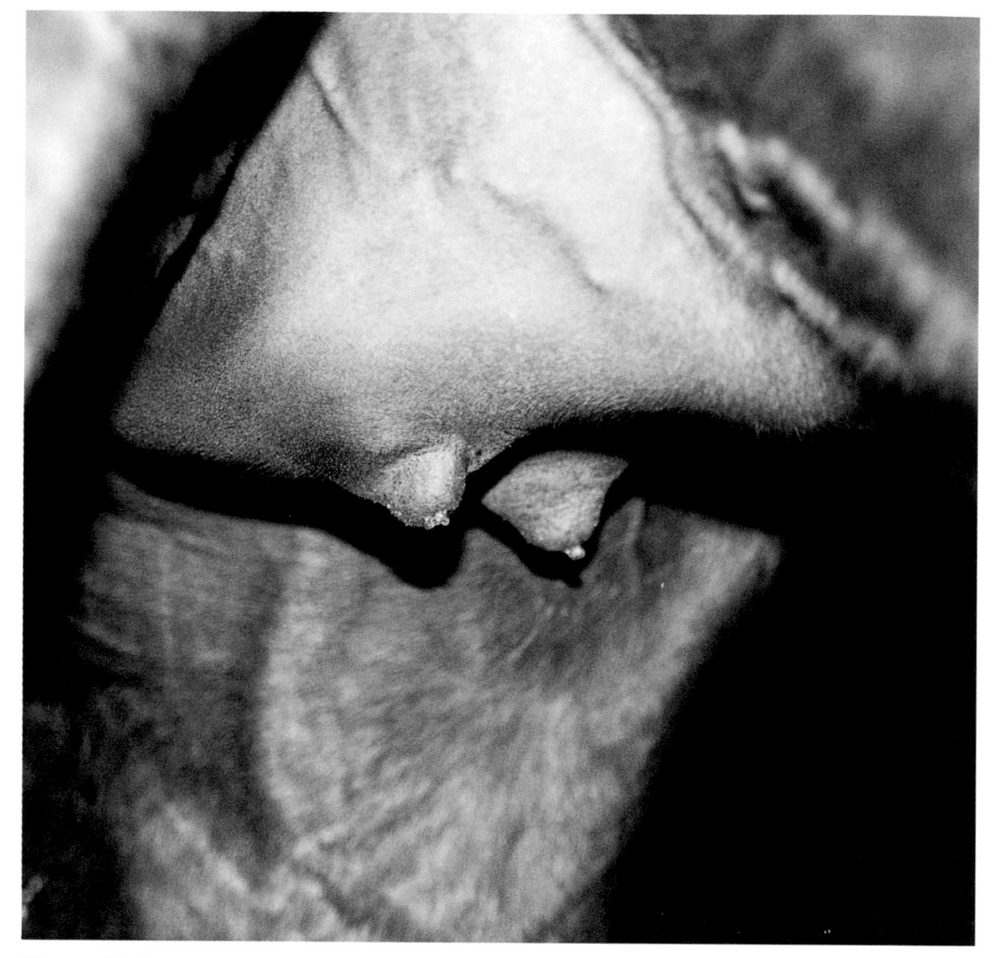

Figure 11.4

Udder development indicative of impending foaling. The udder is well developed and the teats are distended. The presence of colostrum can be seen as waxy deposits on the teats – this is termed 'waxing up'

found in the differing lengths of the periods in which first stage signs are exhibited; some mares may show signs on several occasions at roughly 24-hour intervals before actually entering first stage leading up to foaling itself.

The fact that most foalings occur during the hours of darkness (Figure 11.6) indicates that the mare may have some control over the exact timing of foaling, although the fetus and placenta would appear to have the controlling influence of the length of pregnancy overall.

Second stage

The onset of second stage is heralded by the rupture of the placenta and the escape of allantoic fluid, the so-called 'breaking water' (Figures 11.7–11.14).

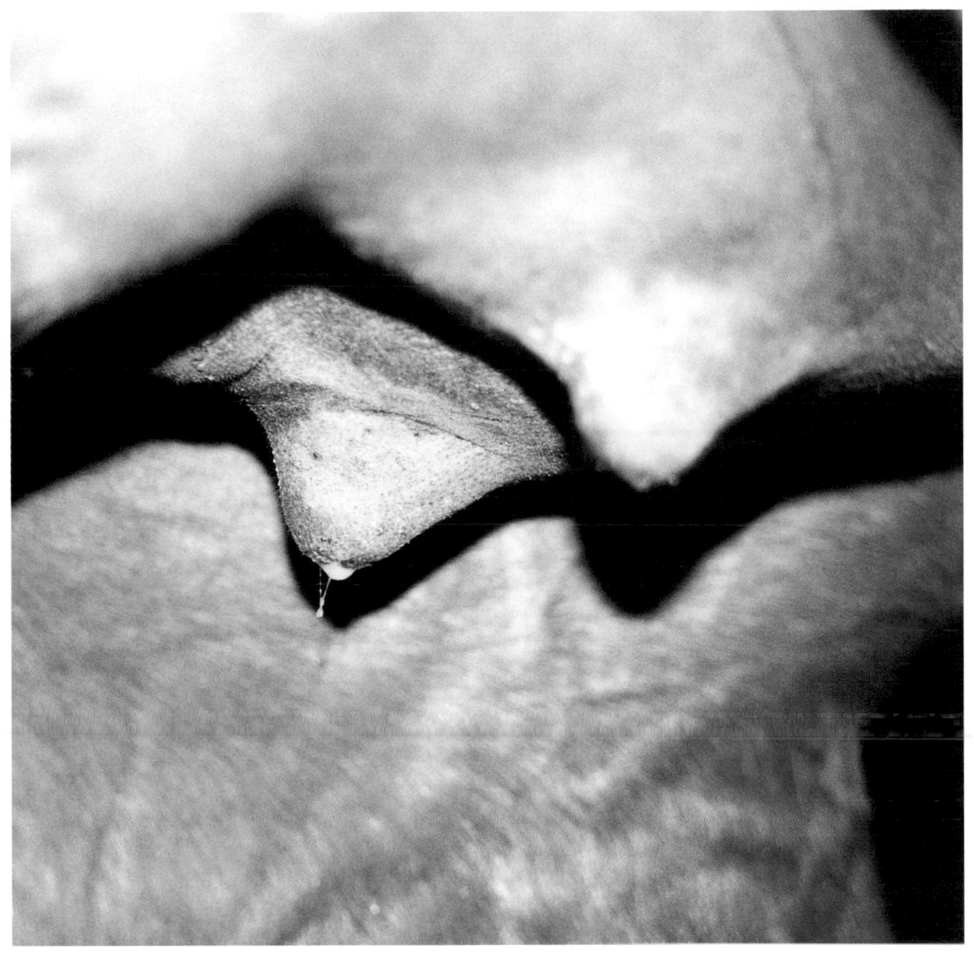

Figure 11.5

This mare has begun to secrete colostrum from her udder. This is commonly termed 'running milk'

Once this has occurred, unlike in first stage, foaling must be completed and the foal delivered. This usually occurs within half an hour but there is some variation depending on the age of the mare, size of foal relative to the mare's pelvic outlet and the strength of the mare's expulsive efforts.

The landmarks of second stage delivery are as follows;

- Rupture of the allantochorionic membrane (placenta) and escape of allantoic fluid.
- Appearance of the amnion at the vulval lips (Figure 11.7).
- The presence of one of the foal's hooves within the amnion (Figure 11.9).
- The appearance of both forefeet followed by the muzzle of the foal's

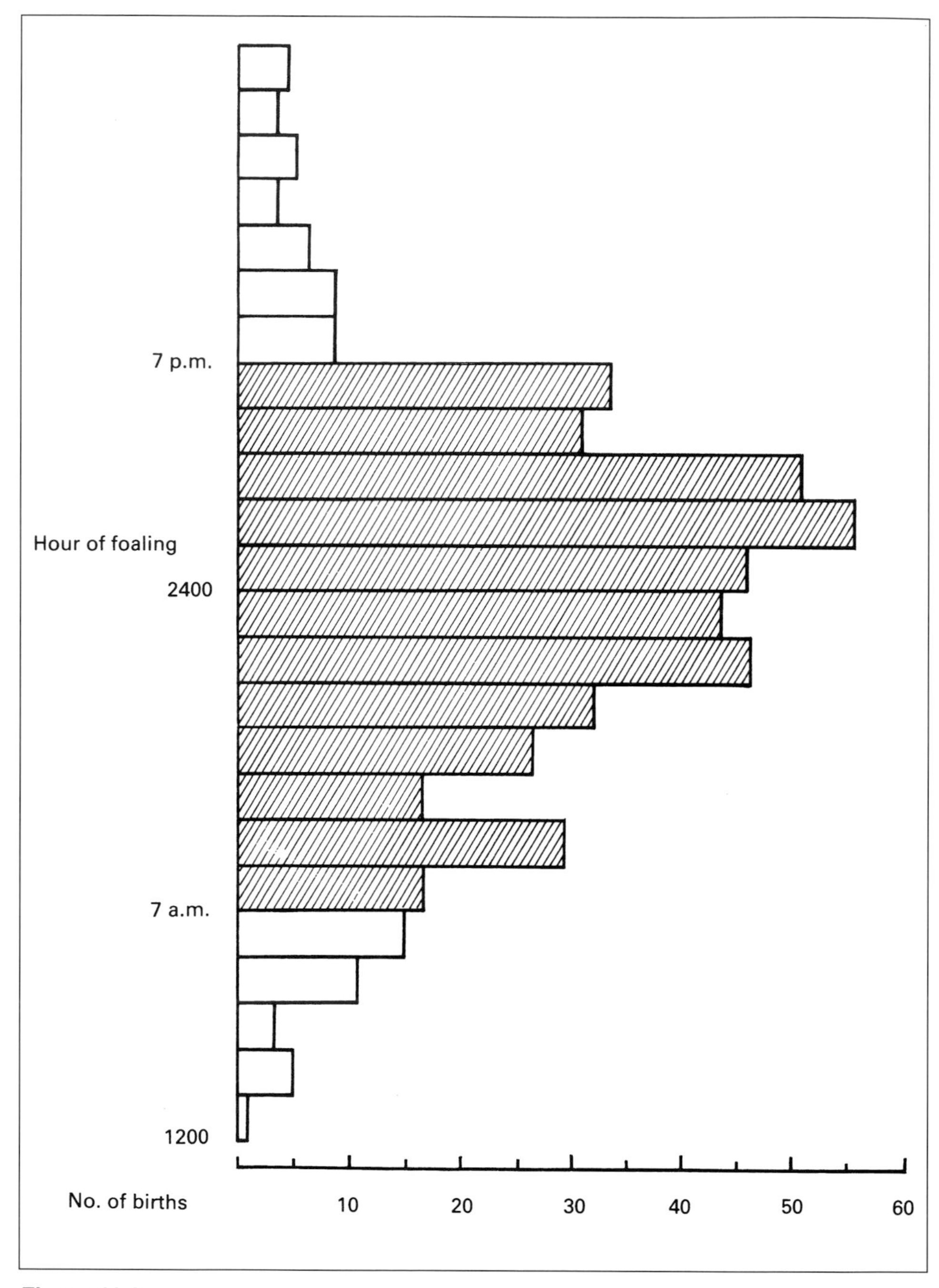

Figure 11.6

Times of foaling recorded in 501 mares. Of the 501 foals born, 90 per cent arrived between the hours of 7.00 pm and 7.00 a.m. (From Rossdale and Short, *J. Reprod. Fert.* (1967) 13, 341–3) head lying above the forelegs (Figure 11.11).

- Passage of the head, neck and shoulders followed by the chest and hindquarters (Figure 11.12).
- The foal is finally delivered with its hind legs to the hocks left in the mare's vagina (Figure 11.13) providing the mare is recumbent as is the situation in most cases at the final stage of delivery.

The behaviour of the mare during these stages of delivery may vary but typically includes the following:

- Breaking the water usually occurs with the mare in the standing position although sometimes as she becomes recumbent at the end of first stage.
- Once the water is broken the mare usually shows signs of voluntary straining. Although these efforts may occur while the mare is standing, they take more force and are more frequent when she becomes recumbent.
- Recumbency is the typical position for a delivery but the mare may rise to her feet on several occasions during second stage before the foal's chest is delivered through the vulval lips. After this stage, the mare does not usually rise to her feet until delivery is completed.
- Shifting from one side to the other would seem possibly to be related to the position of the fetus as it enters the birth canal and a logical action in shifting the alignment, should this instinctively be appropriate.

Third stage

Third stage involves the expulsion of the afterbirth (placenta and amniotic membrane) (Figures 11.15–11.18).

At the end of second stage the mare normally remains recumbent for anything up to 45 minutes. At first the umbilical cord remains intact, and it is most important that this connection should not be severed artificially. The cord breaks either when the mare gets to her feet or when the foal struggles in its attempts to stand. In either event, it breaks at a natural point about 4 cm from the foal's umbilicus.

The placenta starts to separate from its attachment to the wall of the uterus soon after delivery has been completed or, in some cases, before. Separation is usually complete within half an hour and the afterbirth drops away from the mare, occasionally still attached to the newborn foal by the umbilical cord.

Retention of the afterbirth may be due to one or both of the horns failing to separate. In practice, it is generally accepted that veterinary attention should be sought if the afterbirth has not been expelled after 12 hours. Retention beyond this point may lay the mare open to the risk of infection of the uterus and, even, laminitis.

Premonitory Signs

Within about three weeks of foaling, the two mammary glands of the udder begin to enlarge and contain an increasing quantity of milk. In maiden mares the udder may start to spring more abruptly and closer to the event than a mare that has previously had several foals. Beads of milk may form on the end of the teats within 24–48 hours of birth and dry into a wax-like substance which eventually drops off.

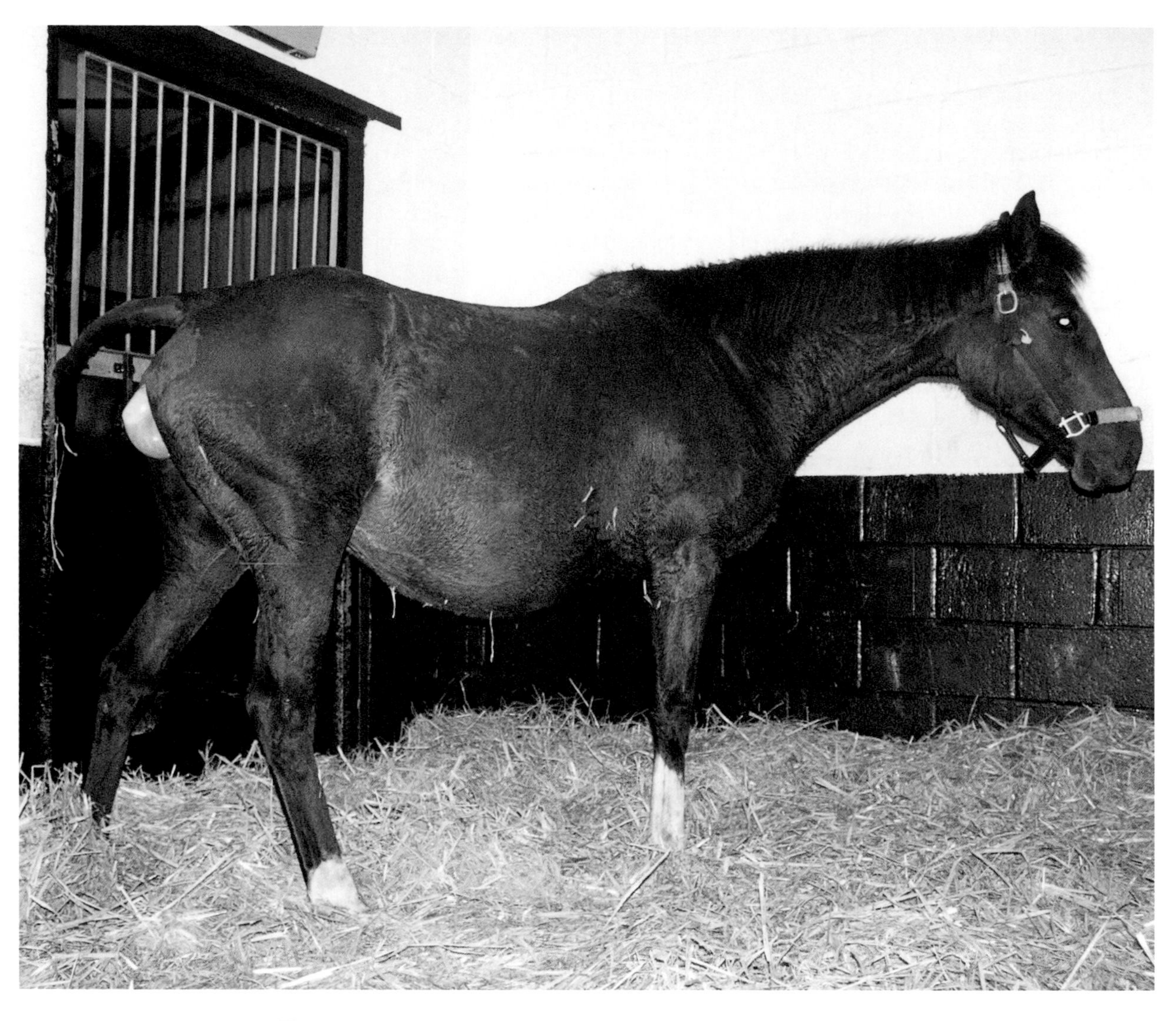

Figure 11.7

This mare is in the second stage of foaling. The amnion appears as a white bag at the vulval lips. Note that her tail has been bandaged up for hygiene reasons

Figure 11.8 (opposite)

This mare was 'opened up' prior to foaling as she had previously had a Caslick operation

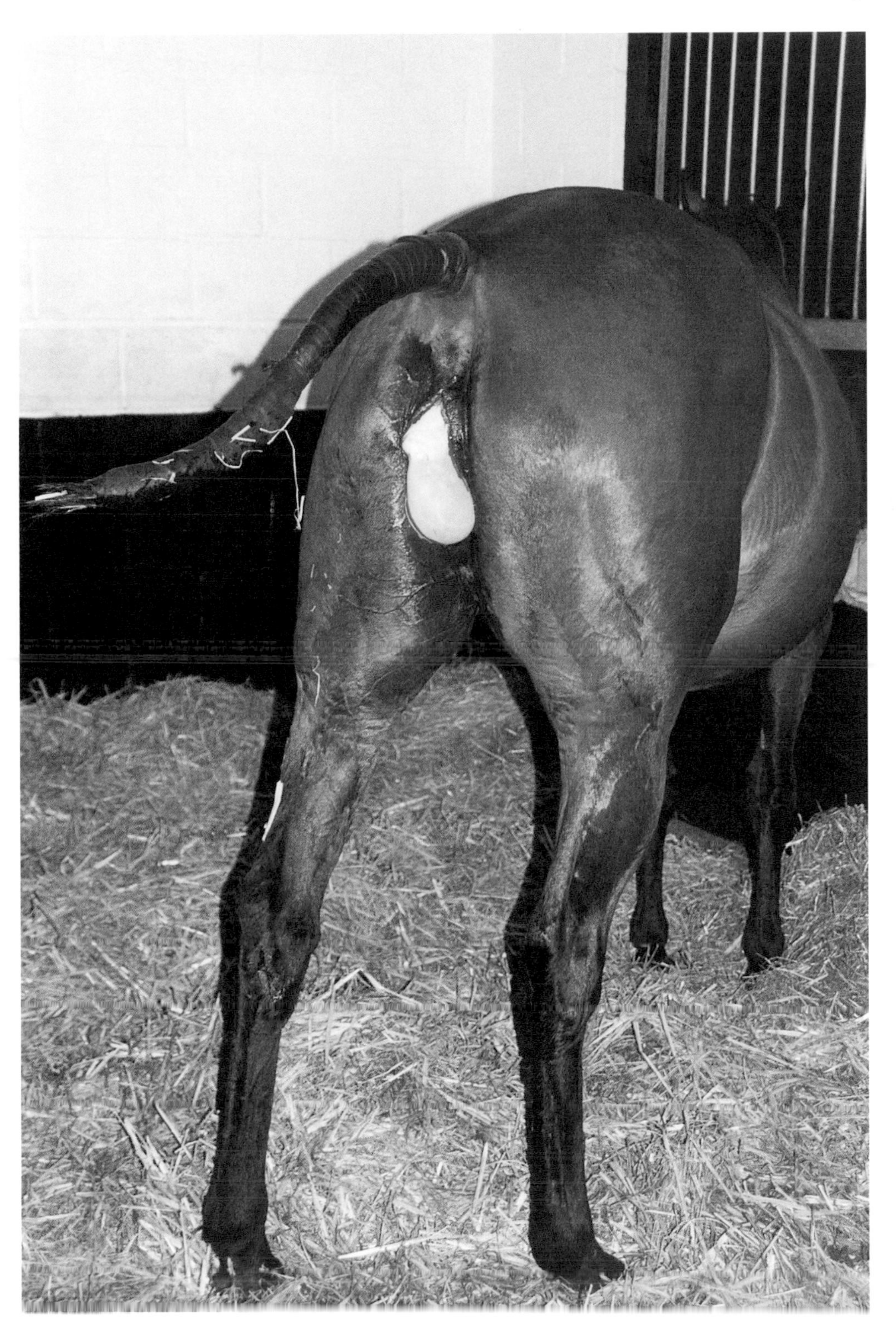

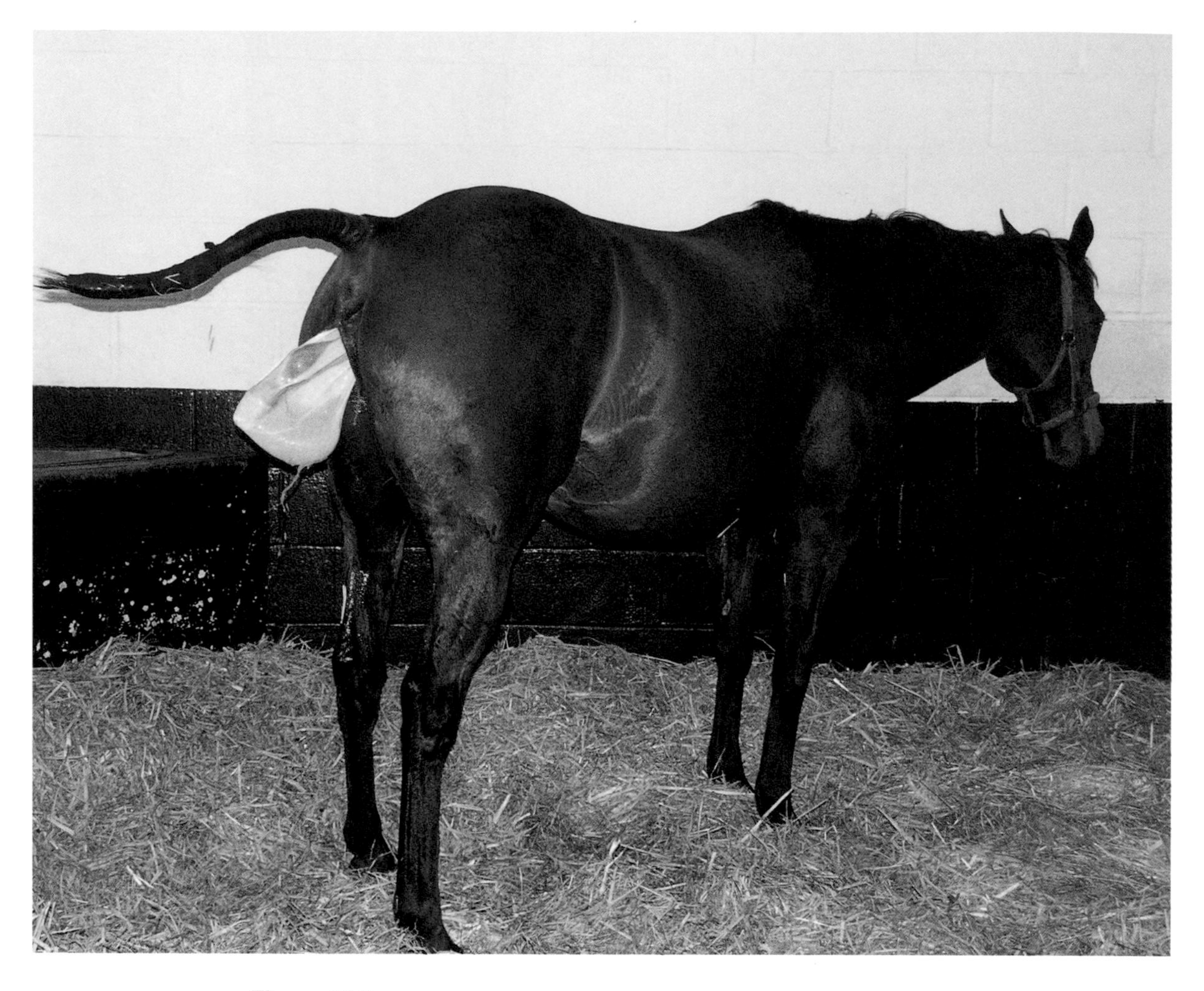

Figure 11.9

The foal's foreleg can clearly be seen still contained in the amnion. One foreleg precedes the other to allow the foal's shoulders to pass easily through the pelvic hoop

Figure 11.10 (opposite, top)

Mares will normally foal lying down, although they may get up and down several times before finally giving birth

Figure 11.11 (opposite, bottom)

The foal's forelegs and head can clearly be seen in the amniotic sac

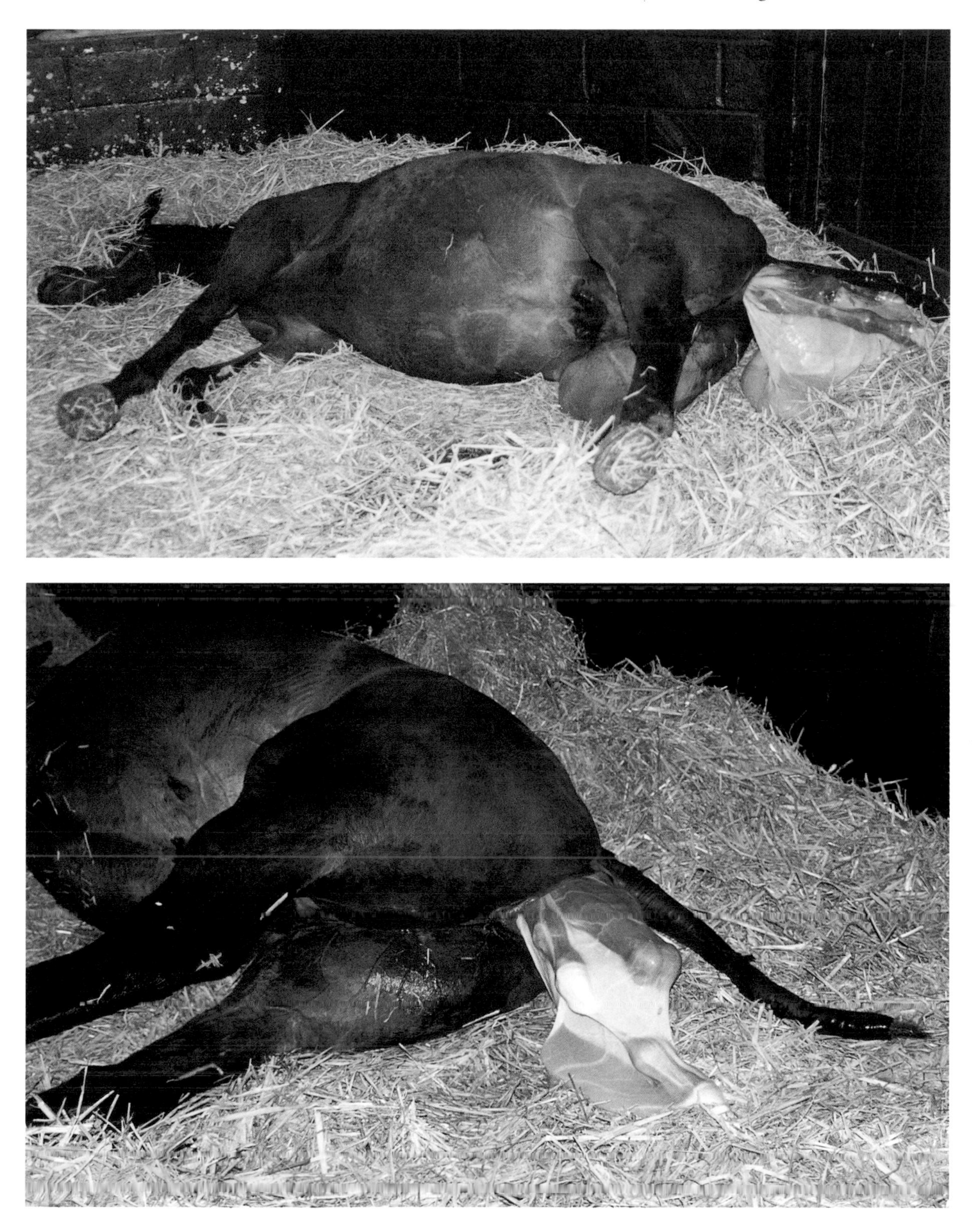

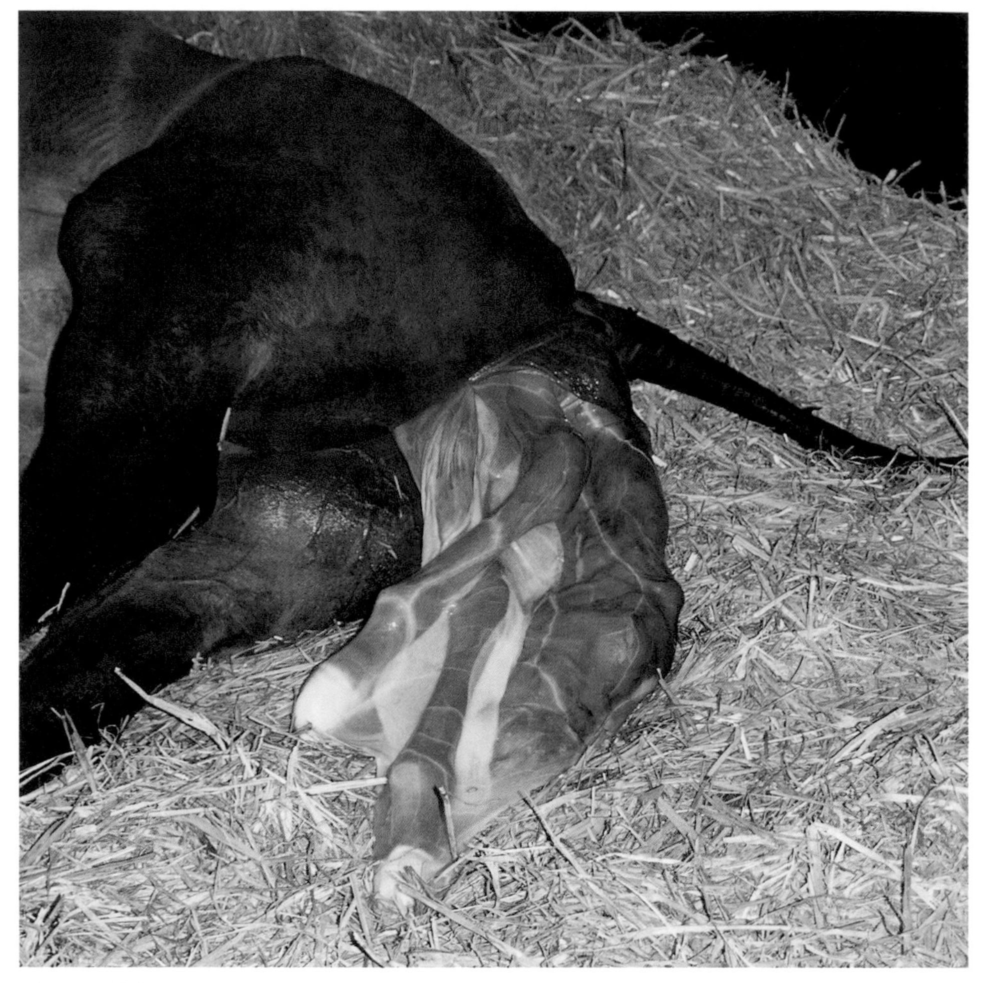

Figure 11.12

Once the foal's shoulders pass through the pelvic hoop, the remainder of the body follows quickly

Figure 11.13 (opposite, top)

At this stage only the foal's hind legs remain in the birth canal. The foal will now begin to breathe and move its forelegs. The placenta can just be seen at the mare's vulval lips. The amnion may be broken by the foal's first movements, or by the foaling attendant; it should be white in appearance and checked for meconium staining, as this indicates that the foal has suffered some distress during the foaling procedure

Figure 11.14 (opposite, bottom)

The foal's hooves have characteristic flaps of soft hoof to avoid damage to the uterus and vagina during pregnancy and birth

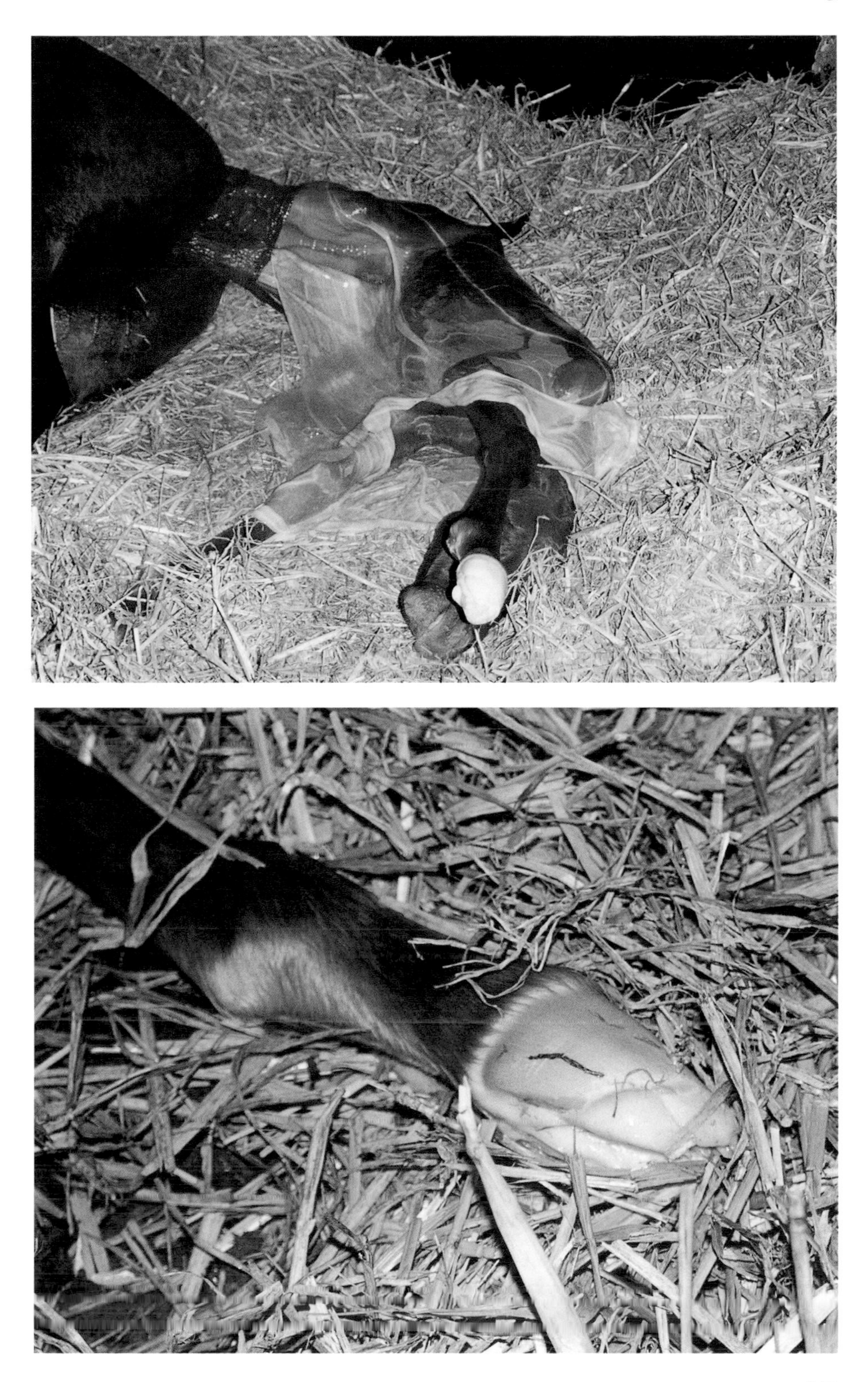

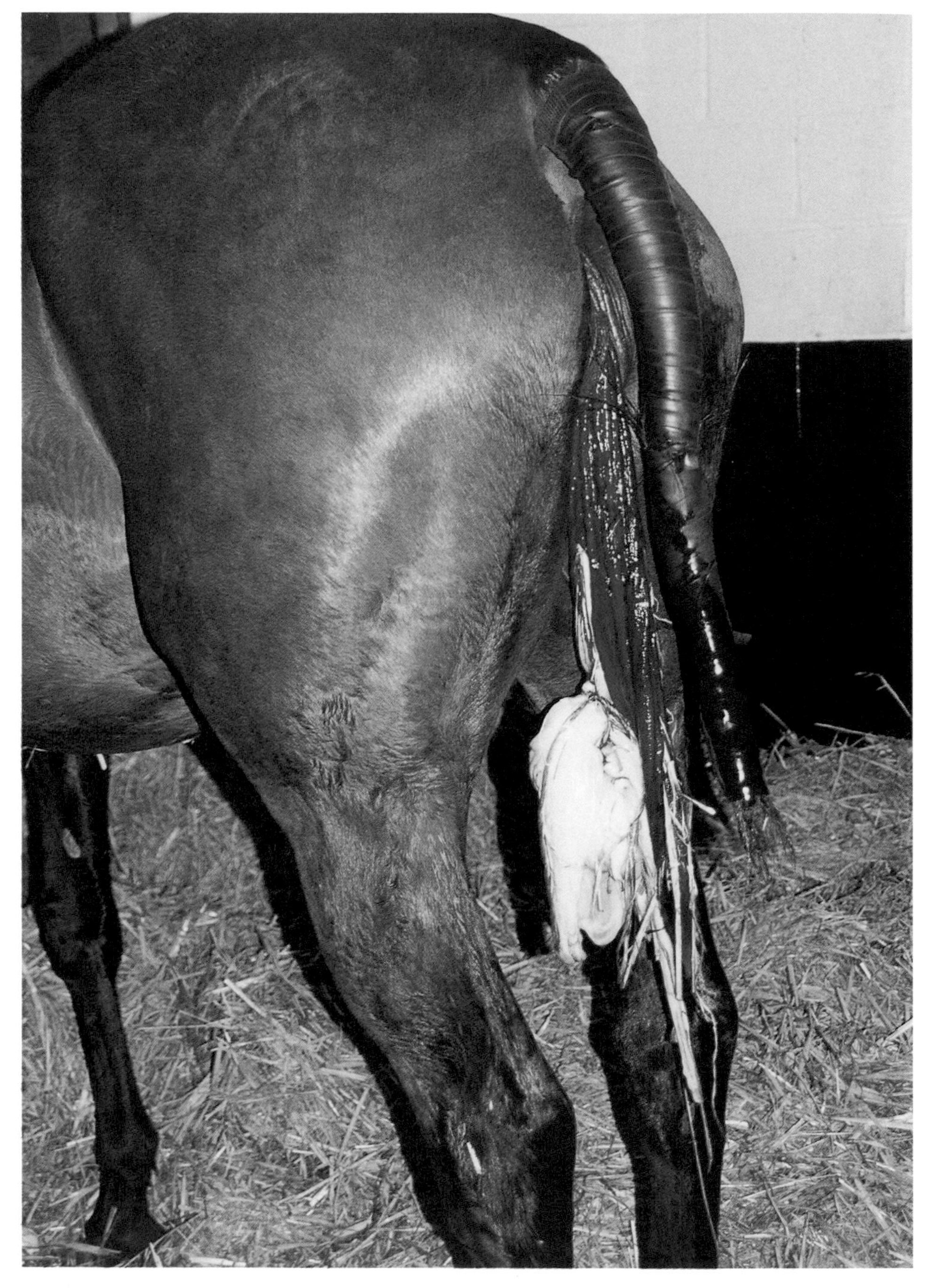

Figure 11.15

The placenta is normally tied up with string after foaling to avoid the mare accidentally standing on it. The placenta or afterbirth is passed during the third stage of foaling

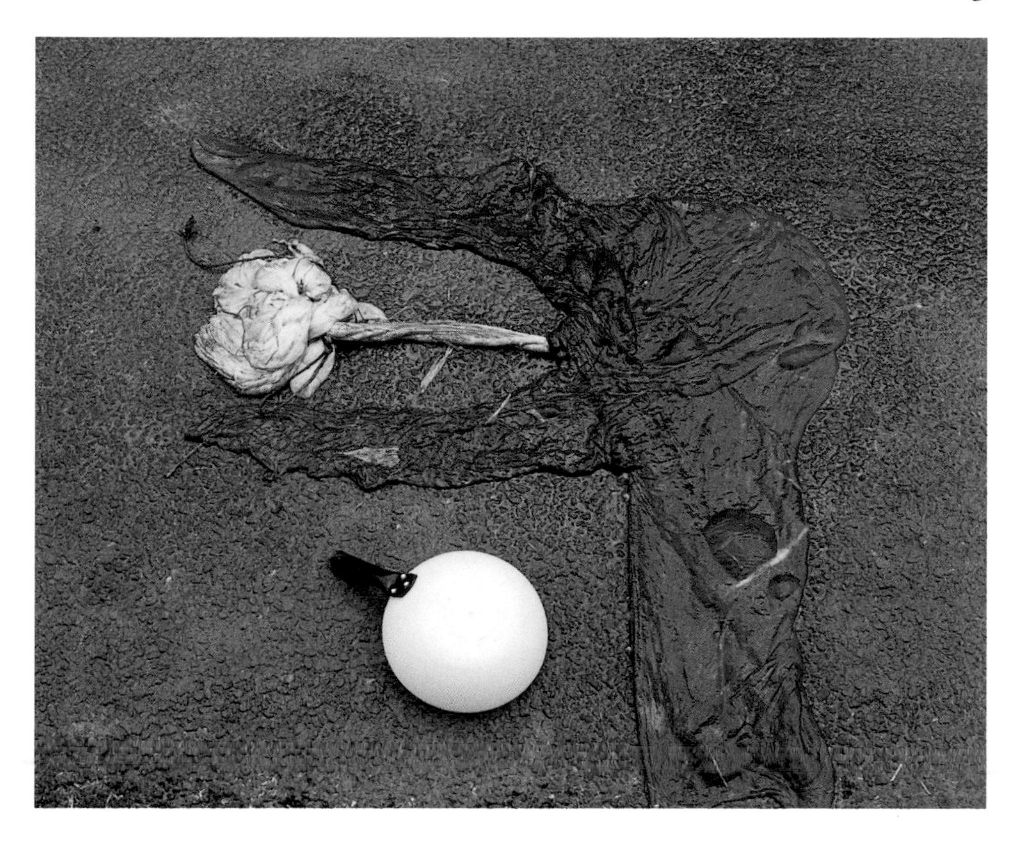

Figure 11.16

The placenta should be examined carefully to ensure that it is complete and to check its condition. This placenta is uterus side out; the velvety red side would have been adjacent to the mare's uterus during the pregnancy. The two horns of the placenta can clearly be seen as well as the amniotic membrane, still tied with string. The pregnant horn also can clearly be seen next to the feed scoop

This waxing-up is not an entirely reliable guide as to when mares are about to foal. Calcium levels in the milk rise at term (to 10 mmol/l) and give an early indication of when a mare is going to foal.

Many mares may run milk for several days before they foal. Hence, the first milk (colostrum) which contains the vital protective antibodies, is lost and the foal deprived of a substantial proportion of its resistance against infective diseases. There is much that still has to be learned regarding the causes of this loss of colostrum before birth. Udder development is linked, to an unknown extent, to the way mares are fed in the latter stages of pregnancy. Insufficient levels of protein in the diet will undoubtedly result in a poorly developed udder, while on the other hand 'steaming-up' might promote the loss of colostrum.

It is important to ensure that mares

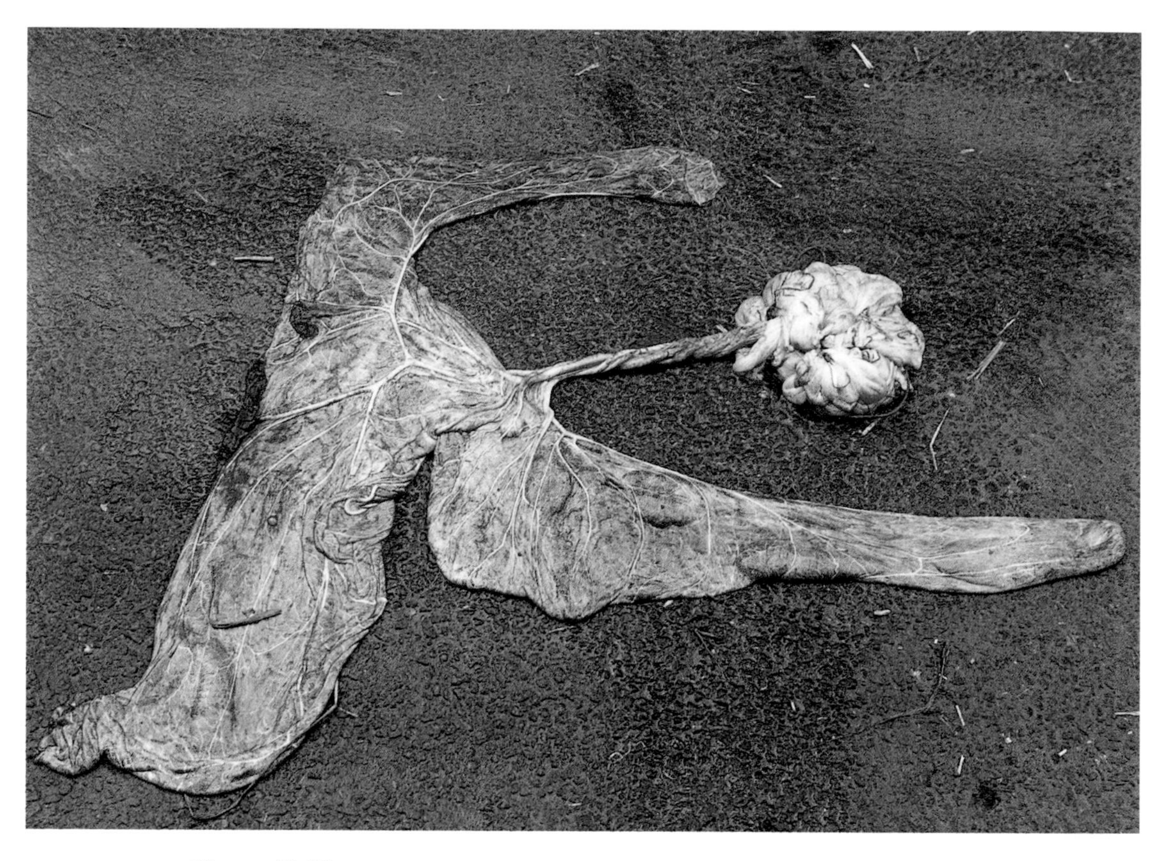

Figure 11.17

This placenta has been turned 'foal side' out – this is the side that would have been next to the foal during pregnancy

close to foaling should be subjected to a regular routine. Consistency in the timing of movements into and out of the paddock and contact with known attendants are factors which add to the stability of the environment and to the tranquillity which helps ensure a normal birth.

In the UK, most mares are foaled in specially appointed stalls. Looseboxes in which mares foal should be at least 4.24 m x 4.24 m and have suitable facilities for observing mares without the attendant having to enter the loosebox. This may be achieved by windows placed on internal walls and/or television monitors.

The floor should be sloping to the drain and its surface roughened to prevent slipping. There should be a doorway placed so that people can enter and leave the loosebox from a neighbouring room or passageway, in case of a veterinary problem with the mare or her foal.

Foaling boxes should be used as infrequently as practical in the context of the studfarm's number of mares due

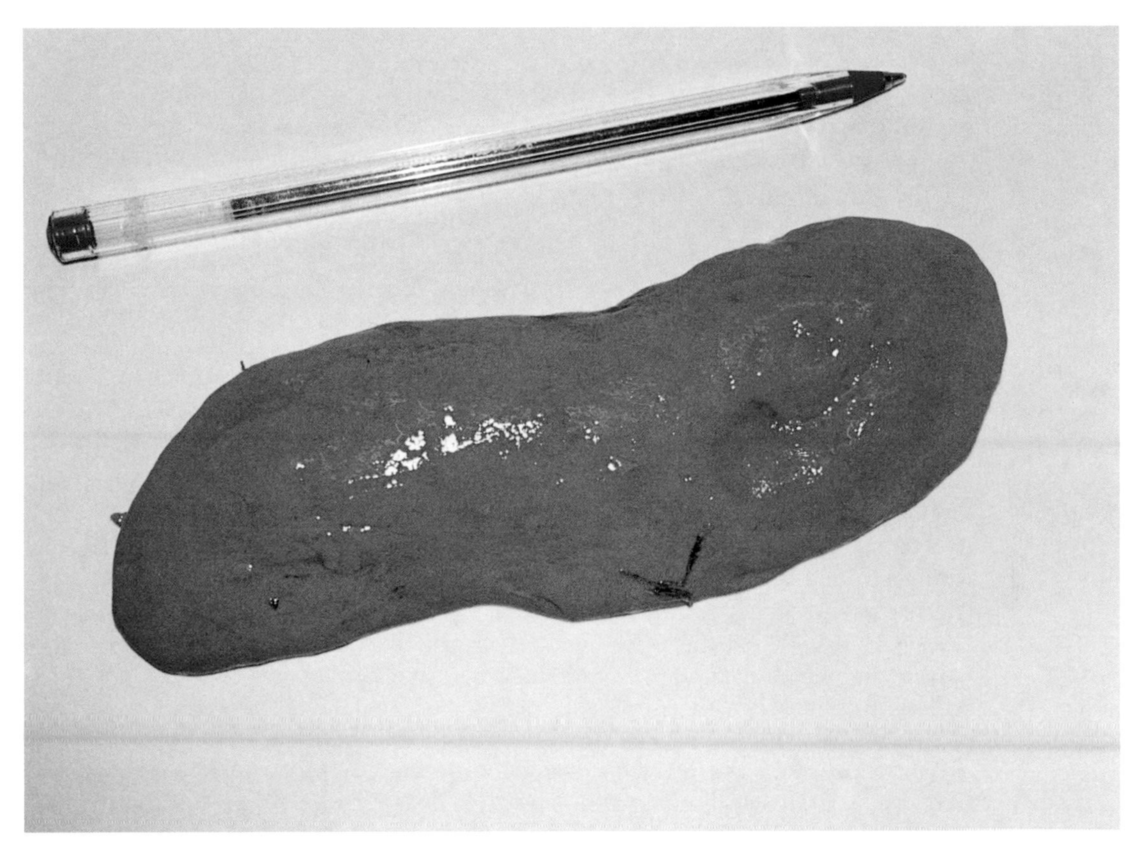

Figure 11.18

The hippomane. This is not always found, but forms in the allantoic fluid during the pregnancy

to foal. After each foaling they should be well cleansed and all straw removed so that a new mare may enter with fresh bedding and minimal risk of infection being carried over from previous incumbents. Adequate lighting, electricity points and running water should be available for routine and emergency use.

Air hygiene is most important and the mare's needs of good ventilation and minimal dust from bedding must be met. Consideration should also be given to the insulation in foaling boxes as most heat lost from the foal is by radiation; that is, through the roof and walls. This can be avoided with the provision of good levels of building insulation.

When first stage signs become apparent, the 'sitting up man' calls the stud groom who has the sole responsibility of the 'midwife'.

First stage signs may become apparent; then the mare may cool off to await another occasion for birth, some hours or even days later. These false alarms need not be regarded as abnormal, although in certain instances, such as when they are associated with the running of milk, they are potentially harmful and may indeed indicate a problem of dystocia (difficult birth).

Duties of Those in Charge of the Birth

When the placenta ruptures and the allantoic fluid escapes, the mare is said to have 'broken water'. In comparatively rare occurrences, the membrane is so thickened by disease that it fails to rupture in the normal manner. In these cases it appears between the lips of the vulva as a red membrane, and should be artificially broken with the fingers or a pair of scissors (Figure 11.19).

The rupture of the placenta represents a critical point as far as management of the foaling mare is concerned, since it marks the beginning of the process of expulsion of the foal. Once second stage has begun, it is essential to ascertain whether the foal is lying in the correct position. This can be done by inserting a hand into the vagina and feeling for the two forefeet and the muzzle of the foal.

The best time for this is while the mare is lying down and within about five minutes of the time that she has broken water. It should be remembered that during the last few months of pregnancy the foal has been lying in the uterus in the ventral position, that is, on its back, and that during the first stage and early second stage of labour it rotates 180 degrees to lie in the normal dorsal position. For this reason, if examined very early in the second stage, the limbs may give the impression that the foal is lying upside down. Providing the muzzle can also be felt, this is unlikely to be the case and, anyway, the normal process of delivery will usually complete the transition from the ventral to the dorsal position.

It is customary for mares to break water when they are in a standing position, but having done so they will very soon lie down and the amnion should then appear between the lips of the vulva. If it does not, or if the mare ceases her efforts at straining, we must suspect that the normal passage of the foal is impeded, perhaps by a malalignment of its limbs or head. This condition (dystocia) must be corrected if the foal is to be born alive.

This is not the place to describe in detail the various procedures necessary to solve problems of dystocia; it is a subject which is best taught by working alongside experienced people.

If the mare has previously had a Caslick operation on her vulva, she should, at this time, be cut with a pair of straight scissors (a procedure called episiotomy). In most cases this is a simple procedure, because the vulva loses sensation during birth. However, some mares may be apprehensive or even so sensitive as to jump to their feet or kick out at the attendant. Some studfarms prefer to have their vet open the vulva under local anaesthetic when the mare shows signs of being close to foaling.

Once the amnion has appeared, the attendant should notice whether it has a normal, smooth shiny appearance through which can be seen a clear-coloured fluid. In certain instances this membrane may be thickened and/or the fluid it contains stained a brown colour. This denotes that the foal has been stressed in the later stages of development and may be unable to adjust properly once it is delivered.

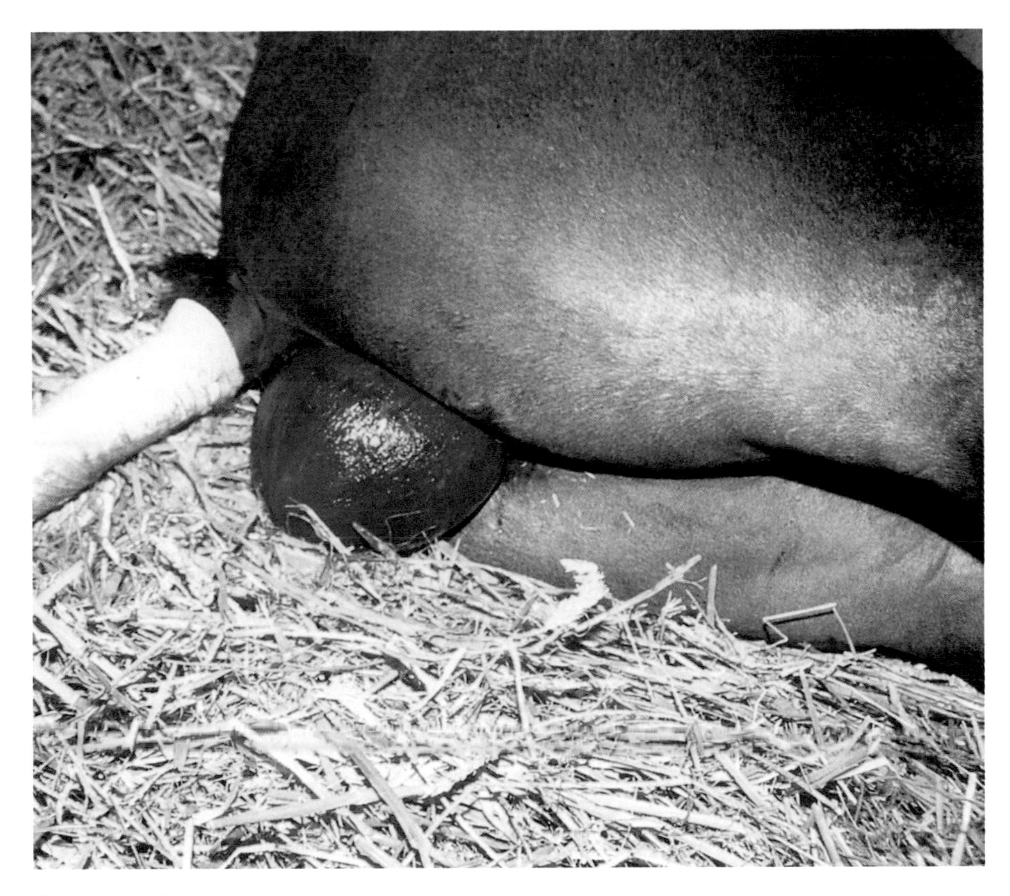

Figure 11.19

The appearance of the allanto-chorionic membrane at the vulval lips is abnormal and must be dealt with promptly. This indicates that placental separation has already begun and that the foal is being deprived of oxygen. As the foal may automatically begin to breathe there is a real risk of suffocation – with the foal literally drowning in the birth fluids it is still contained in. The membrane should be broken immediately and efforts made to ensure that delivery of the foal proceeds as quickly as possible

Delivery should proceed steadily and it is by this estimation that we can judge whether or not help is required during second stage. It is helpful to note the time at which the water breaks so that at any given point of second stage one can judge accurately how long delivery has been proceeding. It is surprising how inaccurate a guess can be in this respect.

If a foal is positioned normally it is unnecessary to pull on the forelegs. As previously explained, the natural course of delivery is that the foal is pushed from behind by the combined forces of the uterine and abdominal muscles. The implication is, therefore, that any traction on the forelegs of the foal would introduce an unnatural force. Nevertheless, it does appear helpful to apply gentle traction on one of the forelegs, especially if the foal's elbow becomes caught up on the mare's pelvis so that one foot is far in advance of the other.

Those attending the birth may have to get the mare to her feet if she is lying with her hindquarters so close to a wall that she cannot pass her foal. Apart from the actions described, it is preferable to watch second stage throughout its completion and interfere as little as possible.

The foal may be delivered retained completely in amnion and when it starts to breathe will break this membrane by striking forward with its foreleg and arching its neck. It is only when the foal has been ill during the latter stages of development or been seriously affected by the birth process that it is essential to break the amnion and raise the foal's head to make sure its nostrils are clear of the fluid when it starts to breathe.

Once the foal has been delivered, it will lie with its hind legs in the mare's vagina. Both mare and foal should, at this time, be left undisturbed. It is not advisable to sever the umbilical cord unless there are compelling reasons for doing so. Chief of these reasons is any evidence that the placenta or amnion are abnormal.

It is usual for those attending the birth to tie the amnion to the cord so that it hangs as a weight behind the mare. If the afterbirth is retained longer than a few hours, it is advisable to consult the veterinarian as to when it should be manually removed. If the afterbirth is left too long, it may set up infection in the uterus and perhaps even cause laminitis. Veterinarians differ as to the exact time they like to remove a retained afterbirth, but in general about ten hours is the maximum allowed to elapse.

Once the afterbirth has come away, it is important to check that both horns are intact and that a portion has not been left in the uterus. After the foal and its membranes have been expelled from the uterus the organ normally contracts quite rapidly. This process is often referred to as involution.

The mare may show signs of after-pains as her uterus contracts and especially before the afterbirth has been expelled. During these pains she may roll and sweat or look around at her flanks. There are a number of complications which can arise at this time and need a skilled diagnosis, so a close liaison between management and veterinarian is advisable. These complications include uterine haemorrhage.

Mares do not often bleed from the lining of the uterus after giving birth as may be the case in women. The difference is due to the fact that the placenta does not invade the uterine lining as it does in human beings. When it becomes detached the risk of bleeding is therefore less.

However, a quite common occurrence, especially in old mares, is for haemorrhage to take place internally from a branch of the artery supplying the uterus. This causes a great deal of pain and a haematoma (blood blister) forms between layers of the peritoneum (the lining of the abdomen which covers the walls and the organs). The mare may lose a substantial quantity of blood in this manner resulting in anaemia and pale membranes together with initial severe pain.

If the blood blister breaks through the peritoneum the mare bleeds to death as her blood escapes into the peritoneal cavity. If mares show evidence of severe pain following foaling veterinary assistance should be sought immediately.

A twitch should not be applied during this first three days after foaling as this will inevitably raise the blood pressure and may precipitate a haemorrhage. Nowadays, there are tranquillising drugs available which are very effective when used to control mares.

Another complication of the after-foaling period is a prolapse of the uterus. In this case, the organ turns itself inside out and protrudes through the vagina. In this event, immediate professional attendance should be sought. While waiting for the arrival of the veterinarian, the mare should, if possible, be kept in the standing position and the organ held in a clean sheet to avoid it becoming damaged or contaminated. Massaging with warm soapy water may help. The longer the organ protrudes, the more difficult it is to restore it to its normal position.

Successful replacement is usually followed by normal fertility, although it may be necessary to rest the mare for a year rather than to attempt to get her to conceive in the months following prolapse.

Management of the Foaling Mare

Up to this point we have been concerned solely with an explanation of the events as they occur during birth. It is now time to consider the significance of these events in relation to modern stud management.

Because of the great value of each individual Thoroughbred, we cannot leave these matters entirely to chance; it is true that 90 per cent of mares will foal without trouble whether or not attendants are there. In the remaining 10 per cent of births, some assistance of a major or minor degree may be necessary.

The essence of good management may be summed up in terms of watchfulness before and during birth, immediate provision of assistance when necessary for mare and/or foal, attention towards the feeding of the newborn and its protection against the elements.

A management perspective

The birth of a foal is the final part of a year-long investment in breeding and caring for the mare. The birth is not a complicated process and problems are rare. However, if a problem does occur it can be life threatening if not dealt with promptly. Knowledge of normal foaling and an understanding of the management requirements for a mare close to foaling are essential.

The selection and design of facilities for foaling deserve special consideration. The type of facilities used will depend on factors such as the size of the farm, the number of mares expected to foal there each year, labour available and climate.

The main areas used for foaling are specially designed stables or outside in specific paddocks. The most important consideration is provision for maintaining a high level of hygiene, as both mare and foal are particularly susceptible to infection after parturition. Secondly, the area must be safe for both mare and foal. Thirdly, it is ideal if the mare has been resident on the farm for at least six weeks prior to foaling to allow her to build up antibodies against those organisms that are present in that area and, therefore, pass on this protection to the foal through the colostrum.

In the UK, most studfarms have specialised indoor foaling units. These allow close supervision of the mare before and during foaling as well as permitting a high level of care and supervision after foaling. As mentioned earlier, the majority of mares foal without needing any assistance and rarely suffer from complications, but most breeders still prefer to have the birth closely supervised. Some breeds are bred early to foal early each year, such as Thoroughbreds who normally foal from January onwards. These mares will obviously need to be stabled at night to provide some protection from the elements and foaling outside would not be a practical consideration. The high value of most broodmares combined with the capital invested in her foal means that every care is taken in their management.

Many foaling boxes are fitted with monitoring devices in the form of closed-circuit cameras, or alternatively the mare may wear a foaling alarm which alerts the attendant to any sign of impending foaling. Although large farms can justify having specially employed staff to monitor the foaling mares, this may not be justifiable on smaller farms. The use of monitors can be useful, but they are no substitute for an experienced night watchman and sometimes monitors such as foaling alarms are not 100 per cent reliable. The advances in modern camera technology are increasing each year and the range of cameras suitable for monitoring foaling mares is now vast.

If cameras are to be used, they should be set up so that it is not possible for the mare to go 'out of range' and not be visible on the monitor; they should also be fitted well out of reach of any horses. Many cameras use infrared technology so that mares can be monitored at night without having to be disturbed with normal lighting. Cameras can be particularly useful as they allow minimal disturbance to the mare, as she is obviously unaware that she is being watched. Some mares may be particularly shy when they are close to foaling and may become anxious at the presence of too many people. Cameras also allow the mare and foal to be monitored safely after birth without any interference.

Foaling boxes may be kept just for the actual foaling with the mare being moved as soon as signs of foaling are imminent and moved back to her own stable the next day. Alternatively, the mare may be moved to the foaling box about two weeks before she is due to foal and will remain there until about a week after foaling. The latter is perhaps the most satisfactory, as it allows the mare to settle in her new surroundings and reduces the risk of infection transfer by moving her from place to place when she and her foal are at their most susceptible.

The stables used for foaling should be larger than average and preferably with rounded corners to avoid the mare getting wedged while giving birth and to avoid the foal getting stuck after foaling. If the stable is constructed of timber, the lower part of the wall should be solid so that there is no risk of the mare and/or the foal being injured, all surfaces should be checked for splinters or loose nails and stable furnishings such as buckets and feed bowls should be removed. Ideally, the stable used for foaling should be constructed of brick with a plaster or sealed wood facing so that it provides a completely smooth surface which can be cleaned easily. If feed and water containers are to be provided then these should be boxed into the corners and be high enough to reduce any risk to the foal. Heat lamps are often used on studfarms that foal mares early in the year. These should be of the type designed for stables and each should be thoroughly checked each year to reduce any risk of electrical faults or fire. Obviously, heat lamps must be fitted high enough to be completely out of reach of the mare and foal. Heat is lost by convection (evaporation), conduction (direct contact with the floor) and radiation (loss to the atmosphere). Radiation is responsible for by far most heat loss in the case of the foal.

Floorings vary from one premises to another. The use of rubber flooring is becoming increasingly common even on smaller studfarms. It is a very desirable surface for foaling boxes as it is warm, non-slip (some old types of rubber flooring were slippery when wet) and easy to clean. Concrete floors are also suitable as they can be cleaned thoroughly, but the box may require more bedding to reduce the risk of bruising or scrapes. Clay or soil floors are more traditional and provide a warmer, safer surface than some man-made types. However, they do need frequent maintenance and are almost impossible to clean properly. This type of flooring is probably more suited to smaller farms who foal a static group of mares and therefore have a minimal infection risk.

Each foaling box should be thoroughly cleaned and disinfected after each mare. This includes removing and changing all the bedding. There should be no compromises with the standard of cleaning of each foaling box and many studs use high-pressure steam washers as well as more standard equipment. The box should be left to dry if at all possible before fresh bedding is put in.

The type of bedding that is used in foaling boxes tends to vary from stud to stud. Straw is about the most common bedding used as it provides a warm, deep bed at a economical price, but it can be difficult for newborn foals to stand and move about in when they are still very young. Shavings or wood chip tend to stick to wet newborn foals and can cause eye irritation but are very useful for foals with limb deviations who are having difficulty in walking. Peat bedding is relatively unsuitable as it can be damp and cold to the skin – it is also becoming increasingly expensive. Whichever type of bedding is chosen, it should be as dust-free as possible – dust entering the foal's lungs may help to set up infection. For this reason, the temptation to rush in after a mare has foaled and shake up clean bedding should be avoided. The dust spores present in almost all bedding materials can also enter the mare's reproductive tract through her still open cervix and cause considerable irritation and inflammation. The environment of the stable should be kept as well ventilated as possible without draughts and it is unlikely that there is ever a need to shut the mare's top door.

The equipment needed for foaling should be assembled well before the first mare is due to foal and kept specifically for foaling. Every foaling kit is different but the basics would include tail bandage or wrap, two buckets (kept just for foaling), bin liners for the afterbirth, etc., paper towel – ideally of veterinary grade on a roll – disposable arm-length gloves for examinations, sharp surgical scissors, antiseptic or iodine for navel dressing, foal enemas, protective washable trousers and overshirt for attendant, wellington boots kept specifically for foaling attendants/or plastic boot covers.

Larger studfarms keep other items such as obstetrical ropes, oxygen cylinders, sedatives and antibiotics but this would depend on the number of mares foaled each year and how close the nearest vet is.

In areas such as Newmarket, where a vet can be in attendance on most of the studfarms within 15 minutes, there is little need to have too much unnecessary equipment; however, in some very rural areas this type of equipment can save lives. After each foaling the kit should be checked and replenished as necessary; all washable items should be cleaned and disinfected.

For each foaling mare a routine management programme will ensure the best possible chance of her producing a live and healthy foal, as well as giving the mare the best chance of returning to breeding as soon as possible after the birth. The mare's vaccination record should be checked to ensure that she has up to date vaccination, particularly for flu and tetanus. As discussed in the Codes of Practice (Chapter Ten), most large studfarms will not permit foaling mares on to the stud without correct vaccination against EHV, so any new arrival's paperwork must be double checked before they are allowed off their transport. Many studs give a tetanus booster to the mare about a month before her due date to give extra protection to the foal via the mare's colostrum – although this is normally supplemented with tetanus antitoxin given to the foal shortly after birth.

The mare's vulva should be checked and if she has been stitched she will require opening with scissors along the line of scar tissue. This procedure can be carried out by the veterinary surgeon once the mare shows signs of getting close to foaling – as this is can be very difficult to predict with accuracy, sometimes the mare may be opened as early as ten days prior to her actual foaling. Other farms have a policy of not opening the mare until she starts to foal and her water has broken. If the latter policy is followed it is essential that an attendant can be present at the mare's foaling – if there is any risk, however small, of her foaling unattended then she should be opened early (Figures 11.20 and 11.21).

Stitched mares that foal alone can do enormous damage to their external genitalia that may preclude them from being bred again that year, and will be prone to reproductive inflammation and infections in subsequent years. This is due to the fact that scar tissue forms each time the mare's vulva is torn and if this is not carefully controlled it may make the vulval seal permanently incompetent. Some mares will tear in several places and some may suffer rectal damage if the foal's feet are forced against the wall of the rectum. Although correctly opened mares will also form vulval scar tissue, it is unlikely, once she is sutured again after foaling, that this will cause any lasting problem. Whichever policy is used, all handlers attending foalings should be familiar with opening mares.

On public studs where many unknown mares may arrive to foal each year, it is helpful to get as much information about previous foalings as possible. Any information such as any difficulties the mare has had in the past, any foals she may have lost during birth, any known behavioural problems with mare or foal after birth, any problems with the mare's milk production and if

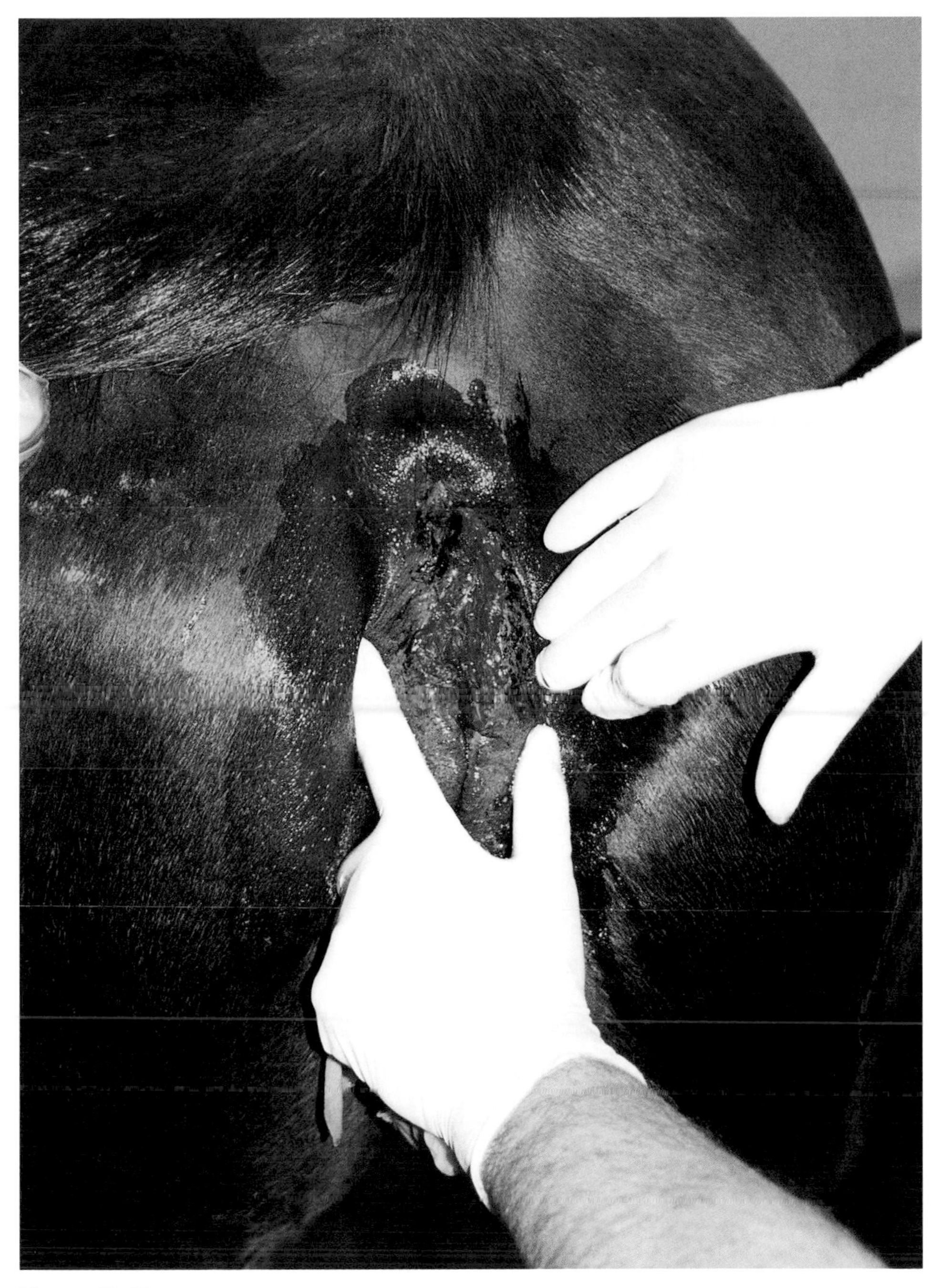

Figure 11.20

This illustration shows the amount of damage that can occur when a mare who has been stitched is allowed to foal without being opened up. This type of damage can seriously affect the mare's future reproductive health by causing the formation of scar tissue and compromising the vulval seal

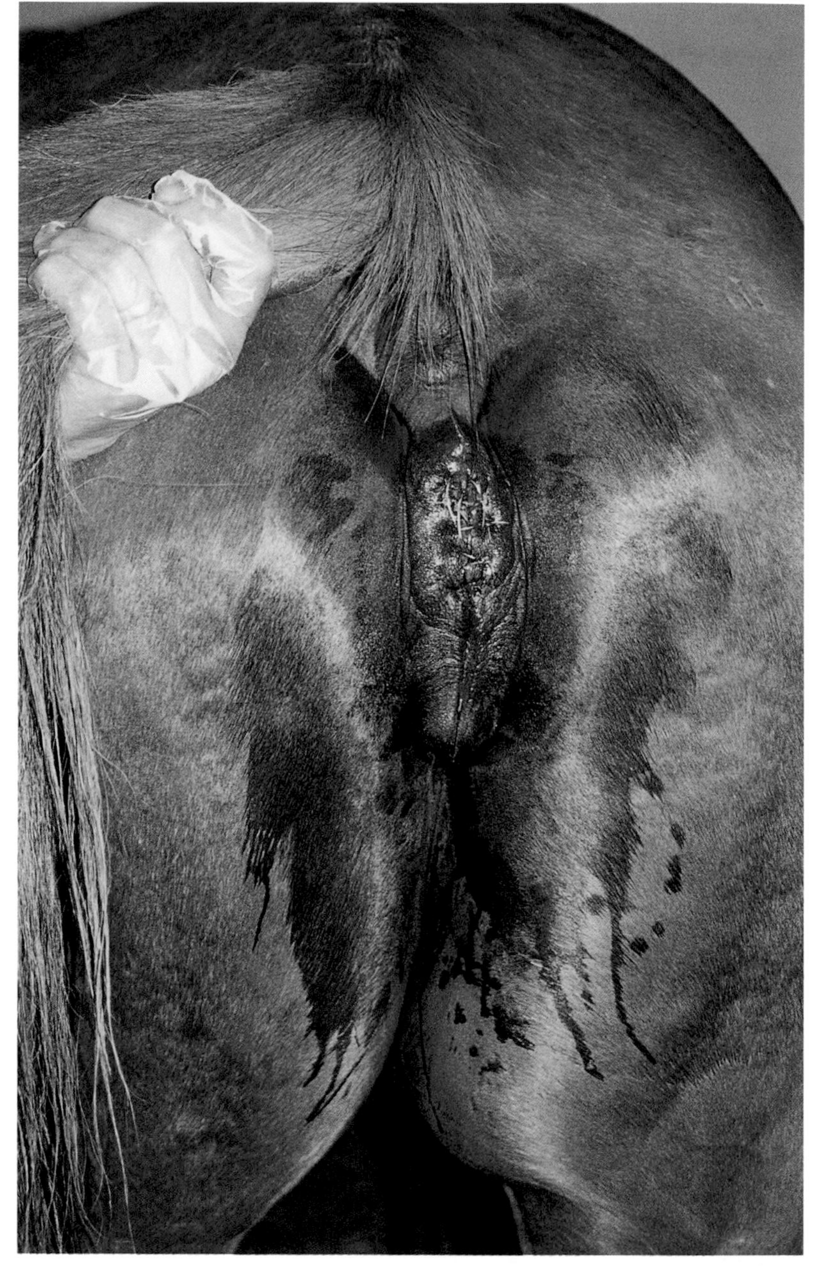

Figure 11.21

A mare who was opened correctly prior to foaling and then restitched the next morning

she is know to be particularly foal proud following birth, should be obtained if possible. Mares that have produced a haemolytic foal in previous years should be tested before foaling to determine if this foal is at risk. If this is not possible, it should be assumed that the foal is at risk and special care plans made (see Chapter Twelve).

Larger studfarms may make comprehensive records of each mare's foaling, including details such as whether she ran milk for long time prior to foaling (foals born to such mares will require supplementary colostrum after birth) and normal signs and times of foaling, etc. Mares will not always follow the same pattern with each foaling, but any information is useful.

Free exercise is important for heavily pregnant mares. As mares get closer to foaling they tend to become more sedentary, due to their increased size and weight. Filled legs can be a problem during this late stage and access to exercise will help to reduce inflammation and stiffness. If mares cannot be turned out for any reason, they should be walked in-hand if at all possible. Any foot problems or old injuries may start to give some discomfort as the pregnancy progresses, so careful and regular farrier assessment is vital.

The mare's nutritional needs at this time also require careful consideration. As the size of the foal increases mares generally begin to lose their appetite and may only pick at their food. It is important to try to provide small quantities of a high-quality ration as well as good-quality forage. Some studs prefer to cut the mare's normal two or three concentrate feeds into several smaller feeds throughout the day, while others try to improve the nutritional intake by feeding forage such as haylage which has a higher protein content than normal hay. Older routines insisted that mares should be deprived of food when close to foaling to avoid the risk of colic or scours after foaling – this is now considered unnecessary. As always, any changes in the mare's diet, whether she is close to foaling or not, should be made gradually.

After foaling the mare will normally stay lying down for some time if she is not disturbed. During this time, she will normally show considerable interest in her newborn foal and respond to its movements by whickering and licking any part of it that she can reach. Moving the foal so that it is closer to her head can be helpful, but some farms feel that this may cause too much disturbance and result in the mare standing up.

This period immediately after birth is a critical time for bonding between the mare and foal. The smell of the afterbirth and fluids seems to assist in stimulating the mare's maternal reaction and any human intervention at this time should be kept to a minimum (Figure 11.22).

Once the mare stands, the umbilical cord will be broken naturally and the afterbirth should be tied up to prevent the mare from standing on it. The afterbirth will be expelled within a hour or so of foaling and the mare may show some discomfort at this time. The stump of the umbilical cord on the foal's abdomen should be dressed with antiseptic powder and then left alone. Once the immediate care has been completed, the mare and foal should be left alone for as long as possible, although they should still be observed from outside the stable or via a camera. Continued observation is important to establish that the mare has expelled the placenta (this should be removed and checked to ensure that it is complete), to establish that the foal is nursing (Figure 11.23) and at what time it had its first drink, and that the foal has passed its first droppings in the form of meconium.

Any abnormal behaviour of either mare and foal should be careful monitored as it is at this time that some abnormalities or complications may become apparent, even though the foaling process itself seemed routine.

The mare is often offered a warm wet

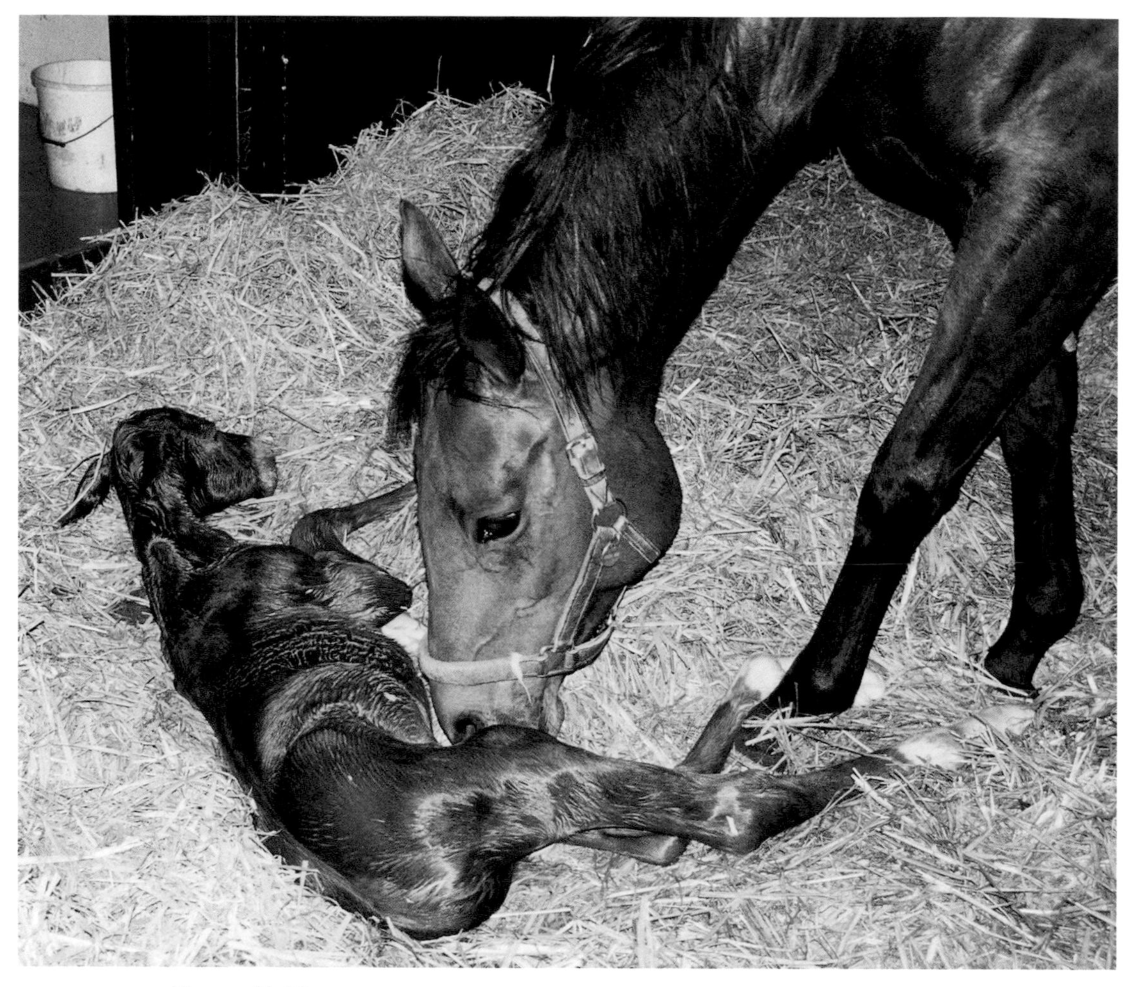

Figure 11.22

The mare begins to bond with the foal immediately after birth by licking and nuzzling

feed after foaling and should have access to water. Some large studfarms give lukewarm water to the mare to drink after foaling, especially if the weather is very cold; however, this is probably unnecessary during the warmer months. Mares may start to eat their beds after foaling and seem to have a need for roughage, so feeding a wet high-fibre mash-type feed is usually appreciated and this will also help to encourage bowel movements even though the sore abdominal and rectal muscles may cause some discomfort to the mare. The foal may be given an enema immediately after birth (Figure 11.24).

Many Thoroughbred studfarms will wash the mare's lower body and legs with warm water and disinfectant solution after foaling before the foal is standing (Figure 11.25). It is now

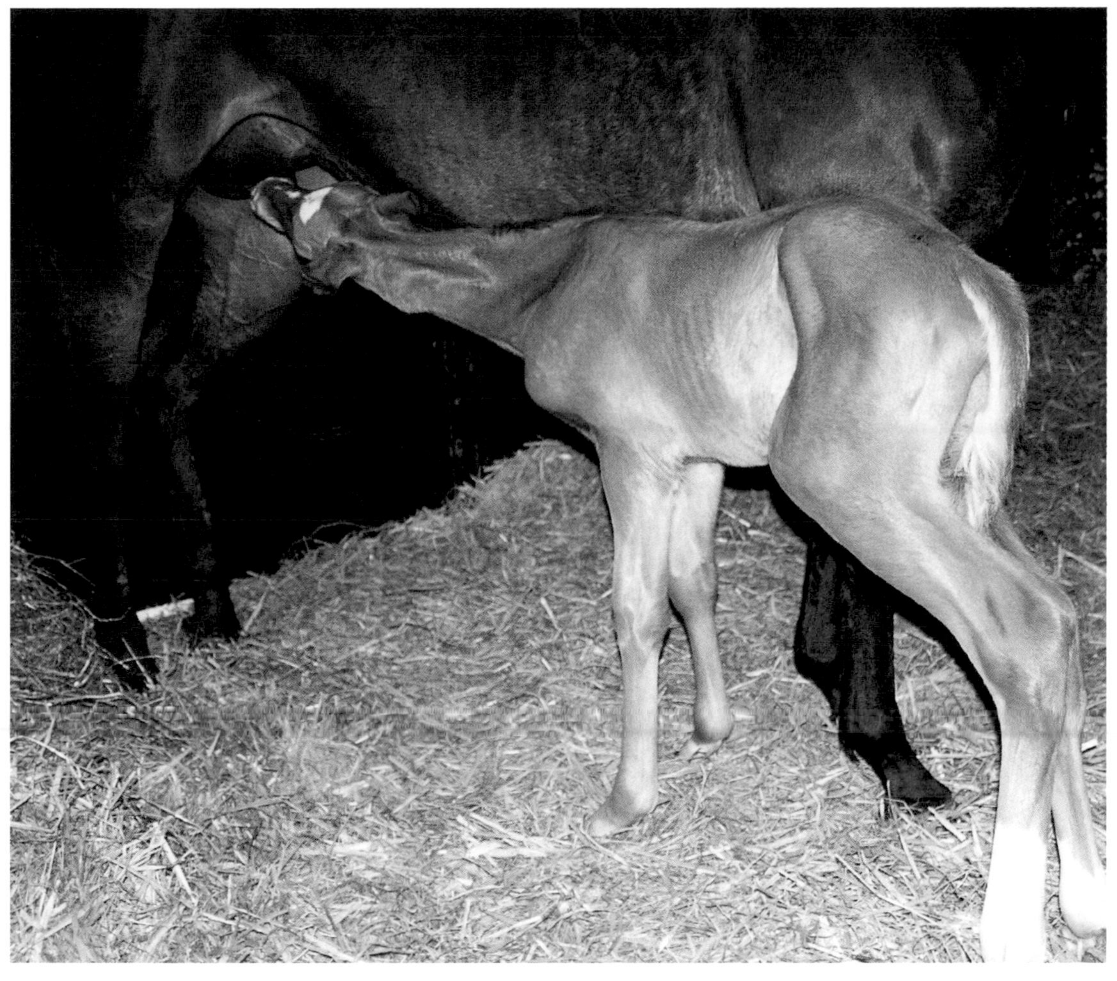

Figure 11.23

The foal's first food of colostrum. The mare rests her opposite hind leg to ease access to the udder for the foal

thought that many of the early infections that can affect foals may be reduced by carrying out this procedure, particularly those causing diarrhoea. Once the foal is standing and starts to search for the udder, he will instinctively seek dark areas and suck at the mare's legs and belly as he makes his way eventually to finding the udder. This may lead to him accidentally ingesting environmental pathogens that could cause illness at this early stage in his life when he is at his most vulnerable. If this procedure is to be carried out, it should be done with the minimum of fuss and as quickly as possible as soon as the mare is standing to avoid interfering with the bonding process. Some mares, particularly those who have foaled for the first time, may not tolerate such a procedure at this time. It is also only commonsense to keep any

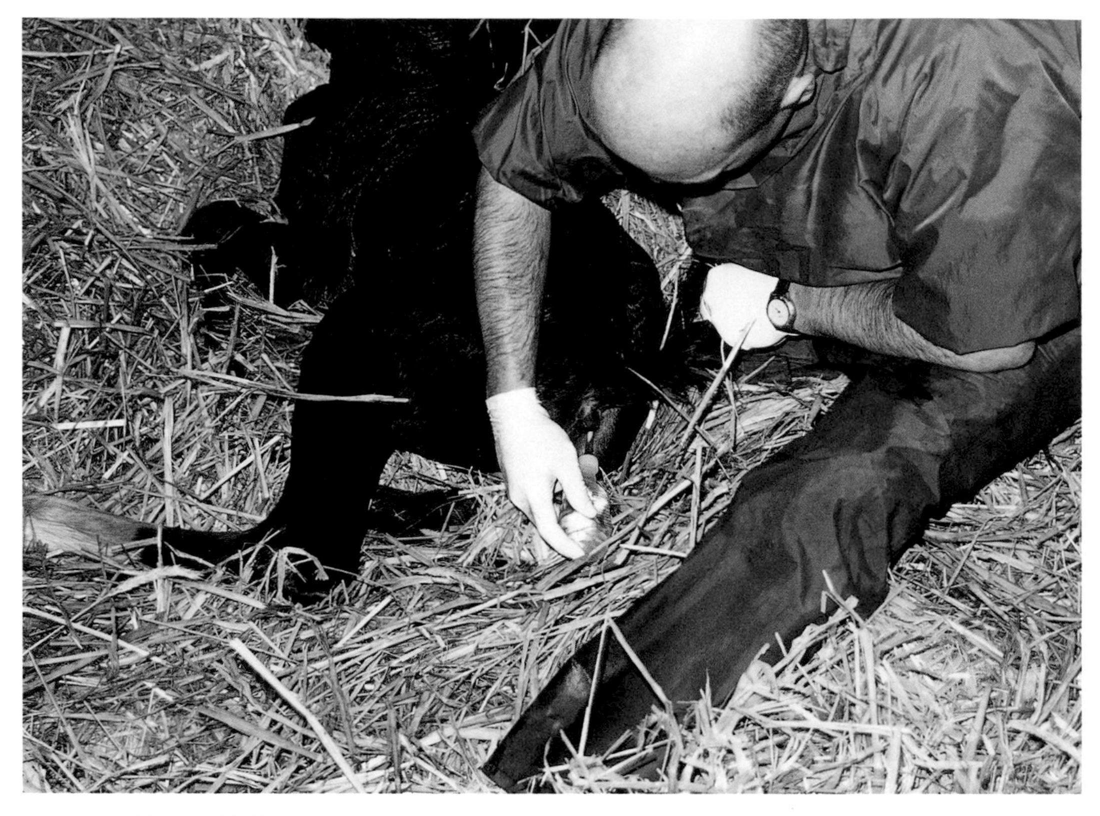

Figure 11.24

An enema is often routinely given to the foal immediately after birth. Note that the attendant is wearing protective clothing and gloves for hygiene

intervention to the absolute essentials if there have been complications during the birth for either mare or foal.

In normal circumstances, the mare and foal will be turned out for a short while from the next day after foaling (Figure 11.26), this duration of free exercise increasing as the foal gets stronger. Exercise assists in stimulating full involution of the mare's uterus and helps her to expel any remaining discharge, as well as strengthening the muscle tone of the foal. The mare and foal should be turned out alone in a small area for the first few days before being gradually introduced back into the group with other mares and foals of similar age after approximately three to four days. Decisions regarding turning the mare and foal out will depend on the individual circumstances and on time of year, condition of mare and foal and any problems the mare may have had with foaling or any physical problems that the foal may have, etc.

As discussed earlier, it is particularly important to give the mare and foal time alone to bond after birth with minimal human intervention. Although nearly every mare has an instinctive

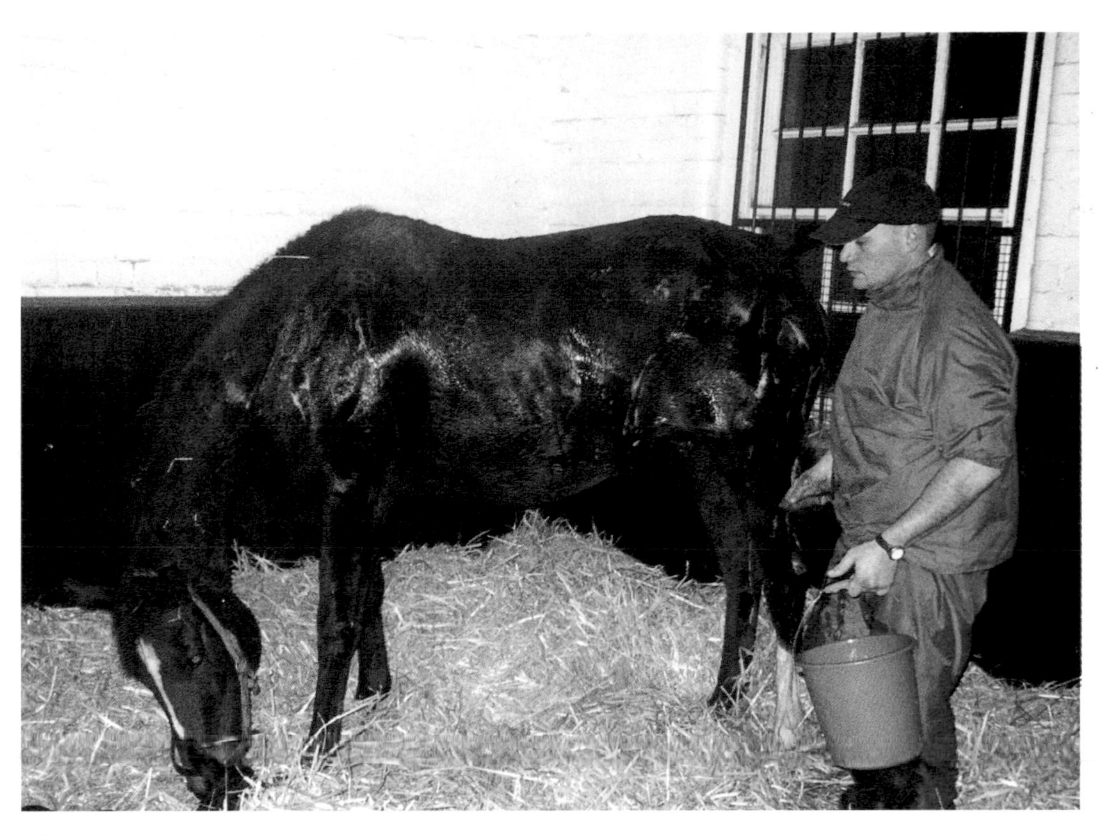

Figure 11.25

The mare is washed with a warm water and disinfectant solution immediately after birth

reaction to protect and nurture her offspring, certain environmental and psychological factors can cause her to reject the foal. The effects of the artificial domestic environment on normal equine behaviour are well researched and some mares' maternal reaction is challenged by these stresses.

In the wild, survival of both mare and foal is compromised during and after birth and both are vulnerable to attack; therefore, throughout their evolution, certain behaviour patterns have developed and become instinctive to maximise survival of both parties. Mares tend to give birth quickly and under the cover of darkness. The foal is encouraged and stimulated by the mother as soon as it is born and the foal soon becomes aware of its surroundings, recognises its mother, achieves a good level of mobility and feeds. Within two to three hours of being born the foal could flee a predator with its mother if the need arose.

Most behaviour, whether maternal or not, is influenced by three main types of factors – instinctive, hormonal and learned.

Mares will instinctively protect and

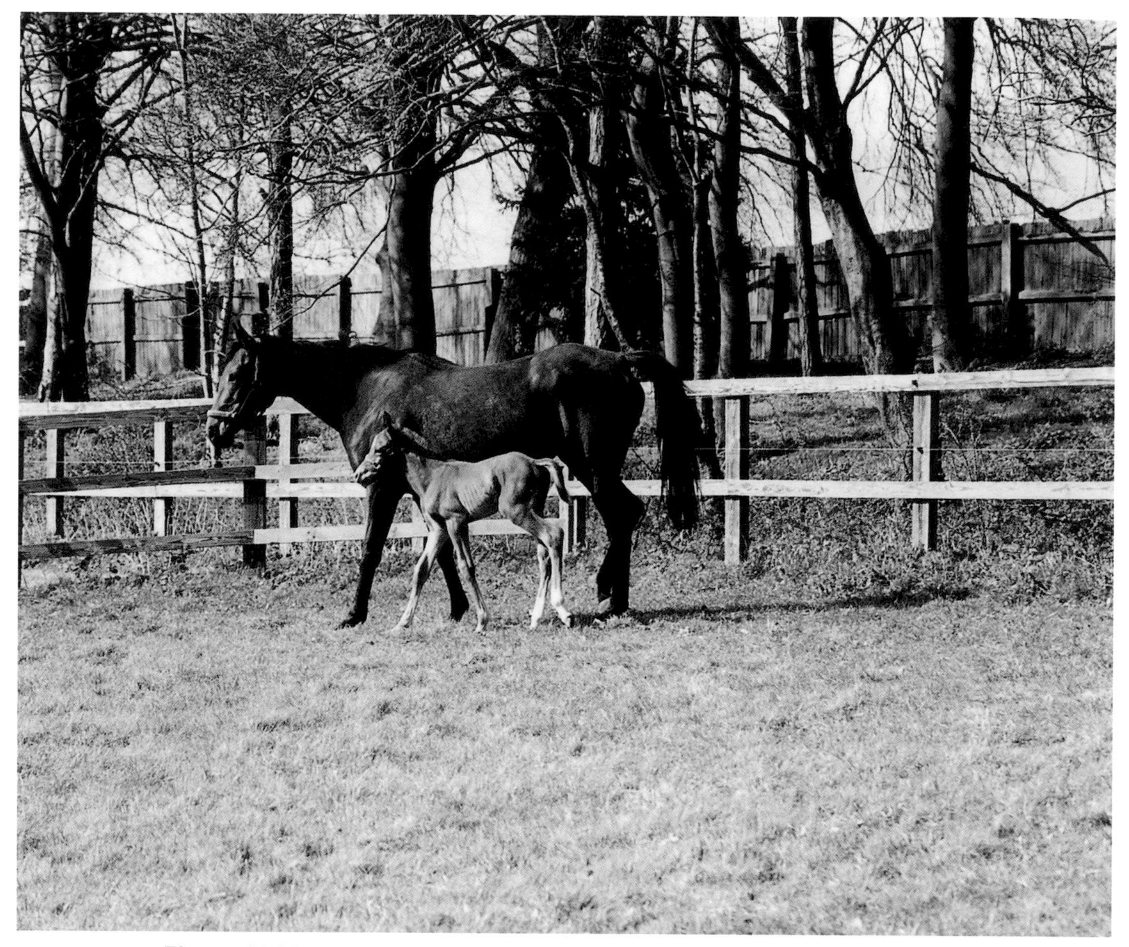

Figure 11.26

The mare and foal are turned out in a small nursery paddock the following morning

nurture their offspring, even if she has not bred before; hormonal influences include, for example, the effect of oxytocin on milk production. In fact, the use of hormone therapy in treating mares that have a negative response to their foals has had some success, similar to therapies used to treat mares that have breeding cycle abnormalities. However, it should be noted that some areas of maternal recognition and reaction are not yet fully understood. Learned behaviour is a difficult area to quantify. Examples of learned behaviour may include that of the mare who associates the foal suckling with discomfort and pain – it may be that she reacted this way with her first foal due to inexperience and perhaps the foal was taken away due to concerns for its own safety – the mare learned that the 'discomfort' gets taken away and she failed to develop her maternal behaviour past this stage. It is likely, therefore, that she will react in the same way with subsequent foals until she 'learns' otherwise. There may be other reasons why this type of behaviour appears – perhaps the mare developed an infection in her udder and associated pain with the foal suckling.

Total rejection of foals is very rare in the wild but relatively common in the domestic environment. As already mentioned, the stresses of the artificial environment can adversely affect the mare's maternal reaction. Mares kept in relative isolation may be very slow to grasp the required behavioural responses, due to a lack of education. In the wild, mares have generally witnessed the rearing of foals within their herd group. Some mares, however, repeatedly and completely reject or savage their foals. Such mares can be difficult to manage and consideration has to be given to their value within a breeding operation; highly-prized mares who have achieved success themselves or through their offspring may be bred from and the resulting foals immediately fostered, but this is not always practical or desirable. Ideally, every possible physical and psychological cause for this abnormal behaviour should be explored before a final decision is made.

A large number of mares are termed 'foal proud'. This is a commonly seen behaviour displayed by the mare during the first few days after giving birth. The mare becomes extremely aggressive towards other horses and handlers, even those with whom she previously had a strong bond. This reaction is thought to be an additional safety factor due to the foal's inability to immediately and completely imprint on its memory its own mother. There is a chance that the foal may become confused and bond with another horse who was just curious, or with an over-enthusiastic handler – the mare's aggressive behaviour avoids this risk and she does not normally relax her protection until a few days after the foal is born, when imprinting has had a chance to occur fully. Mares who react this way are not abnormal – if the aggression was directed towards her foal that would be abnormal, so it is important that her reaction is not misinterpreted.

Milk production in the mare is of prime importance as the foal relies solely on the mare to supply all of the nutrients that it requires. Broodmares are often valued just for their pedigrees and little consideration is given to their ability as mothers. The mare's ability to provide both protection and nutrition to her foal is governed mainly by inherent and environmental factors. In order for the foal to achieve optimum growth during the time that it is nutritionally relying on its dam, it is important that the mare's diet and management is given careful consideration.

Milk production begins during pregnancy with the development of milk ducts within the udder, and the milk is released either just prior to or after the birth (although some mares will 'run' milk for several days prior to giving birth). The first milk or colostrum is formed during the late stages of pregnancy and will be replaced by milk proper after about 48 hours. Colostrum is essential for newborn foals in almost all situations; failure to receive adequate colostrum during the first 24 hours after birth can seriously compromise the foal's chance of optimum survival. Substitutes such as donor colostrum freeze-stored from another mare are ideal, but it may be necessary to use colostrum powdered replacers as the next best alternative. Foals that have been unable to receive adequate colostrum should receive a course of antibiotics to ensure adequate protection. Most larger studfarms will take a blood sample from the foal between 12 and 24 hours after birth to assess the levels of transfer of protective antibodies in the foal's bloodstream. It is common for a foal who may have had a straightforward birth and received colostrum from suckling its own dam, to display a very low level of antibodies in its bloodstream – this is termed failure of passive transfer. There are several reasons why this might occur (see Chapter Thirteen).

Foal's will suck regularly during the first few weeks of life and the nutritional needs of the mare are paramount. Her requirements will increase by approximately 75 per cent for optimum milk production and she should have consistent access to good-quality feeds and, most importantly, constant access to clean and fresh water. Some bodyweight loss is unavoidable during the mare's peak milk production, but too great a loss indicates an immediate problem, particularly if the mare is to be bred again shortly after the birth of this year's foal.

CHAPTER TWELVE

The Newborn Foal

The newborn foal is delivered into an environment and way of life which is quite different from that experienced within the uterus; in utero, the lungs do not function as an organ of exchange for oxygen and carbon dioxide as is immediately necessary once the foal is delivered. The exchange of gases is performed by the placenta and the close apposition of the maternal and fetal bloodstreams.

Nutrients and all the compounds and substances necessary for growth and development of the fetus are, likewise, passed from the mare into the fetal bloodstream and carried to the fetus through the umbilical cord.

Once the cord is severed following delivery, oxygen and nutrients must enter the foal via the lungs and the alimentary tract (intestines). Thus the interfaces of essential exchange are the air sacs of the lungs and the lining of the intestines of the independent individual, compared with the placenta in utero. In effect, within the uterus it is the mare which breathes air and digests food on which the fetal foal depends.

Body temperature is also maintained and regulated by the mare, in marked contrast to the situation immediately following delivery into ambient (surrounding) temperatures which may be many degrees below that experienced in utero. Heat loss experienced after birth requires, therefore, a corresponding increase in energy consumption just to maintain the body temperature of the foal.

Once delivered, the foal meets the pull of gravity, contact with hard surfaces, bright lights and clear sounds; none of which were experienced in utero. Further, there is the need to coordinate and employ neuromuscular activity aimed at rising to the feet, finding the mammary glands of the mare for the source of food and maintaining contact with her even at fast paces within a few hours of birth.

Period of Adjustment (Adaptation)

The foal makes a series of physiological adjustments in order to survive in the new environment. The first and most necessary is that of breathing which must start immediately after delivery. If not, the lack of oxygen causes breakdown of all organ systems and the foal dies within a minute or two of having been separated from the placental circulation.

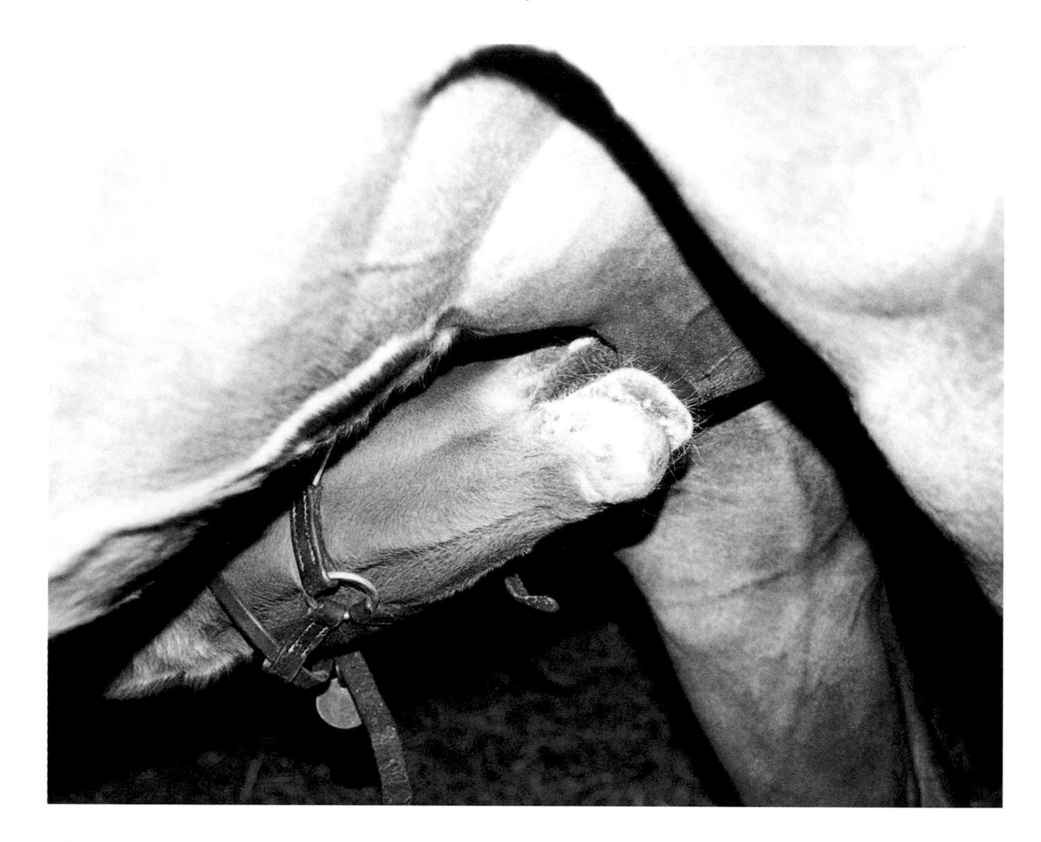

Figure 12.1

Sucking colostrum is an important element in adaptation

The next adjustment is concerned with bonding with the mare on the basis of getting to the feet, which requires neuromuscular coordination and balance, and sucking from the mammary glands. Sucking colostrum (Figure 12.1) is also an important element of adaptation, because it is by this means that passive immunity is transferred from mare to foal.

The period of adjustment may be completed within a few hours, but clinically it is often regarded as covering the first four days after foaling. The reason for this is that it is during this period that the major consequences of failure to adjust, become apparent.

However, adjustment from the fetal to the newborn cardiovascular status is essentially a change occurring in the circulation. In the fetus, blood passes in sequence from the fetal heart into the placenta and back into the heart where it is pumped out by the heartbeat to continue in this circle.

In the independent individual, blood is pumped from the left side of the heart to the body and extremities returning to the right side, where it passes through the lungs and back to the heart. There are, therefore, two circulations after birth existing in parallel to one another.

In the fetus, there are two bypasses, one at the entry to the heart (foramei ovale) and the other which carries blood issuing from the right side of the heart into the aorta rather than into the lungs. This communication is called the ductus arteriosus.

These bypasses close within hours of birth and completely by the second day after foaling.

The Challenges of the Environment

Survival of the newborn depends upon successful responses to the challenges of the new surroundings which include, as already indicated, the immediate need to breath air, to overcome the effects of gravity and to keep the body temperature within normal limits. In general, a foal born normally and which has undergone a healthy development in utero has no difficulty in adjusting and overcoming these challenges. But those disadvantaged by birth trauma or an unhealthy pre-natal existence may not be able to meet the challenges of the external environment at all or without a measure of critical care.

Behaviour

Essential information on the health and well-being of the foal is provided by the way it behaves. Those with experience can generally judge from the foal's reactions whether or not the process of adjustment is normal or if there is cause for concern.

The patterns of behaviour are fairly stereotyped and, for this reason, they can be presented in the sequence in which they appear from the moment final delivery is complete.

The position of final delivery leaves the foal with its hind legs in the vagina of the mare and the cord intact (Figure 12.2). When its chest is passing through the birth canal the foal may gasp (a breathing movement in which air is sharply drawn into the air passages through the mouth while the head and neck are arched), but regular breathing movements (a respiratory rhythm) are established within a few seconds to, at the very most, a minute of final delivery.

As breathing begins so the lungs are expanded and filled with air for the first time. In consequence, the concentration of oxygen in the bloodstream rises enormously and this enables the foal to exert the energy necessary for moving and standing in the world outside the uterus; inside the mare it had little or no need for any such activity.

Within two or three minutes of birth, the foal raises its head and then begins to right itself onto its brisket. This causes a reflex action – the hind limbs are withdrawn from the vagina so that they are underneath the foal's body in the preliminary position for getting up and standing.

Within five minutes of delivery, the sense of suck develops and the foal shows typical sucking movements of the tongue. The senses of sight and hearing are also active, although at this stage the foal may not interpret all visual and auditory stimuli that it

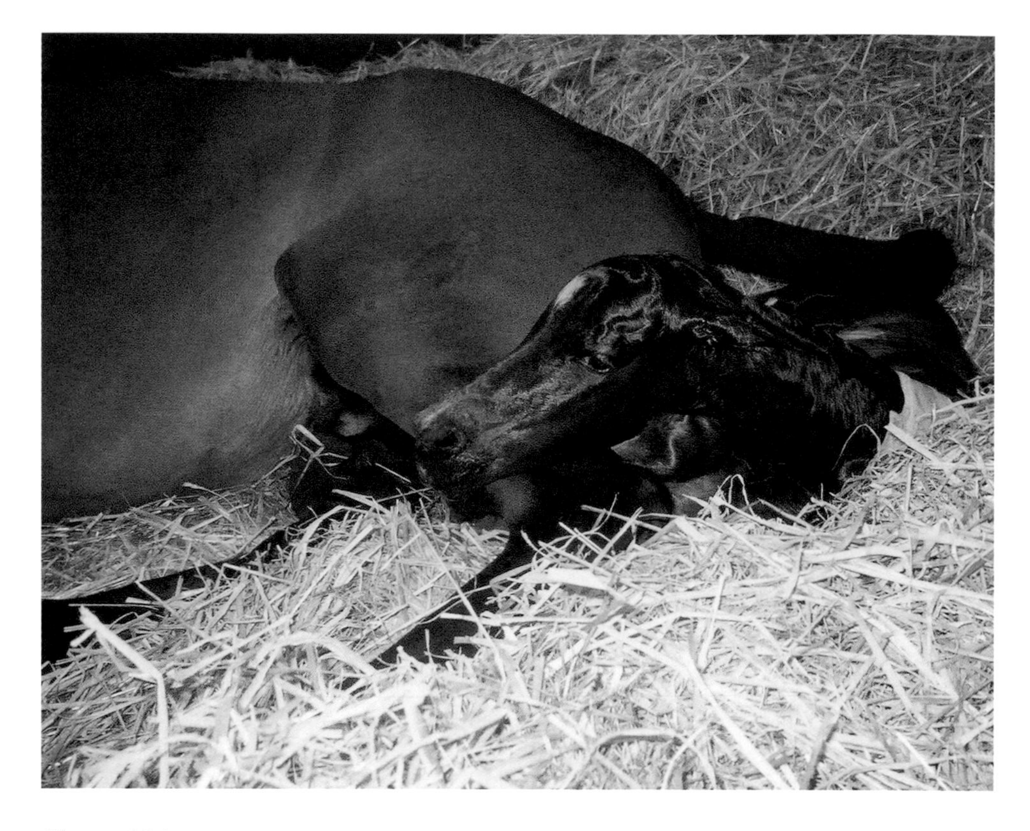

Figure 12.2

The position of final delivery leaves the foal with its hind legs in the vagina of the mare

receives. It may whinny and move its ears towards any sound. Another feature is the way the foal uses its muscles for shivering. This is part of the mechanism for keeping its body temperature within normal limits.

As the foal becomes progressively stronger so it increases its efforts to stand. In the first instance it may have difficulty in getting to the standing position necessary for raising its body; that is, with the forelegs stretched out in front and the hind legs drawn underneath its body.

Its early struggles place an increasing tension on the umbilical cord (Figure 12.3) and eventually this ruptures at a point about 4 cm from the umbilicus. This is a natural breaking point and there is no need to sever the cord artificially or, apart from exceptional circumstances, to tie it. Even if a small amount of haemorrhage occurs from the stump after rupture it is generally sufficient to pinch the vessels with two fingers for a matter of a minute or so and the bleeding will cease.

Many people still use iodine to treat the umbilical stump after the cord has separated. Others use antibiotic or anti-

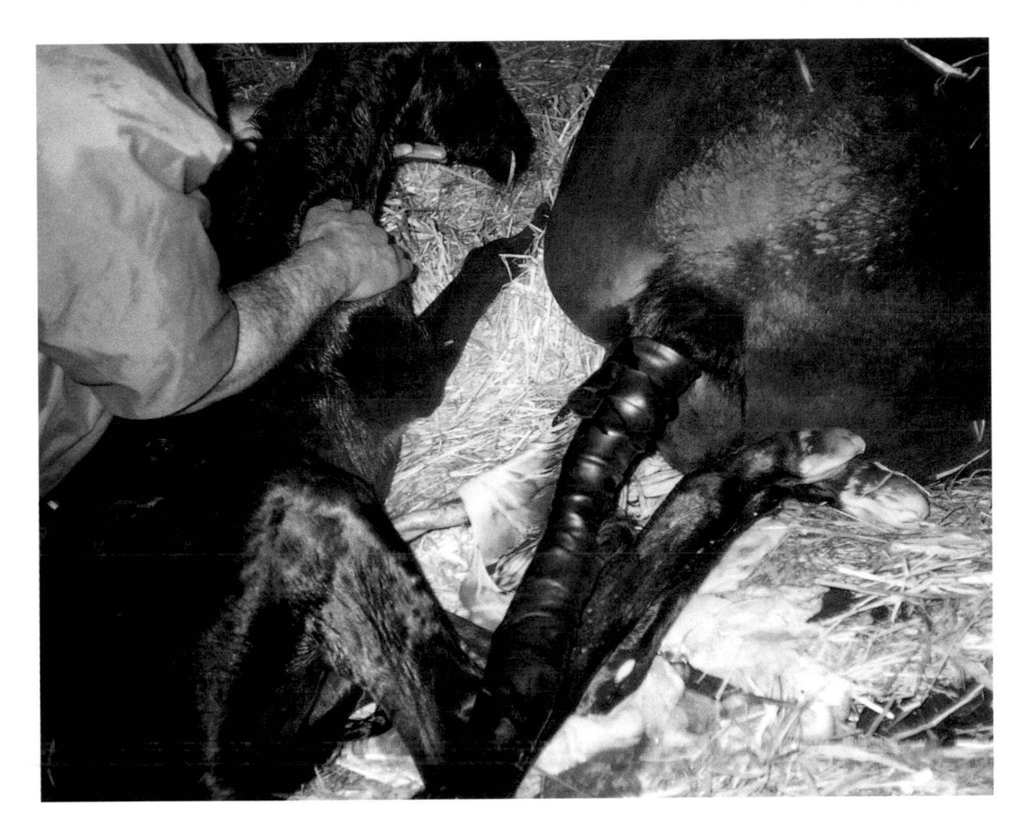

Figure 12.3

The umbilical cord remains attached until it is ruptured when the mare stands or the foal breaks it with its movements

septic powder. However, the most important consideration is that the cord should be left and not severed artificially. Natural separation seals the stump more effectively than can be achieved with artificial severance with scissors or with any preparation to the outside.

Another way the cord ruptures naturally is by the mare rising to her feet. Most mares lie down for many minutes after they have delivered their foal and it is important to disturb them as little as possible during this period. It has been shown that early severance of the cord may deprive the foal of as much as a third of its blood volume compared with severance in a natural manner some minutes after delivery (Figure 12.4). If the foal is so deprived then there may be few or no drastic consequences but, on the other hand, the foal will suffer anaemia and disturbances in its circulation as a consequence of leaving part of its blood in the placenta. This may be of no consequence to a strong, healthy foal but may seriously affect one that has been weakened by illness while in the uterus or damaged by the birth process.

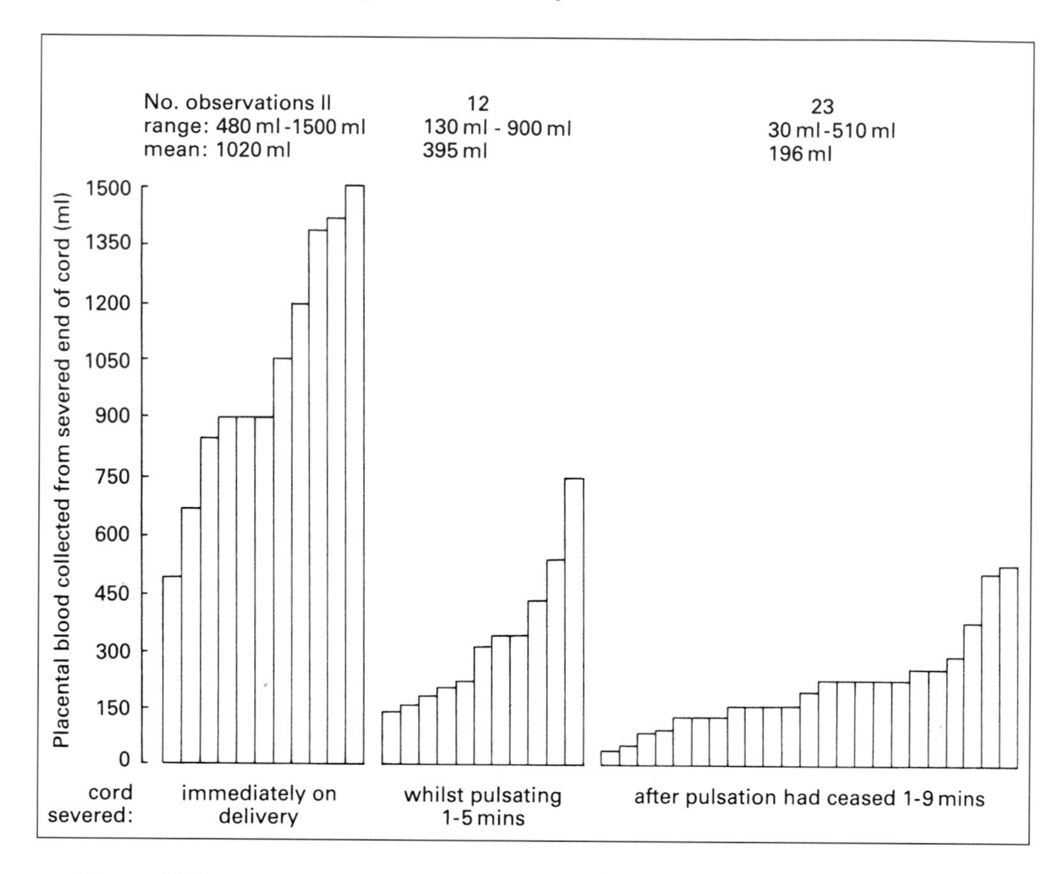

Figure 12.4

The chart shows the amount of blood that can be collected from the severed end of the umbilical cord at varying times after delivery is complete. (From Rossdale and Mahaffey *The Veterinary Record* (1958), 15 February)

After several unsuccessful attempts a foal will eventually gain the standing position about 50 minutes after delivery. The foal's ability to get to its feet for the first time gives us an overall indication of its health and well-being; any individual which has failed to stand within two hours of birth must be regarded as abnormal and possibly in need of veterinary attention.

Once on its feet a foal soon develops an affinity towards the mare and within about two hours of birth should have found the udder and sucked for the first time.

In its search for the teats, a foal follows a well-defined pattern of behaviour. Contact with the mare's body usually begins in the forepart around the brisket and front legs and thence along the flanks to the stifle, at which the foal may suck quite vigorously for a time (see Chapter Eleven). Eventually it turns its attention to the region of the udder and then attaches itself to one of the two teats. Of course, progress is not continuous and the foal may wander around the box and even suck at the wall or manger before eventually reaching the correct position. The instinct for direction appears to be stimulated by shadow, so that the foal is attracted by areas of darkness such as that between the mare's hind legs.

The presence of attendants or other factors in the environment may disturb the mare and cause her to walk away from her foal, so delaying the time when the first suck is taken. By contrast, attendants may hold the mare and guide the foal directly to the udder which, in many cases, speeds up the process.

Young mares may be ticklish and instead of resting one hind leg to expose the udder, they kick or otherwise jostle their foals as they sniff round the mammary region. In these cases, it may be helpful to hold the mare and perhaps raise one of her forelegs; where a mare is particularly resentful of her foal it may be necessary to administer a tranquillising drug. It is not advisable to apply a twitch to the mare since this may raise her blood pressure and thereby increase the risk of post-foaling haemorrhage.

Once a foal has sucked for the first time it will seek the mare's udder at regular intervals and with increasing sureness. Bouts of sucking become longer and less frequent as the foal's age increases. One of the best methods of observing the well-being of a young foal is to cause it to get to its feet; it should rise without difficulty and suck without undue delay. If it does not get up with ease and/or shows no interest in sucking, we must suspect that all is not well.

Maternal Instincts

The mare recognises her foal by its taste and smell. At birth, the foal's coat is saturated with amniotic fluid and it is contact with this which stimulates maternal instinct and provides the mare with a method of distinguishing her own foal from others. When a mare has recognised her foal, which normally she does within minutes of its being born, she will accept no other, unless there are special circumstances; for example, where an orphan foal is introduced to a foster mother.

Establishing a Steady State

The body is said to be in a steady state when its various parts function at a particular level and do not alter within certain small and well-defined limits. In general terms, this means the limits of normality. For example, we recognise normality through such indicators as rectal temperature, rate of breathing, heart rate and so on; and internally by means of laboratory tests which provide information about the concentration of sugar, minerals, salts, acids of the blood, etc.

Whereas the fetus possesses a steady state at a certain level, the newborn foal has to establish one at a much higher level of activity. It achieves this state within 12–24 hours of birth and the intervening period must therefore be regarded as one of transition. Foals that do not successfully achieve this transition display signs of illness which are characterised by disturbances in their behavioural patterns.

Two particular functions by which the newborn steady state may be recognised are standing and sucking. There are others; for example, the foal normally has no difficulty in maintaining its rectal temperature between 37.3°C and 38.3°C.

Although a foal breathes very rapidly in the first half hour after birth, the rate falls so that once the foal has sucked for the first time the number of respirations is in the range of 30–40 per minute.

Heart rate can be felt quite easily on the left side of the foal's chest; at birth the rate is normally in the region of 80 beats per minute, rising to 140 beats per minute when the foal tries to get to its feet and returning to about 100 beats per minute by the time the foal is a day old. Of course, when either breathing or heart rates are measured we must be careful to distinguish those recorded while the foal is at rest from those recorded after exertion or struggling.

During the first 12 hours, profound changes occur in the composition of the foal's blood. These are complicated and necessarily lie in the province of the veterinarian, so only one of great practical importance needs to be mentioned here. This is the increasing concentration of protein substances know as immunoglobins (Ig) (antibodies). When the foal is born it lacks these substances and they are provided in the colostrum or first milk. The foal sucks for the first time at about age two hours and the protective substances pass from the milk into the foal's bloodstream after being absorbed through the stomach lining, thereby giving the foal a passive immunity (that is, an immunity based on protective substances supplied from outside, in this case the mare, in contrast to active immunity in which the individual itself develops antibodies). The most obvious example of active immunity is that stimulated by vaccination.

There are a number of situations in which this passive immunity fails to develop (failure of immune passive transfer) so that the foal has a reduced resistance to infection. This may happen if the colostrum is deficient in antibody because the mare has run milk prior to foaling. It may be that the foal does not receive a sufficient quantity of colostrum, or that it fails to absorb antibodies.

The antibodies are only absorbed from the lining of the intestines up to age about 24 hours and after this they will not be available to the foal, however high the concentrations of antibody in the colostrum.

If it is suspected that the colostrum of the mare has been lost because she has run milk, donor colostrum may be given. On Thoroughbred studfarms small quantities of colostrum are taken from mares with surplus quantities and stored deep frozen for this purpose. The quantity that is necessary for such circumstances is about 400 ml. This must be administered from a bottle or via a stomach tube inserted by a veterinarian before the foal has sucked any other milk and before it is age 12 hours.

If there has been failure of passive transfer, a condition that can be diagnosed only by measuring the IgG in the blood at age 24 to 48 hours, levels may be supplemented by intravenous serum therapy under veterinary supervision. Before the foal has sucked, blood levels of IgG are zero, increasing after suck-

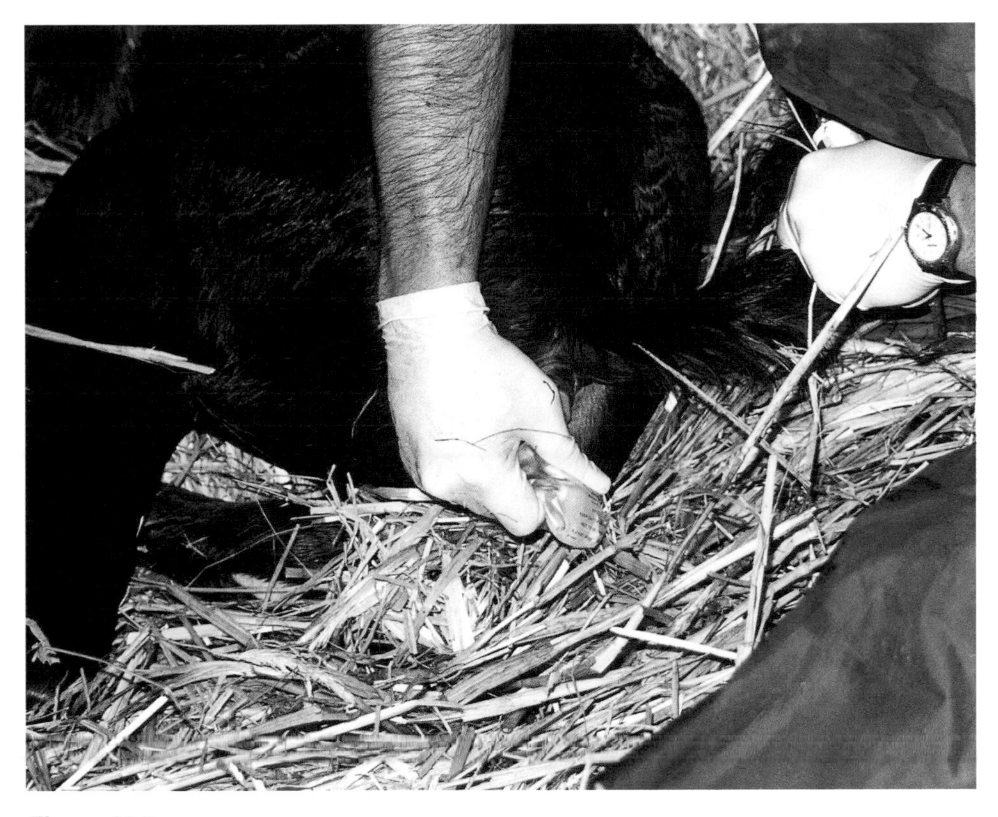

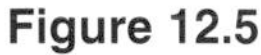

Figure 12.5

An enema is administered to ease the passage of meconium

ing to more than 8g/l in most cases. The level of failure may be set at 4g/l.

An important aspect of the steady state is the ability to pass meconium. This is the dung stored during fetal life as green, black or brown pellets. Except in abnormal circumstances, it is not evacuated until after the foal is born, when it must be voided before the first milk can pass along the gut in the normal manner. All the meconium is usually expelled by the time the foal is two days old. Failure to pass meconium in the usual manner is often associated with signs of colic.

Foals suffering from meconium retention can be helped with an enema (Figure 12.5). It is inadvisable to administer large quantities of fluid at one time. As a rough guide, about 50 ml can be used when the foal is about eight hours old and it may be useful to repeat the enemas every three or four hours until the meconium has passed and the yellowish 'milk dung' appears. Special enema packs may now be employed for foals and can be used in the first hour after foaling and repeated at intervals, hourly or two hourly.

On establishments where many foals are born each year, it may be necessary to give antibiotic injections during the

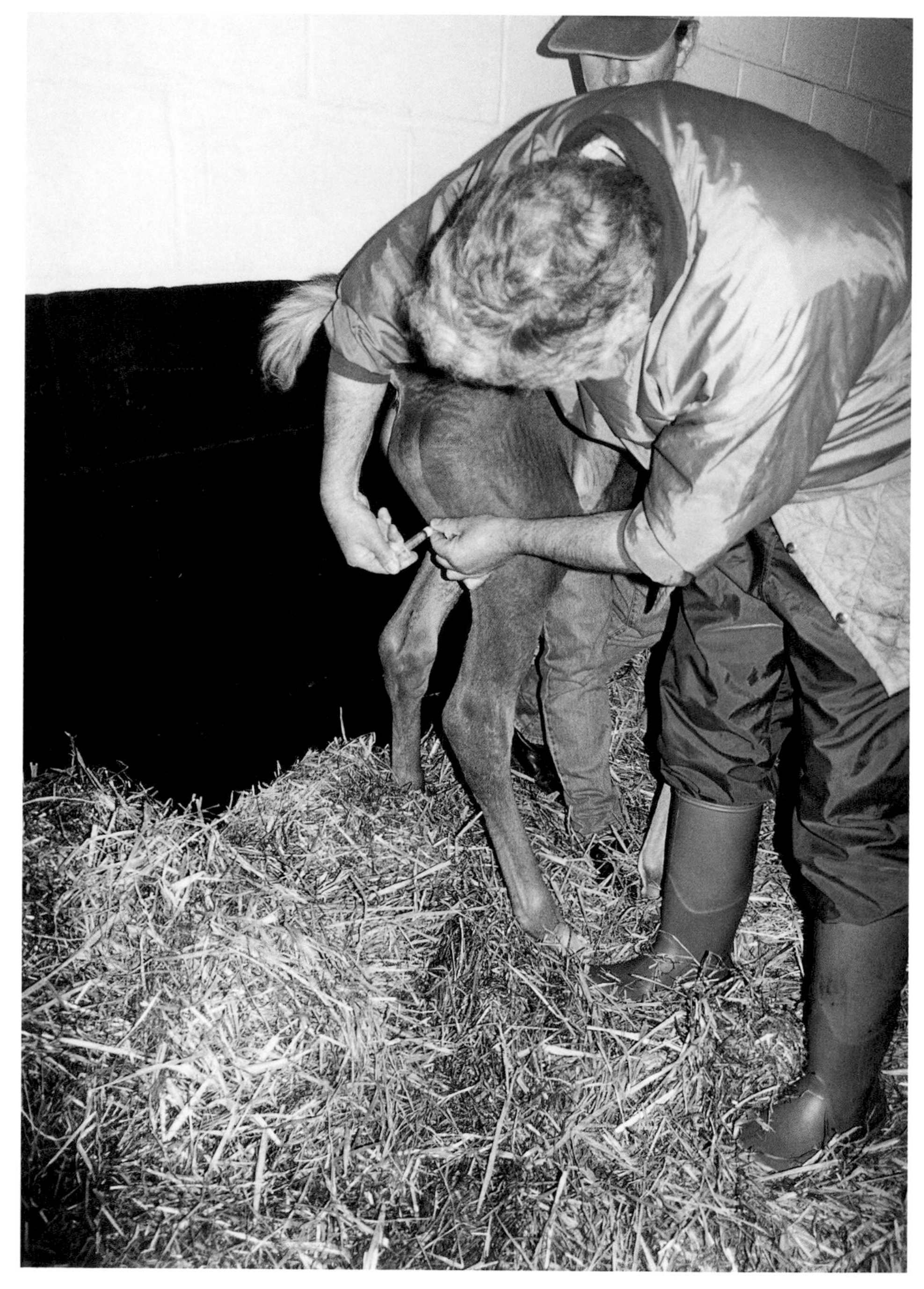

Figure 12.6

On larger studfarms, foals may be given a course of prophylactic antibiotics during the first few days of life first few days, to supplement the foal's natural resistance to infection. This decision is made by the attending veterinary surgeon (Figure 12.6).

Iron is also important if a foal has been deprived of its placental transfusion of blood, such as when a mare foals in a standing position or when the cord is severed immediately after delivery. In addition, foals that are born early in the year so that they have to spend much of their time confined to a box may benefit from vitamin and mineral supplements, but owners should rely on veterinary advice in their particular circumstances.

Handling the Young Foal

In all circumstances, young foals should be handled with care. Every effort should be taken to avoid rough handling in the early hours after birth when mare and foal are establishing a bond.

Young foals should be caught and handled with one hand placed in front and one hand behind. They should never be lifted with the hand underneath the chest as this will put pressure on the rib cage and possibly displace or even fracture a rib.

A leather headcollar may be placed on the foal when it is about one day old and it should taught to lead at an early age. Some mares may resent or even attack their foals if they smell a soiled headcollar, so it is important to fit one which is clean and does not smell of other horses.

Newborn foals should be housed in stables as free from dust as possible, well ventilated and sufficiently insulated to prevent undue heat loss. It is not necessary to raise the air temperature above 20 C. Normal foals can withstand zero temperatures quite easily, but it is a different matter if a foal is sick. They may then require special measures.

Orphan Foals and Fostering

The sad loss of a mare during foaling or shortly afterwards can be a real blow to any breeding operation regardless of the size or type. However, a foal may also be termed an orphan when its mother rejects it or is physically not able to rear it. A newborn foal depends on its dam not only for immunity to infection through the colostrum, but also for the development of normal behaviour. Orphaned foals can suffer serious physical and psychological setbacks at an early and critical stage in their development; therefore, it is vital to plan a proper supervised care programme to reduce the additional stresses that the foal will have to cope with. They are also more prone to infections, and extra consideration should be given to their early management.

The immediate needs of an orphan foal will vary enormously depending on age and circumstances. The first most important factor is immunity level. If the foal has been orphaned at birth it will not yet have received any colostrum. This first milk contains the immunological protection that is vital for its welfare for approximately the first three months of its life. Even if the mare has died during parturition, it may still be possible to use her colostrum and bottle-feed it to the foal. This has produced very good levels of passive immunity in a high percentage of orphaned foals. However, most studfarms keep a spare supply of colostrum frozen for emergencies should milking the foal's dam not be possible. Colostrum can be kept in this way for up to five years, but care does need to be taken when defrosting it for use; overheating can cause damage to the delicate proteins it contains and reduce its quality accordingly.

A small percentage of mares are lost each year during parturition due to conditions such as ruptured uterine arteries, torsion and twisted intestines. The orphaned foal may have suffered some level of compromise during a traumatic foaling and may require special care in the immediate period following birth. Weak or depressed foals will normally require tube feeding initially, or injected antibiotics, as well as an enema to encourage normal evacuation of the bowel. Stronger foals will normally readily accept a bottle and can be put onto a regular feeding routine immediately – colostrum in the first feeds changing to a suitable mare's milk replacer as appropriate.

As with any other foal during the immediate period post-parturition, careful monitoring is essential – perhaps more so with an orphaned foal who has already suffered additional stress.

Mares may reject a foal for a variety of reasons. Some mares having their first foal can become frightened and react aggressively to their offspring in their confusion; some repeatedly reject their foals year after year. As discussed in earlier chapters, it is essential to keep human intervention to a minimum during the initial period following foaling – particularly with a maiden foaling mare. The bond that is formed between mare and foal during this period is vital. A mare who has required attention following foaling, or perhaps her foal has required special care, may not form a strong bond and subsequently fail to maintain a sufficient interest and level of care towards her foal. There are many factors that can inhibit the normal maternal response to her offspring and great care should be taken to avoid a pattern of behaviour becoming established.

A very small percentage of mares may savage their foals – some causing very serious injuries. In these situations the foal should be removed for his own safety and the mare suitably restrained. Some mares seem to have a delayed acceptance of their foals, initially being aggressive and then becoming protective – this may be due to factors such as udder tenderness which is relieved once the foal has had adequate chance to nurse. In the case of the aggressive mare, it is worth trying to get the mare to accept her foal by similar procedures to that used when getting a foster mare to accept an orphan, as this is reported as successful in a good number of cases. If a mare is showing signs of increasing irritation and lack of interest in her foal, all possible checks should be carried out to ascertain whether there is a simple reason to explain her behaviour. Mares can 'learn' to react aggressively towards their foals and, particularly with Thoroughbreds, this conditioning may result in her reacting in the same way with every foal resulting in her never being able to raise her own foals.

Orphaned foals need to be fed at least once every two hours, day and night, during the first week. Hand rearing is extremely time consuming and, if there is no alternative, some handlers will try to get the foal drinking milk from a bucket or bowl very early on. Most foals will master this technique quite quickly, but this technique should only be used if fostering has been decided against. There are many reasons why hand rearing may be the only option – the foal may be too weak or ill, a foster mare may just not be available or the owner may be determined to hand rear the foal. The ideal method for raising an orphan foal is to find a suitable foster mare. Hand rearing is perfectly possible, but is not ideal as the foal will thrive better with a mare to feed and care for it, and may become too humanised and ultimately difficult to train. Fostering of a foal can be time consuming and immensely frustrating during the early stages, but is the best possible alternative to his own dam.

Advertising for a foster mare can be done via specialist press or, as used by many Thoroughbred studs, by contacting racing programmes on television for announcement during a televised race meeting. There are organisations such as the National Foaling Bank in Shropshire, who may be able to put the studfarm in touch with a mare owner who has lost a foal, as well as offer considerable advice and assistance. There are also people who specialise in providing foster mares for studfarms. This is usually on the basis of payment of a fee for the mare and the request that the mare is returned in foal when the fostered foal is weaned. These mares are normally of native or mixed breed and are kept specifically for fostering foals. In fact, some large studfarms keep one or two 'nanny' mares (Figure 12.7) for fostering should the need arise. On occasion a studfarm may prefer to keep a valuable foal at home when its dam goes away to stud, particularly if this is overseas, to reduce the risks of injury or infection and the foal will be fostered on to one of the native mares.

Choosing a foster mare may not be easy, as it will very much depend on availability of a suitable mare at the right time. The most important factor is to try and find a mare that seems to have the right temperament for fostering. Some mares that have lost their own foals will not accept another as a replacement and can be extremely aggressive towards the new foal. The breed of the mare is immaterial if her temperament and attitude is suitable, but normally native or heavier breeds tend to adapt best. Size of the mare may also need to be a consideration – fostering a large breed of foal onto a pony mare may be fine for the first few months, but we all know how quickly foals can grow. Feeding from a very small mare may become difficult for the orphan within a few weeks and the foal may need to be weaned considerably earlier than planned.

The other vital consideration in looking for a foster mare is to establish her health status and why her own foal was lost. Any risk of disease needs to be treated very seriously to avoid the risk of bringing any infection onto the stud. Normally, as it may take between seven and ten days to obtain full laboratory results of tests, a foster mare is kept in isolation with the orphan foal until confirmation of her status is available. If isolation facilities are not available it is worth arranging for the orphan foal to be moved to a suitable place with the mare, away from the studfarm, until results are known. As most foals are born during the breeding season it is commercial suicide to allow such a mare contact with the main stud until full results are available. Obviously not all foals die due to infection and, if it can be established that the foal died or was

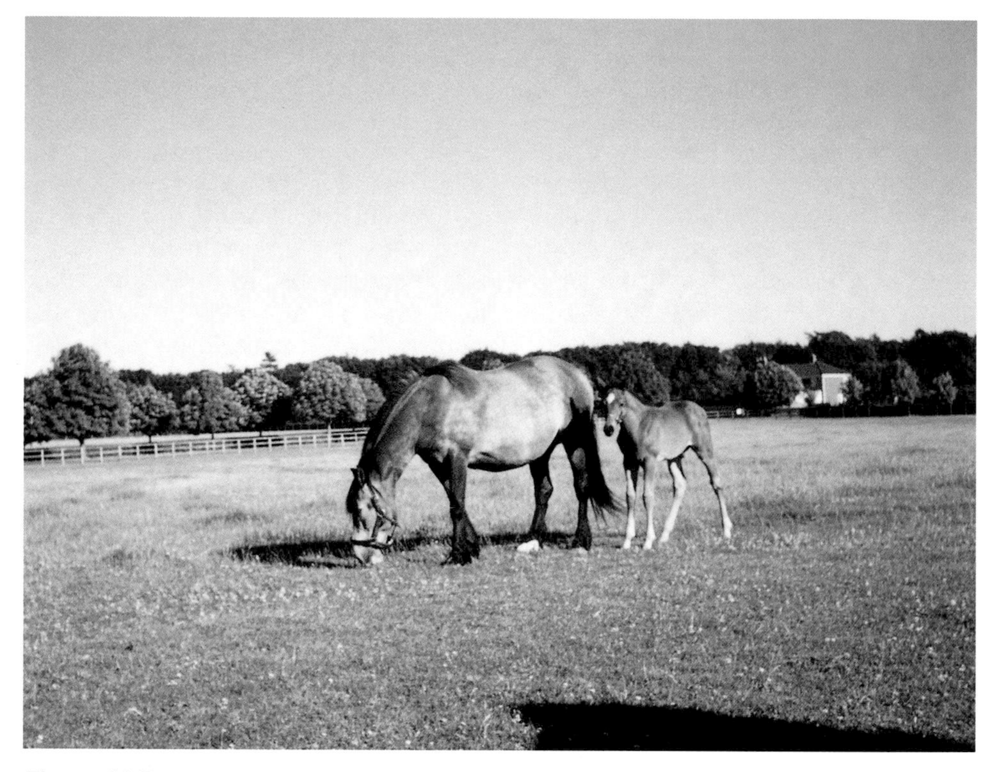

Figure 12.7

On larger studfarms, native breed mares may be kept as 'nannies' for fostering should the need arise

euthanased due to a non-infectious cause such as physical deformity, then of course the risk is reduced. However, it is important to allow time for the normal tests to be carried out for infections such as EVA and CEM. All horses coming onto the studfarm should be tested for EVA and all mares, regardless of whether they are to be bred or not, should be tested for CEM. In such situations, the advice of the stud's veterinary surgeon should be sought.

The old practices of putting the dead foal's skin on the orphan foal or covering the orphan in the mare's birth fluids or urine are thankfully no longer used. Not only are such practices unnecessary, they exacerbate the stress the orphan foal is already suffering as well as increasing the risk of secondary infections.

Once the mare is available for the foal, the next most important factor is maintaining the safety of the foal at all times and providing a suitable quiet environment to allow fostering to take place. In the ideal situation, use of a fostering pen will allow the foal safe access whilst the mare is restrained in a small stall and can safely get used to the foal's presence.

Some foster mares need little or no

introduction to the orphan foal as their maternal instinct is very strong – careful observation will give the handlers some idea as to how the mare is likely to react. It is vital not to take any chances at this early stage and to be certain that the mare is never given the opportunity to harm the foal in anyway. Successful fostering needs a handler that is able to judge the fine line between not allowing enough contact between the mare and foal and allowing too much and putting the foal at risk. It should go without saying that successful fostering usually needs a good team of experienced staff. If a fostering pen is not available then hay or straw bales can be used to make a makeshift barrier but, as before, safety of the foal must be given priority.

The orphan's age will also affect the way that fostering can be set up. A very young foal may be slow to latch on to the mare, especially if bottle feeds have been necessary while a foster mare was found. A young foal may also be at more risk of injury by an impatient mare, as it may be clumsy in its attempts to obtain milk direct from the udder. This is a time when the patience of the handler is vital. Forcing the foal to suckle will only confuse it further, as will using sweet substances on the mare's udder to encourage it to suck. The foal will instinctively learn to suckle properly, but it can take some time to establish and fostering is very labour intensive at this stage. If the foal is becoming very weak and has yet to suckle, it may be necessary to give it a supplementary feed; but it is worth bearing in mind that this may work against the fostering if the foal is then not hungry enough to want to try to suckle.

A young foal should be encouraged to go to the mare very regularly during the first few days and nights and encouraged to suck. The mare should be adequately restrained at this time, but if possible allowed to see the foal and, if she is quiet, to touch it. Allowing the mare contact with the foal will encourage bonding to take place and reduce the levels of stress on the mare; however, she must not be allowed free access to the foal at this stage unless she can be completely controlled should she react aggressively towards him. Mares can cause horrific injuries to foals and should be closely monitored at all times during the early stages of fostering.

The whole fostering procedure can take up to a week, to allow the mare time to fully accept her new foal. If the mare has shown only interest in the foal and is happy for it to suckle from her unrestrained, then they should be allowed relatively free access to each other in the stable. It is wise to continue to have some form of control over the mare until it is certain that she will not attempt to reject the foal – once she displays protective behaviour towards the foal the adoption can be considered successful and it is unlikely that she will reject it from now on. Once this stage has been achieved then mare and foal should be left alone to further the bonding process. Closed-circuit cameras can be invaluable in a situation like this as too much human interference may affect the success of fostering. The mare and foal can be safely monitored with no knowledge that they are being watched and their behaviour and reactions will be more natural. It is essential that they are still observed as much as possible; there have been occasions when a mare will be happy with the foal when people are present but reject it as soon as she thinks she is left alone.

As soon as the mare and foal are settled together, it is useful to try putting them out in a small nursery paddock

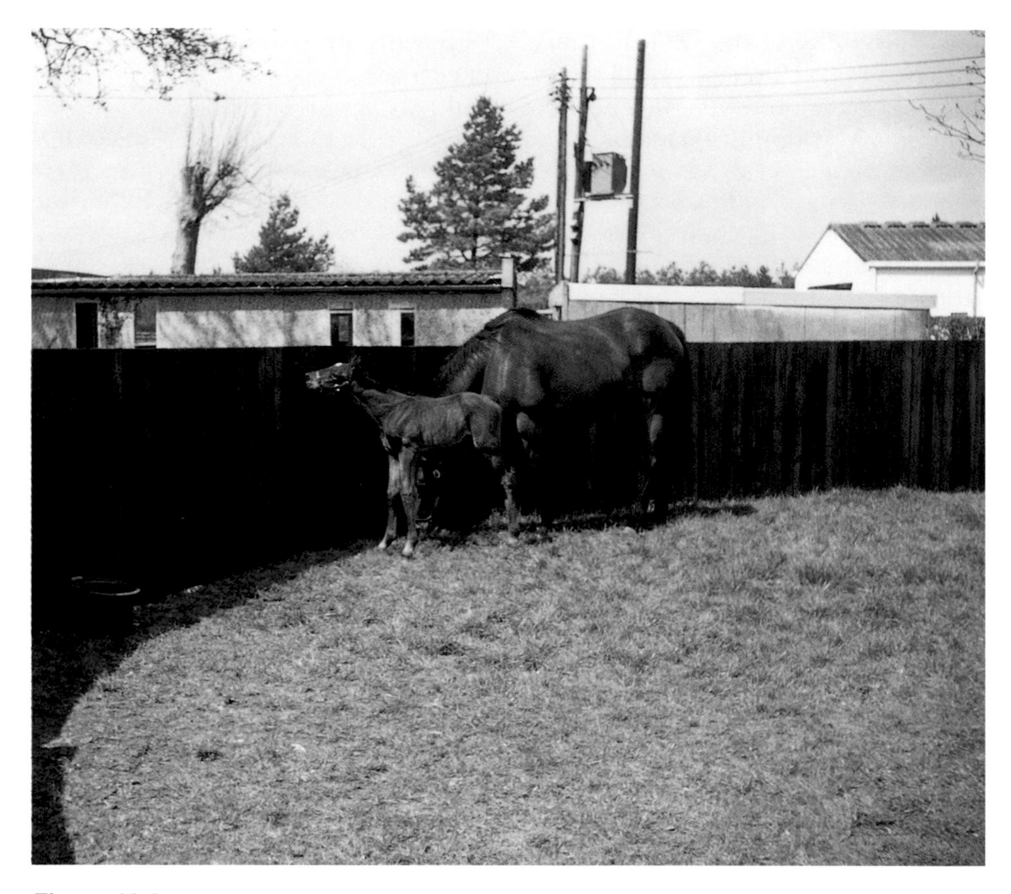

Figure 12.8

The mare and foster foal may be turned out in a small nursery paddock once they are settled together

together (Figure 12.8). Even if the mare and foal are cleared from any need for isolation, it is important that they are not put out with other mares and foals at this stage – foster mares can sometimes be less protective of their foster foals and there is a danger that the foal may wander to another mare and be hurt.

The normal behaviour of the mare towards the foal - calling to it, allowing suckling and keeping it close to her, etc., can be monitored in a safe paddock. This allows the handlers to get some idea of how the mare will be with the foal when she is ready to be turned out with others.

There are no set time limits for fostering – there are too many variations. Some mares will accept an orphan foal completely and immediately, making all of the precautions and procedures detailed at the beginning of this section totally unnecessary. Others may take three or four days before they will allow the foal to suckle unrestrained. Some mares are determined not to accept the orphan even with the best efforts of the handler. These mares cannot be left alone with the foal as they will attempt to force the foal away even when a handler is present. It is worth trying for two to three days if the foal can suckle from the mare, but if she still shows little to no interest then it is probably best to cease trying. Sadly, not all fostering is successful; however, if another mare is available, it is worth trying again.

The most important factor is that a suitable mare is found as soon as possible after the loss of the foal's own dam. The longer the foal is hand reared with bottle feeds, the more difficult it can be to get it interested in suckling from a mare. Suckling is instinctive behaviour, but if the foal has imprinted onto a human with a bottle it can be hard work to change its mind. Suckling from an udder is also more difficult for the foal than suckling from a bottle and it may be reluctant to put the effort into trying, causing irritation to the mare. Try to keep handling of the foal to a minimum during the waiting period for a foster mare to become available; this will help to reduce the strength of bond that the foal will form with its human attendants. Some studs will only tube feed newborn orphan foals to avoid any further confusion, although obviously this is normally a short-term option only. It is worth noting that foals born prematurely may require tube feeding, as they usually display an insufficient suck reflex to feed from a bottle. Orphan foals that are hand reared can become notoriously difficult to handle as they start to grow. They have usually been over-humanised and lack the normal equine social skills. In the ideal situation, the hand-reared orphan is kept with an equine companion; old ponies are wonderful at this role and will educate the young foal. However, again there are no set rules; some studs report (Figure 12.9) remarkable success with goats, sheep and even chickens as companions! However, another horse will help the foal develop the social skills it will need when it is old enough to be turned out with a herd.

Hand rearing will also mean that the foal will have to rely on milk formulas rather than mare's milk. There are some very good milk replacers on the market, but none can match the real thing. Some hand-reared foals develop some level of digestive upset when fed milk replacer and such individuals need extra care to reduce the risk of gastric ulceration occurring. Normally, hand-reared foals are introduced to milk pellets and creep feeds as soon as possible, but as with all diet changes this will need to be done gradually and such feeds are not always suitable for the very young foal. Many of the creep feeds available, such as Dodson & Horrell's Foal Creep or Bailey's Foal Starter, are reported to be suitable for supplementing a foal's milk feeds from approximately two weeks of age, but milk should still form the majority of the foal's diet for at least the first 6–8 weeks.

Foals will generally not consume very much grass or hay in the first few months of life. It is important that any food they are offered is easy to digest, as their digestive systems are still developing in every sense of the word. Setting up a creep feeding system in the foal's paddock or stable will enable the gradual change from milk to concentrates.

Regardless of the circumstances that resulted in the foal being orphaned, careful consideration should be given to the foal's psychological well-being. The

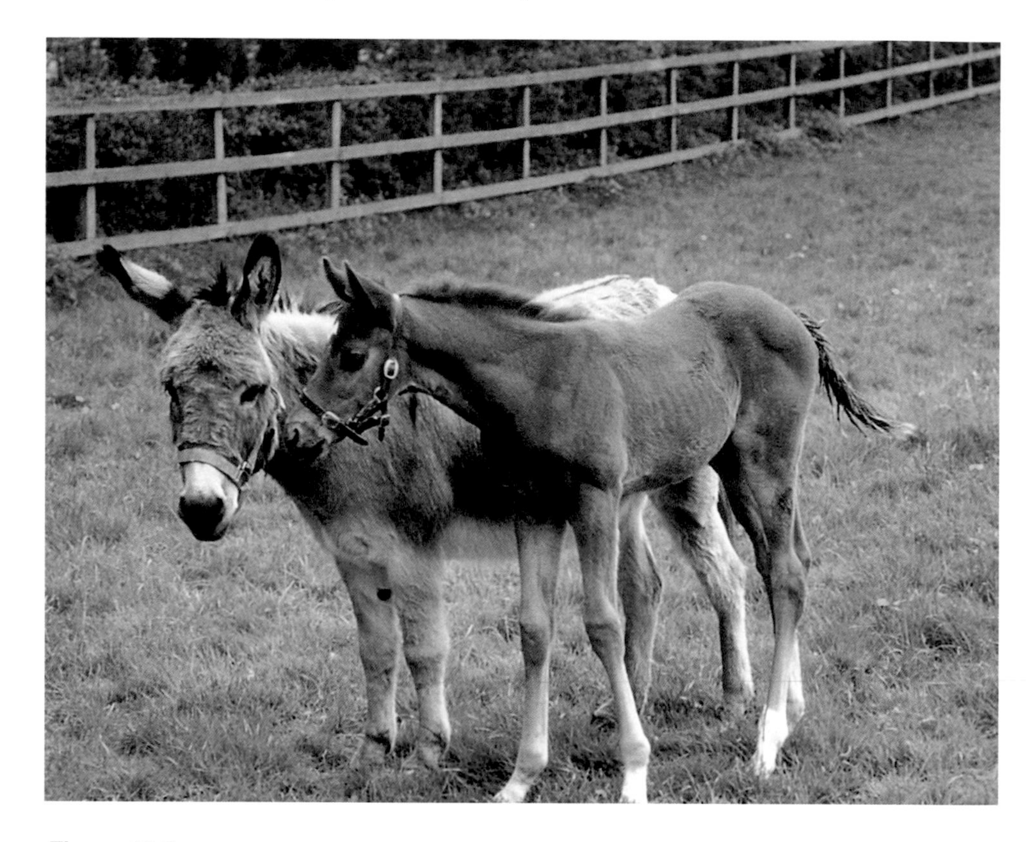

Figure 12.9

Hand-reared orphan foals thrive with companions

foal may have been bred to be at the top of a chosen sphere – be it as an elite athlete racing or eventing, or as a show horse. Therefore, it is vital that every care is taken to ensure that the fact that the foal has been orphaned will not affect its potential in the long term.

The best lesson any handler or manager can give to an orphaned foal is to encourage them to be a horse. If the foal has been hand reared, it may have little or no idea of the complex social behaviour expected when it is in the company of other horses. Some displays, such as biting, kicking and rearing, are natural forms of equine behaviour and, as orphans tend to treat humans as their peers, they can become dangerous if not disciplined from an early stage as to what is acceptable behaviour and what is not. Even if it has not been possible to foster the foal onto a mare, it is vital that every effort is made for it to have a suitable equine companion – ideally of a similar age, so that the foal can learn to develop normal equine social behaviours and attitudes as early as possible.

CHAPTER THIRTEEN

The Foal's Struggle for Survival

The first four days following birth is a critical period of adjustment between pre- and post-natal life. It is during this period that the majority of conditions and diseases peculiar to a newborn foal first make their appearance.

These conditions range from the very mild (slowness in achieving a standing position or successful sucking from the mare) to the most severe (convulsions, weakness, jaundice, etc.).

The health status of the individual is based on a healthy life in utero and a smooth passage through the birth canal without suffering physical or chemical trauma.

In this chapter, let us consider the untoward happenings which may affect newborn health and survival.

The term 'ready for birth' is used to denote that the fetal foal has reached a point of maturity where its body systems are primed for extrauterine and independent life. Premature is a term used to describe the individual that is delivered before this maturity has been reached; and dysmaturity a term denoting some derangement in the process of maturity. The two terms cover conditions which cannot, strictly speaking, always be distinguished as separate entities.

Those attending foals suffering from prematurity or dysmaturity must expect to encounter at least some of the following signs:

- Weakness, expressed in difficulty in standing and/or holding the position of sucking.
- Structural weaknesses of the musculo-skeletal system, usually evidenced by hyperextension at the fetlock joints (Figures 13.1 and 13.2), hyperextension of the knee joints, or an unusually silky coat.
- A suck reflex of varying strength, often diminishing in association with a general weakness and deterioration of the foal's condition.
- In foals that survive, suck reflex may improve in association with strengthening of musculo-skeletal performance and vigour of the individual.
- Rectal temperature may become subnormal and diarrhoea or pasty faeces may be passed (Figure 13.3), often influenced by type and method of feeding (from the mare or artificially

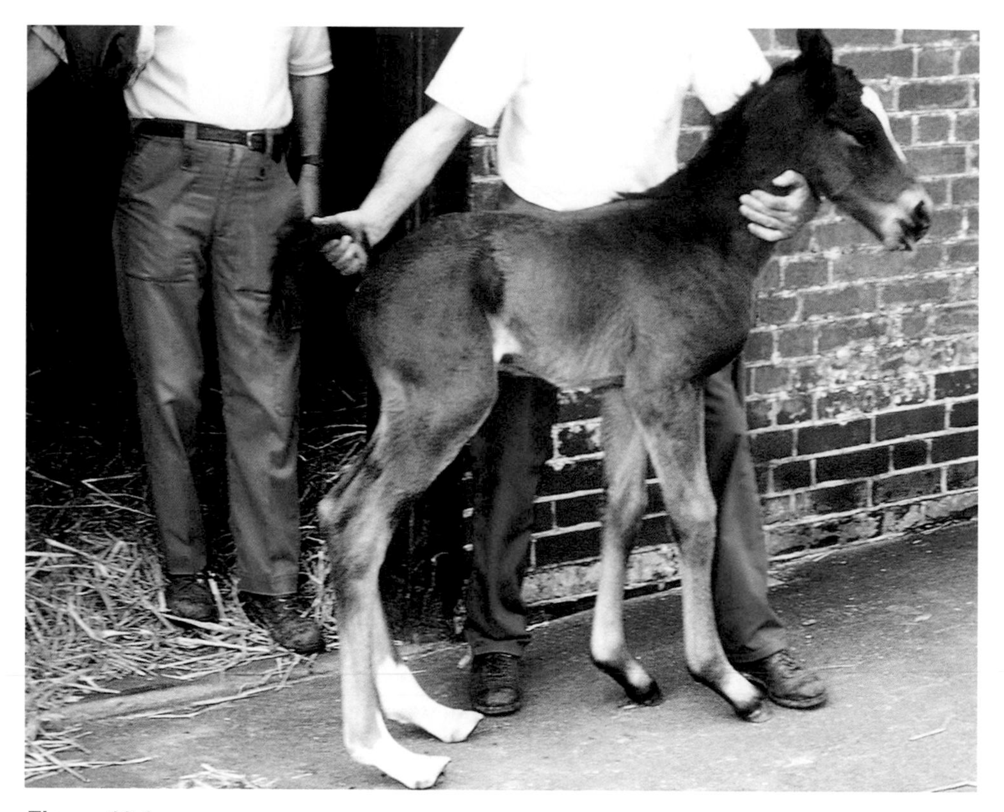

Figure 13.1

Weak or flaccid fetlock joints are relatively common in early developing breeds such as the Thoroughbred

constituted milk, sucking from a bottle or administered via stomach tube).

- Failure of passive immune transfer; that is, low blood levels of IgG may occur and secondary infections, pneumonia, infected joints or septicaemia may develop.

In summary, foals suffering prematurity or dysmaturity have experienced a disadvantaged development at some stage during pregnancy (Figure 13.4). The problem may have involved some of the conditions described in Chapter Eight, of a placental and/or circulatory origin. These conditions, in medical and veterinary parlance, are described as stress or insult to the fetus (Figure 13.5).

The period of stress or insult may be short (acute) or prolonged (chronic), and the time-frame that it occupies in pregnancy is all-important to the outcome; that is, the problems it imposes on development. In general, the earlier in pregnancy it occurs, the more severe the effects because of the accelerated rate of development, at least prior to day 300 of pregnancy.

Further, organs and tissues undergo

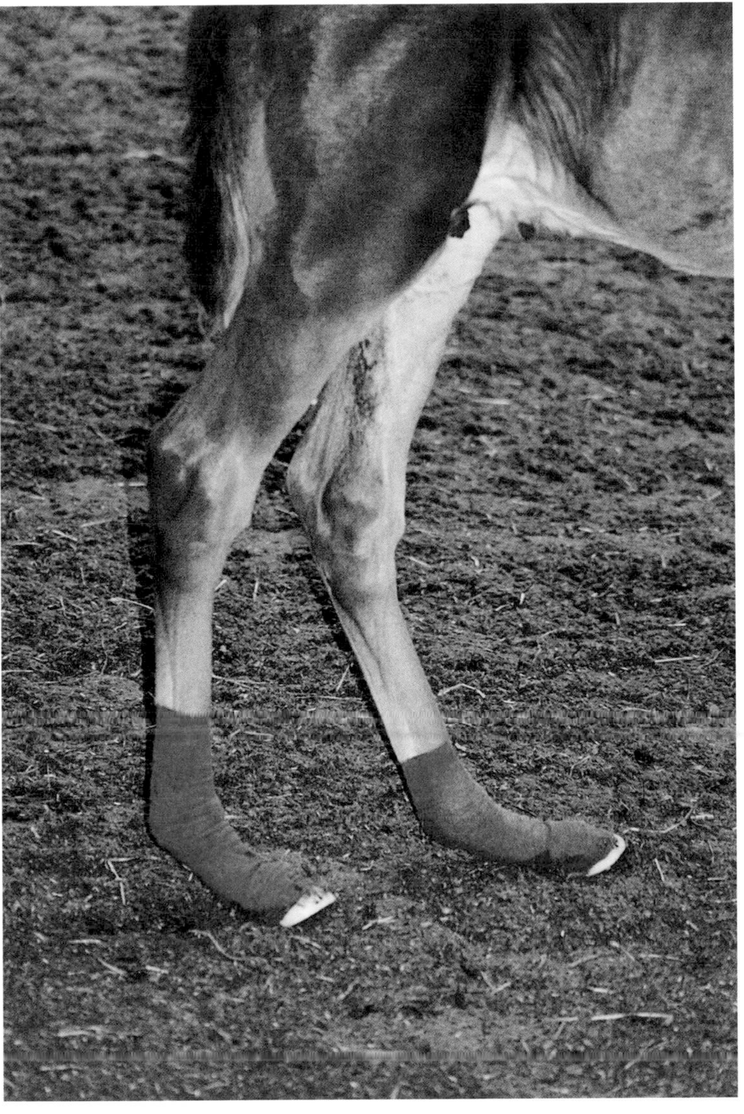

Figure 13.2

Protective bandages are applied to reduce the risk of concussive damage to the fetlock joint and heel bulbs

what are termed growth spurts that occur at differing periods of pregnancy. Thus the growth spurt for the lungs may be at a different time from that of the heart or brain.

Stressful situations have greater impact during these growth spurts and, therefore, the overall outcome has a differential effect depending upon the period in which it occurs. Because of the importance of the lungs in sustaining post-natal life, the effect of stress may be particularly apparent following birth, when it has affected the lungs.

Intrauterine Growth Retardation

This term has been used in human medicine to describe the damage caused

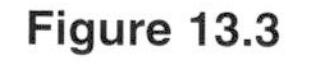

Figure 13.3

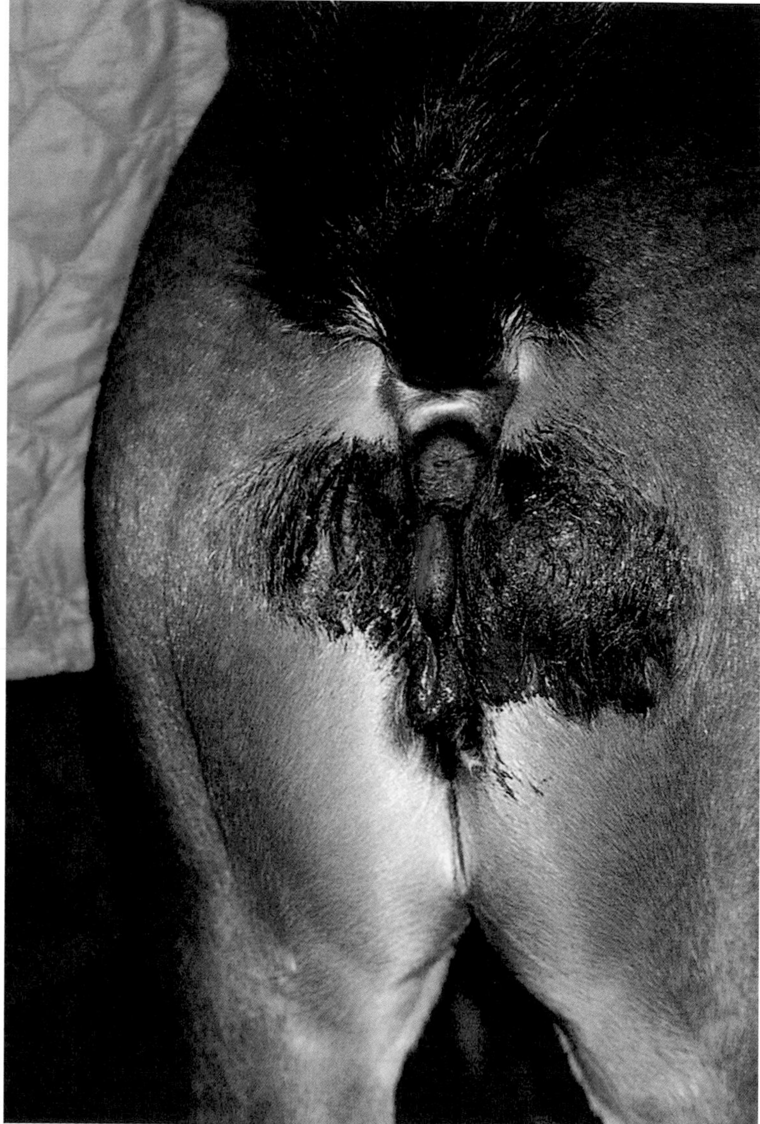

A foal with typical mild diarrhoea. It is essential that the diarrhoea is washed off the foal daily as it is extremely irritant. A suitable barrier emollient (such as Vaseline) should be applied to avoid scalding of the skin or, in the case of this foal, scalding of the vulval lips

by stress or insult to the fetal infant. It has been shown, during the past decade, that the effects may be quite subtle but extend into adult life, resulting in conditions such as heart disease. This is because the microstructure of many organs is complete by the end of pregnancy and no more units of the microstructure develop after birth. They grow in size but not in number.

For example, the kidneys contain units that act as a filter for the blood, so that urine is formed of substances selectively eliminated into the urine as the waste products of the body's metabolism.

Each unit consists of a glomerulus and nephron, the latter consisting of a small tube down which the fluid originating in the glomerulus passes on its

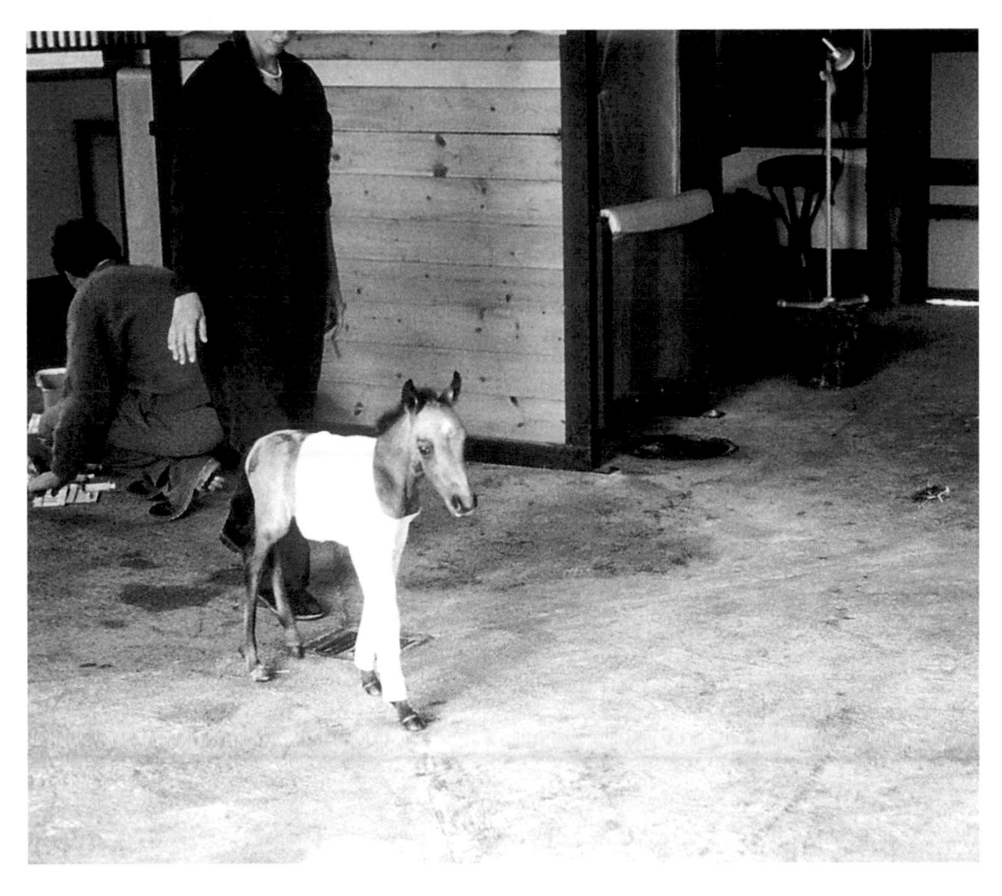

Figure 13.4

A premature foal; he had not developed the ability or a sufficient coat to maintain his body temperature and, as he was extremely small, a jumper was used instead of a foal rug

way to the bladder. The number of glomeruli in the newborn kidney remains the same throughout life; no more are produced. Retarding effects during in utero growth may therefore limit the number of units per kidney in any given affected individual.

The same principle applies to the number of terminal air ducts in the lung. In the horse, there is some evidence that these units (terminal bronchioles and alveoli) in the lung do increase in number for a limited period after birth. This is unusual compared to other mammalian species, and current studies in Newmarket and Northwick Park Hospital for Medical Research are investigating this phenomenon.

Limitations of organ development during human pregnancy have been shown to have a relationship with conditions such as coronary heart disease, asthma, sudden infant cot death and high blood pressure. Whether or not

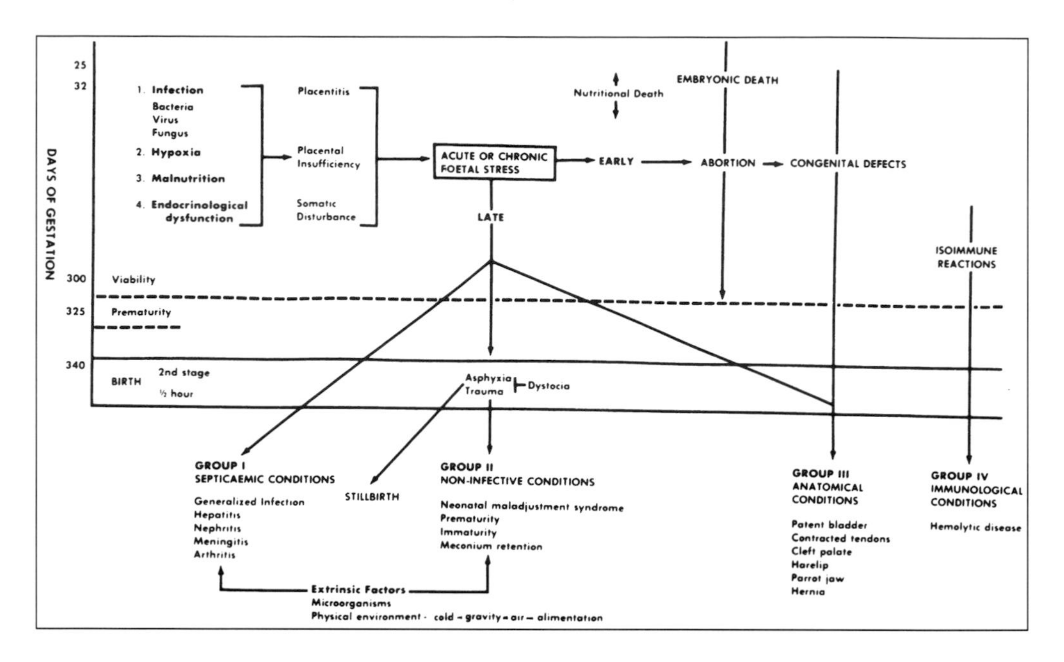

Figure 13.5

Summary of the factors which predispose to diseases of foals in the first four days of life following birth. Four groups of conditions are recognised

similar relationships exist in the horse is also under study, but so far there are no results to demonstrate a cause and effect relationship.

Birth Trauma

Passage of the fetal foal through the birth canal presents a number of specific challenges with risk of injury, traumatic or chemical. The forces of birth in which the foal is pushed through the pelvic hoop of the mare (see Chapter Eleven) are considerable. Pressure brought to bear by contractions of the uterine muscle is supplemented substantially by the voluntary contractions of the mare's abdominal muscles. At the peak of these efforts, corresponding peaks of blood pressure in the foal's jugular vein have been forced to rise to 400 mmHg. Injury to the chest may result from contact with the mare's pelvis in such a way as to fracture a rib or cause considerable bruising to the heart.

In the human infant, it is the head which is most at risk from physical trauma but, in the foal, it is the chest. This is because, in the foal, the chest presents the largest cross-sectional area, whereas in the human infant the largest bulk is that of the head.

In addition, a foal's chest, with its keel-like shape, is particularly vulnerable to becoming wedged against the mare's pelvis if its alignment is not in keeping with the plane of greatest diameter of the pelvic hoop (see Chapter Eleven). Further, the keel of the chest is quite pliable, due largely to the attachment of the lower end of the ribs with the sternum by means of what are termed the costochondral junctures. These attachments are relatively fragile and can become fractured by the forces of delivery.

The heart lies at the lower end of the keel-shaped chest and, as anyone who has felt a newborn foal's heart beating against the chest wall can readily appreciate, the heart itself is exposed to the risks of bruising.

The forces of birth may therefore cause considerable circulatory problems as the heart is exposed to the pressures exerted on the chest wall. In severe cases, where much damage is done, even including fracture of the ribs, the individual cannot survive for more than a few days, exhibiting signs of convulsion and collapse. In less severe cases, circulatory disturbances may lead to loss of blood supply to the brain, with signs of convulsion or other behavioural disturbances.

The same type of symptoms (convulsions, coma, failure to bond with the mare) may be the result of chemical damage; that is, increased acidity of the blood, lack of oxygen and excess carbon dioxide. As the foal passes through the birth canal, the efficiency of the blood circulation in the cord diminishes. If the foal starts a breathing rhythm immediately after delivery, the lungs take in air and oxygen diffuses into the bloodstream in the normal way. However, if for any reason the cord becomes compressed before the foal breathes, there may be a period of lack of oxygen (hypoxia). This results in a substantial accumulation of lactic acid and the pH of the bloodstream may fall from a normal 7.4 pH units to below 7 pH units.

This situation is extremely injurious to body cells, especially those of the brain, kidney and liver. Recovery from this damage may not occur; in these cases, the foal may live for several days, if assisted, but will eventually succumb to the nervous and metabolic effects of the damage to these organs.

The consequences, as seen via the symptoms and behavioural disturbances displayed, depend both on the amount of damage and the organs that are damaged selectively. For example, if the brain is involved, the foal will show neurological signs varying from convulsions to coma and loss of awareness of its surroundings, including apparent blindness. If it is the kidney that is damaged the symptoms are those of kidney malfunction, which include lethargy and coma associated with developing uraemia. If the lungs and/or heart are affected, we may expect circulatory and respiratory signs based largely on failure of the blood to deliver oxygen to various organs and tissues. This, in turn, gives rise to symptoms associated with the other organs involved; if this includes the brain, convulsions and/or coma or maladjusted behaviour due to ischaemia (reduced supply of blood and therefore of oxygen to the tissues) and/or hypoxia (reduced supply of oxygen).

The following conditions are recognised as distinct or semidistinct entities.

Prematurity/ Dysmaturity/ Maladjustment

We have already considered the origin of these conditions which may be described in one of three ways, yet each represents an interrelated situation.

The term dysmaturity is probably the one that should be used insofar as it means bad maturity or, to express it more simply, failure of the normal processes of intrauterine development and post-natal adjustment.

The symptoms are typically those of a foal which is physically undersized and/or shows evidence of dehydration and malnourishment, including weakness of the musculo-skeletal system and general weakness which diminishes the foal's strength in rising to its feet and in sucking from the mare. The suck reflex is generally present in these cases but diminished in strength. The foal's gestational age may vary from 280 days to 360 days (Figure 13.6). In the case of those with shortened gestational length, the stress of placental damage or other factors may switch on the adaptive processes before birth which enable the foal to survive, given varying degrees of critical care.

Maturity of the adrenal cortex gland, which produces cortisol, is essential for survival of the newborn foal. If the stress before birth has 'switched on' this gland to a similar extent as in a normal full-term foal, there is a chance of survival whatever the gestational age.

There may be one of two outcomes to these cases. There are foals which become increasingly stronger over the first few days of extrauterine life; and those which deteriorate, particularly from day 2 onwards. These latter foals have been described as suffering from the second-day syndrome. This is because the deterioration usually starts on the second day and involves a weakening of the foal's behavioural responses, from its ability to stand to the strength of its suck. Neurological signs develop, including spasms of the limbs, head and neck and eventual coma and death. These changes are usually associated with decreased lung function, in which the lungs become virtually airless leading to hypoxia (lack of oxygen) and acidaemia (increased acidity of the blood).

The airlessness of the lungs may be due to loss of residual air to keep the lungs expanded as the foal lies on its side and the mechanics of breathing are

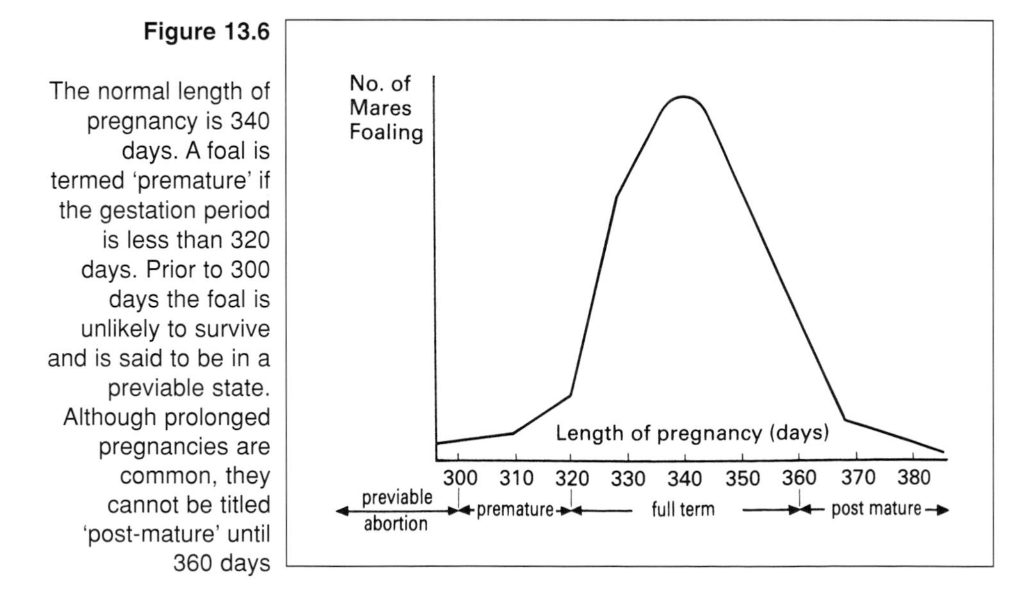

Figure 13.6

The normal length of pregnancy is 340 days. A foal is termed 'premature' if the gestation period is less than 320 days. Prior to 300 days the foal is unlikely to survive and is said to be in a previable state. Although prolonged pregnancies are common, they cannot be titled 'post-mature' until 360 days

disturbed as a result of position and general weakness. However, in dysmature foals the lungs are sometimes underdeveloped and some areas never expand, so that loss of air after birth adds to the situation of airlessness and an increasing lack of oxygenation of the blood as it passes through the lungs.

Neonatal Maladjustment Syndrome

The term neonatal maladjustment syndrome (convulsions, barker, wanderer or dummy) was coined to describe foals which suffered neurological signs after birth due to damage in the central nervous system (Figures 13.5, 13.7 and 13.8).

These foals are usually born at full-term, may have a rapid delivery and often appear normal for a few hours after birth. They are then struck down with convulsions or other major behavioural disturbances, such as wandering or inability to find the mare and suck. The suck reflex is usually suddenly abolished in these cases rather than, as in dysmature foals, diminishing gradually.

The outlook for these cases is quite good if the foal is given substantial crit-

Figure 13.7

Foals with brain damage, as here, may convulse or suffer from increased extensor tone in their muscles

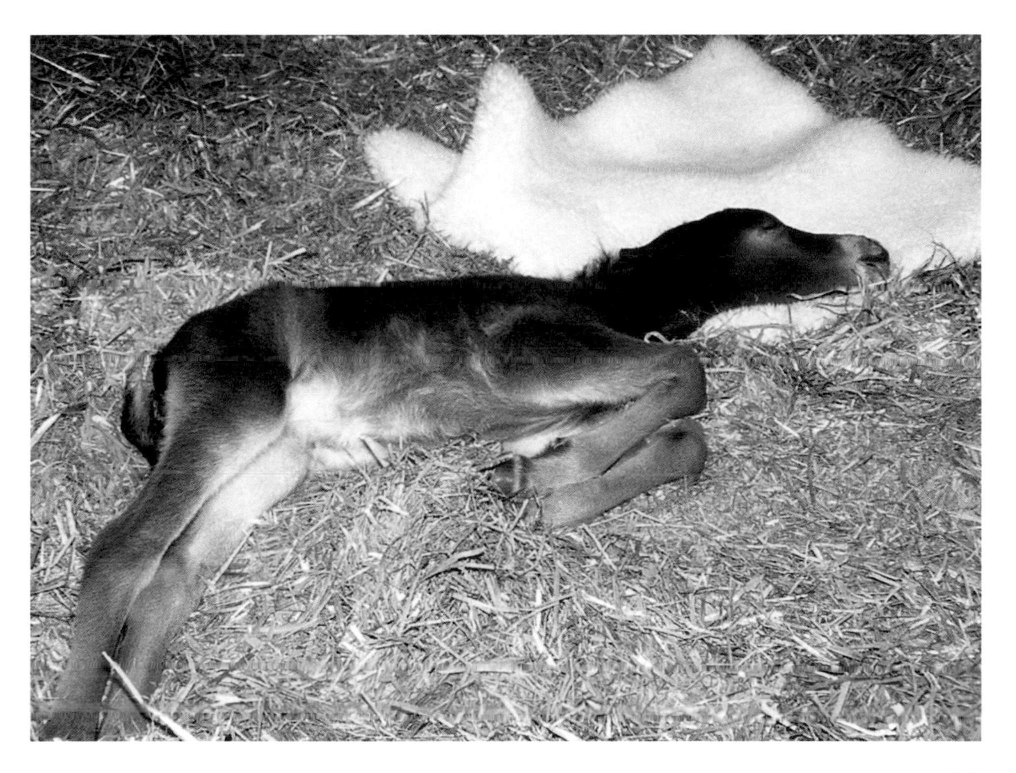

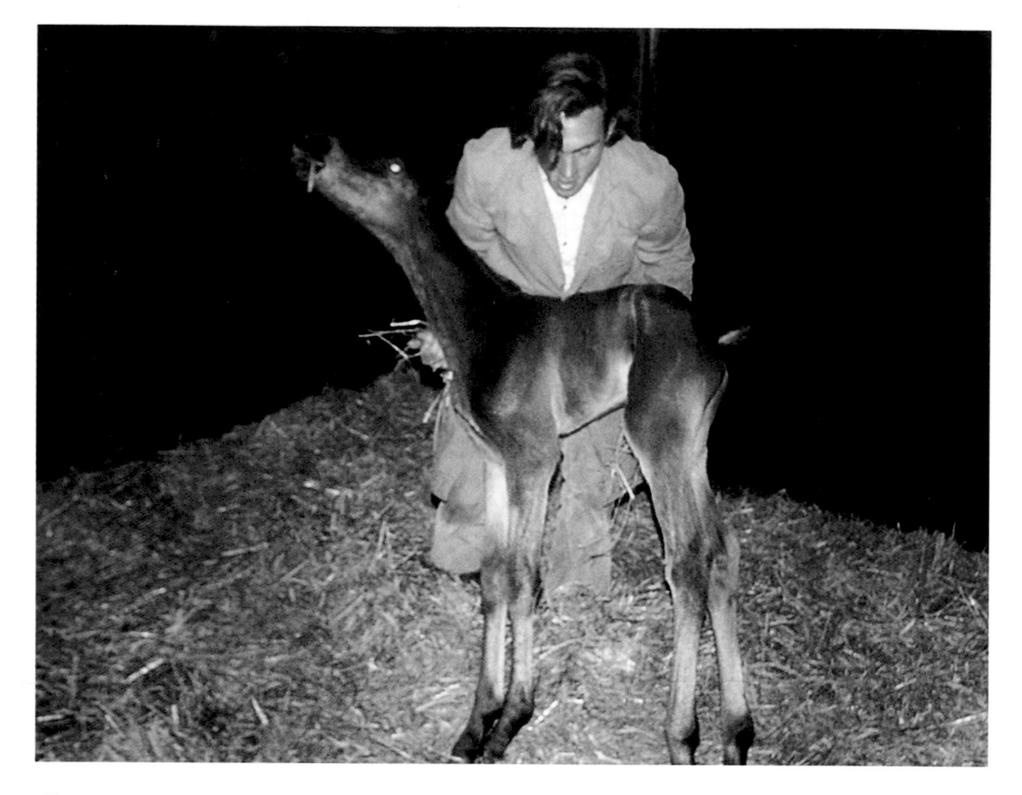

Figure 13.8

This brain-damaged foal is standing with head pulled back and limbs held stiffly

ical care, including artificial feeding, sedation and intravenous fluids.

Septicaemia

Septicaemia is a term used to describe a generalised infection; that is, one that is spread via the bloodstream to most if not all organs and tissues of the body.

The infection may arise from any infectious agent, bacteria, virus or, occasionally, arteritis virus.

Symptoms include gradually developing weakness manifested by an inability to rise to the standing position, diminished strength of suck reflex, dehydration (evidenced by non-pliable skin and sinking of the eyeballs into their orbits) and diarrhoea (Figure 13.9).

Rectal temperature may increase, as would be expected in infectious disease, or paradoxically decrease, which is a feature of young animals insofar as they cannot respond to the challenge of infection in the way that older animals do. Temperature cannot, therefore, be used as a diagnostic sign in the newborn.

The same diagnostic caveat has to be observed when considering the white

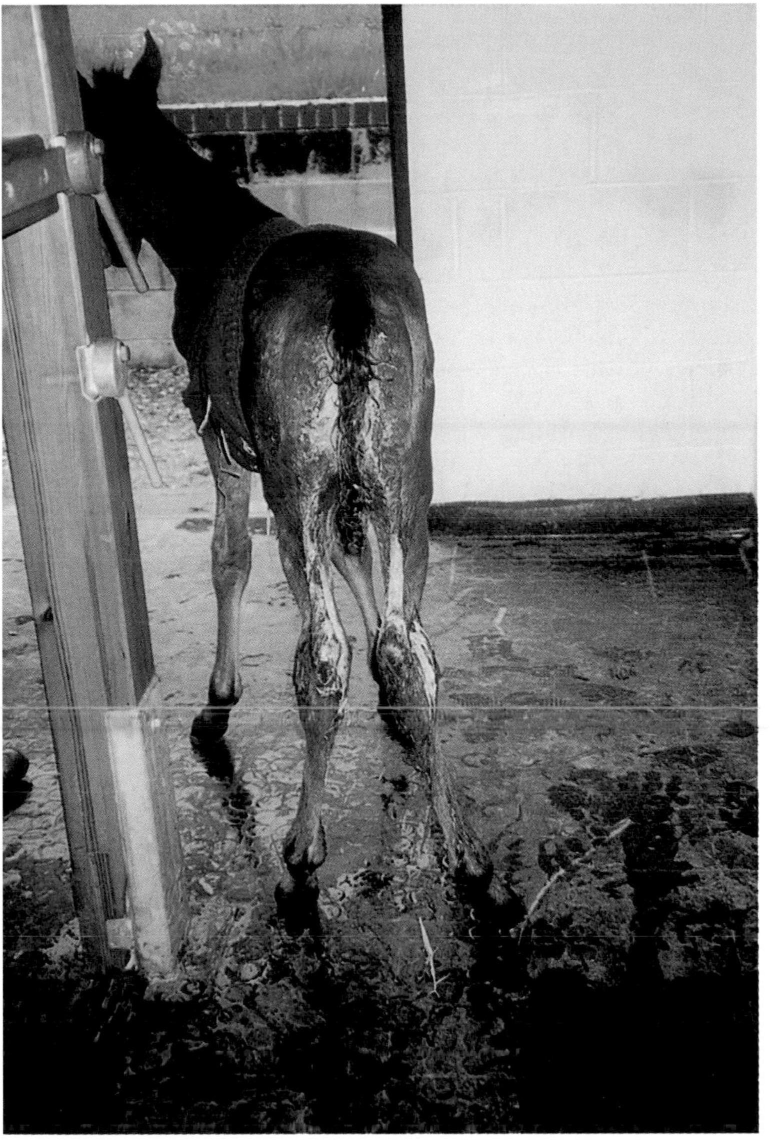

Figure 13.9

A foal with rotavirus. Rotavirus is perhaps one of the most significant infectious causes of diarrhoea on Thoroughbred studfarms in recent years

cell count that generally increases in bacterial infections but may actually diminish in the newborn. An increase (leucocytosis) is not, therefore, necessarily present in newborn septicaemia.

Virus causes a substantial decrease in white cell numbers, both lymphocytes and leucocytes. This leucopaenia is characteristic of EHV-1 infection, which represents a major need for differential diagnosis in newborn foals because of its infectivity to pregnant mares.

Infection

Localised infection may be encountered in a newborn, particularly with respect to infected joints (joint-ill;

infective arthritis). The kidneys are often affected. Micro-abscesses may develop from the kidney cortex due, often, to an organism known as *Actinobacillus equuli*. *Klebsiella* and *E. coli* are organisms which may also affect the kidney.

Infection may also be localised to the lungs (pneumonia, pleurisy) or the brain and its surrounding membranes (meningitis, encephalitis). The gut may become infected, especially with *E. coli* or *Klebsiella*, resulting in enteritis (inflammation of the gut) or peritonitis (the peritoneum). The symptoms displayed by the foal in these circumstances are related to the organ involved. In the case of the lungs, these include an increased breathing rate and abnormal sounds heard on listening through the stethoscope (auscultation). If the brain and its membranes (meninges) are infected, then convulsions may develop and, in the case of the kidneys, uraemia (increased blood urea content) and consequent lethargy and coma are possible symptoms.

Meconium Colic

Meconium is the faeces stored during intrauterine development in the large bowel of the fetal foal. After birth, this has to be voided before the milk dung can pass the entire length of the gut. During fetal life, meconium is expelled only in abnormal circumstances, usually associated with hypoxic episodes (deprivation of oxygen to the gut). However, once delivered, defaecation is a natural means of expelling waste material. The chain from inactive to active gut action (peristalsis) is yet another example of the dramatic change occurring between fetal and newborn life.

On occasions the fetal pellets of meconium may become impacted in the rectum and the foal has difficulty in passing them. This may be associated with colic as the gut goes into spasm and tympany (air) stretches the gut wall.

The signs of colic are rolling, lying in awkward positions and pointing the muzzle towards the flanks. There may be sweating and inappetance during the painful episodes that occur at intervals over several hours, sometimes days.

The condition is alleviated by injecting pain-relieving drugs, administering paraffin emulsion by stomach tube and enemas per rectum. Modern enemas consist of special preparations that lubricate and help to break up the meconium pellets. These are administered routinely following birth (see Chapter Twelve).

Ruptured Bladder

Foals suffering from meconium retention often strain. This stance may also be a sign of a ruptured or patent bladder.

In these cases, urine escapes from the bladder through the bladder wall and accumulates in the peritoneum in large volume, a condition sometimes referred to as uro-peritoneum. Symptoms of ruptured bladder develop from about the second to the fifth day after foaling. In the first 12 hours after birth, the foal does not generate much urine and, in the succeeding 36 hours, the quantity is insufficient to cause swelling of the abdomen.

This is not as common a condition as

meconium colic, but is an important differential diagnosis because, if untreated, it will be fatal. The bladder wall may be breached because of rupture during delivery, because of an anatomical defect in which the two sides of the bladder wall do not unite in embryonic development or due to the bladder wall at the fundic end to which the umbilical vessels are attached becoming pliable and infected.

The symptoms of a ruptured bladder are similar to many of those described for meconium colic. In addition, the abdomen swells increasingly due to the accumulation of urine in the peritoneal cavity. If not alleviated this causes pressure on the diaphragm and, eventually, compresses the lungs and prevents breathing movements occurring so that the foal is literally asphyxiated.

Diagnosis is made by ultrasound examination and treatment is by means of surgery under general anaesthetic to open the abdomen, siphon off the urine and suture the breach in the bladder wall. Providing the case is diagnosed reasonably early, an affected foal usually recovers uneventfully.

Umbilical Problems

The umbilical stump consists of the severed ends of the two arteries and vein, together with that of the urachus. In most cases, the umbilical stump becomes sealed with a small amount of blood clot and shrivels over a period of about two weeks. In some cases, where

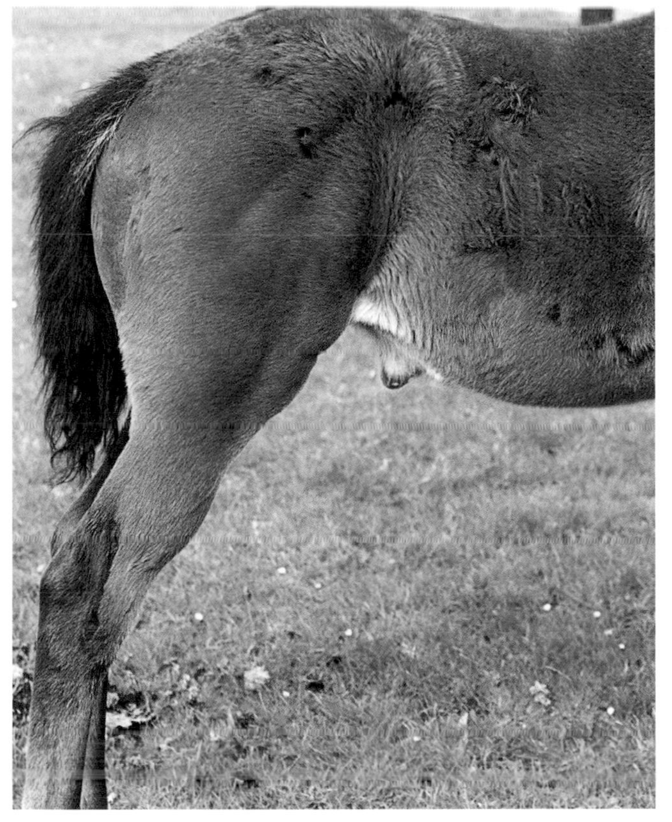

Figure 13.10

An umbilical hernia in a Thoroughbred foal. Umbilical hernias are relatively common in foals and may resolve spontaneously with maturity, but large ones may require surgical repair. Any umbilical swelling in foals should be examined by a veterinary surgeon as there is a risk of strangulation of the protruding intestine the cord is thickened and substantial, the process of shrivelling and retraction takes longer. Some of these cases become infected or the stump produces proud flesh at the tip. This formation of proud flesh extends along the stump up into the abdomen towards the attachment with the bladder wall. These cases may be treated by removing the scab at the end of the stump and treating this with a caustic such as copper sulphate solution or formalin. However, in severe cases, surgery to remove the stump may be advisable.

As the foal gets older, the ring in the abdomen wall at the umbilicus may not close as it should, and a hernia may develop (Figure 13.10).

Veterinary advice should be taken as to how the hernia should be dealt with; it must be distinguished from an abscess, which may give the same appearance.

Haemolytic Disease

Haemolytic disease (haemolytic jaundice) is an example of the situation where, under special circumstances, natural mechanisms can have harmful effects. In this case, the fetal foal invokes an immune response in the mare, probably the result of a few of the fetal red cells passing from the placenta into the mare's bloodstream. Normally, this happening would not provoke any response but, in rare instances, the mare produces protective substances (that is, antibodies) against her own foal's red cells.

At the time of birth, these antibodies are concentrated into the colostrum and, after the foal has sucked, they pass into the foal's bloodstream. Here they destroy the red cells, causing severe anaemia which, if not treated, may be fatal. The red cells causing this problem are of the group R or S. Therefore, if a stallion is R or S, the fetal foal inherits this composition and the red cells act on the mare in a similar manner to a vaccine injected into her. If the mare has a corresponding R or S antigen to that of the stallion, this situation does not arise.

The R and S groups are the most virulent and potentially fatal; the A or Q groups are less virulent but may also cause anaemia, although not always fatal.

Symptoms of jaundice include yellow colouration of the whites of the eye, gums and vagina. The heart and respiratory rates increase, particularly on exertion, as the red cells in the blood are destroyed by the action of the antibody absorbed from the colostrum. This takes at least 12 hours to develop but, from this age onwards, the destruction of red cells increases rapidly, particularly when the R and S group are involved. Symptoms may therefore be seen as early as age 12 hours but, more often, appear on the second day after foaling.

Diagnosis is made via blood tests to identify the anaemia and to establish the presence of antibodies causing the destruction (haemolysis) of the red cells.

Treatment consists of infusing red cells into the foal's bloodstream in order to replace those destroyed.

These red cells may be taken from a suitable donor or the dam's red cells may be used, but it is then essential that they should be washed free of any antibody present in the mare's blood serum (the fluid that suspends the cells of the blood). This requires a mega centrifuge by which the cells are washed free of serum, a process repeated two or three times.

Preventative measures include identification of the blood grouping of stallion and mare in any given mating. This information may be obtained by request from the Animal Health Trust Jockey Club Typing Unit in Newmarket, where all blood groups are recorded.

An on the spot test can be made by examining the mare's blood for antibody in the days leading up to parturition or by cross-matching the mare's colostrum and the foal's blood prior to the foal being allowed to suck for the first time.

Congenital Abnormalities

In the intricate development and growth of the organs during fetal life, it is perhaps remarkable that in the great majority of cases the process is completed without any defects. There are, however, a number of well-recognised congenital (present at birth) defects. For example, button eyes, in which the eyeball is so small as to be virtually non-existent, may occur on one or both sides; deformities of the head include twisted jaw and cleft palate; the limbs may be unable to extend due to the flexor tendons being contracted. The latter condition may affect one or both forelegs as well as the hind limbs. The fetal foal develops lying on its back or side with its legs flexed. The ligaments allow a degree of flexion of the joints, which is exaggerated partly as a precaution against the limbs accidentally causing damage to the mare. However, as full-term approaches these structures become firmer and, because of the pliability of the limbs during fetal development, they may be shaped at odd angles, which is apparent when the foal is delivered. Faulty development of the bladder and developmental failure of the gut, in which part of the colon or rectum is missing, may also be observed at this stage in newborn foals.

The causes of the abnormalities are generally unknown, but probably include such factors as:

- Viral infection and drugs received by the mare during the first few weeks of pregnancy at a time when the organs are being formed.
- Nutritional influences.
- Inheritance.

Nursing of Sick Foals

The responsibility of studfarm personnel towards the care of foals is the same as that towards horses of all ages, namely observation and attention. It is the studfarm personnel who are the first to diagnose that something is amiss. Their close association with numerous healthy individuals provides them with an ideal background to spot symptoms in the early stages of disease.

This is particularly important with a very young foal, because problems are apt to develop very quickly and the foal's condition will deteriorate unless professional assistance is given.

Observation is not a habit or skill confined to the professional veterinarian. Rather, it is a faculty that can be developed by anyone. All that is required is a study of normal behaviour with a knowledge of the timing of changing patterns (for example, when the foal first gets to its feet or when it sucks for the first time). The manner of getting to the feet and of sucking are crucial elements for observation as, of course, are breathing and heart rates, rectal temperature and the general physical appearance of the individual.

Every stud hand should make a point of becoming acquainted with the normal individual in such aspects as physical appearance, the way of walking, feeding, passing dung and urine. Any departures from the normal can then be noted and reported to the attending veterinarian. The treating of sick animals is a matter of teamwork, in which studfarm personnel play an enormously important role.

The physical support and assistance for a weak, maladjusted foal forms an essential ingredient of any veterinary treatment. When the adaptive responses (see Chapter Twelve) are in any way disturbed, survival depends on our giving suitable assistance, such as that detailed below.

- If unable to stand, the foal must be maintained in a gentle and purposeful manner. Restraint should be minimal and those handling the foal should appreciate that struggling is often the result of deranged nervous activity, which may be quietened by action on the part of the handler. For example, if the foal is too weak to enable it to turn from a fully recumbent position to sit on its sternum, turning it into this latter position may be helpful. The same applies to a foal which is trying to stand; gently raising it to its feet, with support, may help the foal to achieve its objective. Restraint in the form of holding the legs or forcing the foal to lie on its side may be counterproductive, in that these actions actually cause the foal to struggle more. In doing so, it expends valuable energy and resources of carbohydrate and oxygen on which activity depend.
- Sick foals may have difficulty in maintaining their body temperature and measures to assist thermal regulation are essential. The majority of body heat is lost through radiation with less through convection (draughts) and conduction (contact with the ground). Radiation loss is countered by improving insulation, particularly that of the roofs and walls of the stable in which a foal is kept. However, this is insufficient for foals with serious problems of temperature regulation and applying foal coats or blankets may be essential (Figure 13.11). Placing bandages on the limbs may also help to avoid heat loss. Laying the foal that cannot stand on its own on soft material helps to reduce bed sores and further insulates the foal from loss of heat through contact with the ground. There are, nowadays, special blankets that help to absorb moisture, which can be used effectively. However, contamination by urine and faeces is always a problem in foals unable to stand.
- Positioning of the foal is an important contribution to its well-being. If foals lie flat on their sides, their oxygen pressures decline compared with standing or sitting on their brisket. Turning the foal from one side to the other is often advocated, although it has yet to be determined objectively as to whether or not this approach is helpful. When the foal lies on one side, blood tends to circulate in greater quantity in the lower

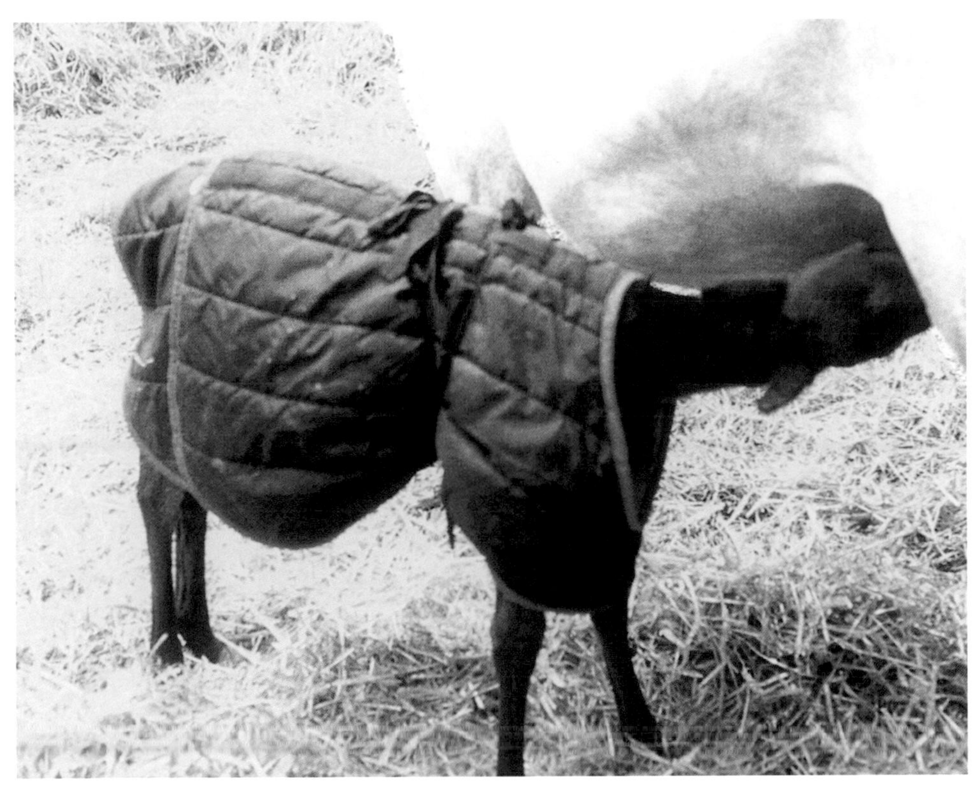

Figure 13.11

Sick foals may have difficulty regulating their body temperature and applying a foal rug is essential

lung while the upper lung expands with air more than the lower lung. There is thus a mismatch between the bloodstream and the air. However, although theoretically turning the foal from one side to the other may help to counter this process, there is at present no evidence as to the actual effect or the frequency with which turning to one side or the other is effective.

- The foal's head should be maintained slightly above the level of its body so as to reduce the risk of milk being regurgitated and being passed into the lungs. The head should be at a natural angle for breathing and not flexed to any marked extent.
- Feeding should be regular and in small quantities. Vets often insert a tube into the stomach or oesophagus and fix this on the head so that small quantities of feed can be administered at frequent intervals of, say, 20–30 minutes. This is a more physiological approach than bolus feeds at hourly or bi-hourly intervals.
- Maintaining a regular evacuation of faeces is another important responsibility. This may be achieved by performing regular enemas.
- Critical care of young foals is largely

symptomatic and a continuing process of adapting measures in response to changes in the foal's health status. Therefore, those attending the foal should be prepared to keep a detailed record of how the case is proceeding. The major landmarks that should be noted down are:

- Rectal temperature.
- Heart and respiratory rates.
- Frequency of passing urine and its colour.
- Frequency of defaecation and the nature of the faeces.
- Frequency and strength of sucking (if foal has not lost the suck reflex).
- Frequency of getting to the feet and standing and of sucking from the mare, if these faculties are present.

CHAPTER FOURTEEN

Schooling for Independence

The first year of any foal's life is a critical time for development and growth. It is important to remember that, from a management point of view, this period begins long before the foal is weaned from its mother and becomes independent.

The mare is the main influence on the young foal. She provides all that it needs in terms of food and security and she teaches the foal essential equine behavioural patterns (Figure 14.1).

As the foal matures it begins to interact with other foals in its peer group and with other older horses it may be in contact with. Proper management and care during this first year can make the difference between a yearling with quality and potential and just another yearling.

Behaviour

The foal forms its first close relationship with its mother. Most of the behaviour displayed at this stage is play orientated, with nibbling/biting, kicking, cantering in circles close to the mare, etc. By two or three weeks of age the foal will begin to move a little further from the mare and mutual grooming of foal and dam is often seen. Once contact with other foals begins, the foal starts to become less dependent on its mother and starts to play further away from her with other foals. If the foal is kept away from other foals, it will continue to play with its mother long after this behaviour would otherwise have been replaced. Foals kept in a herd environment with access to a peer group tend to spend less time in solitary play by the time they are eight weeks old. Additionally, it is worth noting that first-foaling mares may be excessively protective of their foals and nervous of other mares, resulting in their foals becoming shy and reluctant to play with others.

Young foals, as with most other babies, spend a lot of time lying down and sleeping. Normally this is in short periods interspersed with short periods of feeding and play. Prolonged periods of sleeping or lying down are not normal and may be the first signs that something is wrong. Foals that are found lying upside down or in any awk-

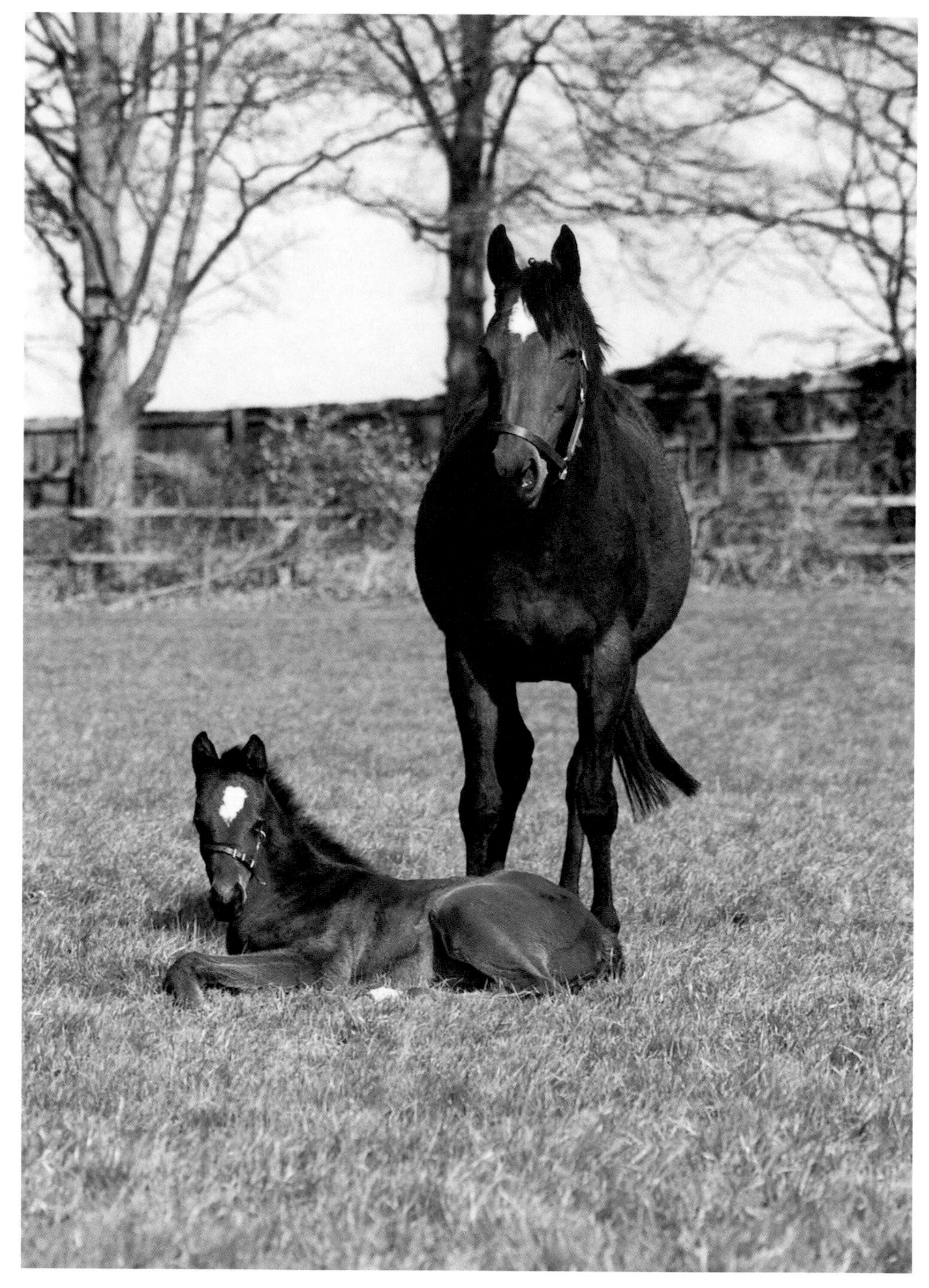

Figure 14.1

The mare is the main influence on the foal during the first few months ward positions are behaving abnormally and this may indicate pain caused by conditions such as colic. Normal sleeping/resting positions are stretched out on one side or up on its chest.

Some foals remain lying down even when approached, so this should not be considered abnormal. The usual abnormal signs include rapid or shallow breathing, rolling, excessive sweating or shivering and lethargy.

Young foals typically nurse feed frequently in short periods, normally every 30–60 minutes. As the foal grows older the nursing will become less frequent – this continues until the foal is essentially weaned (Figure 14.2). In the natural state, foals are normally weaned as late as a few weeks or even days before the mare gives birth again. This late weaning may maintain the bond between the mare and her offspring

Figure 14.2

Young foals typically nurse very frequently during the first few weeks and rarely move far away from their dams

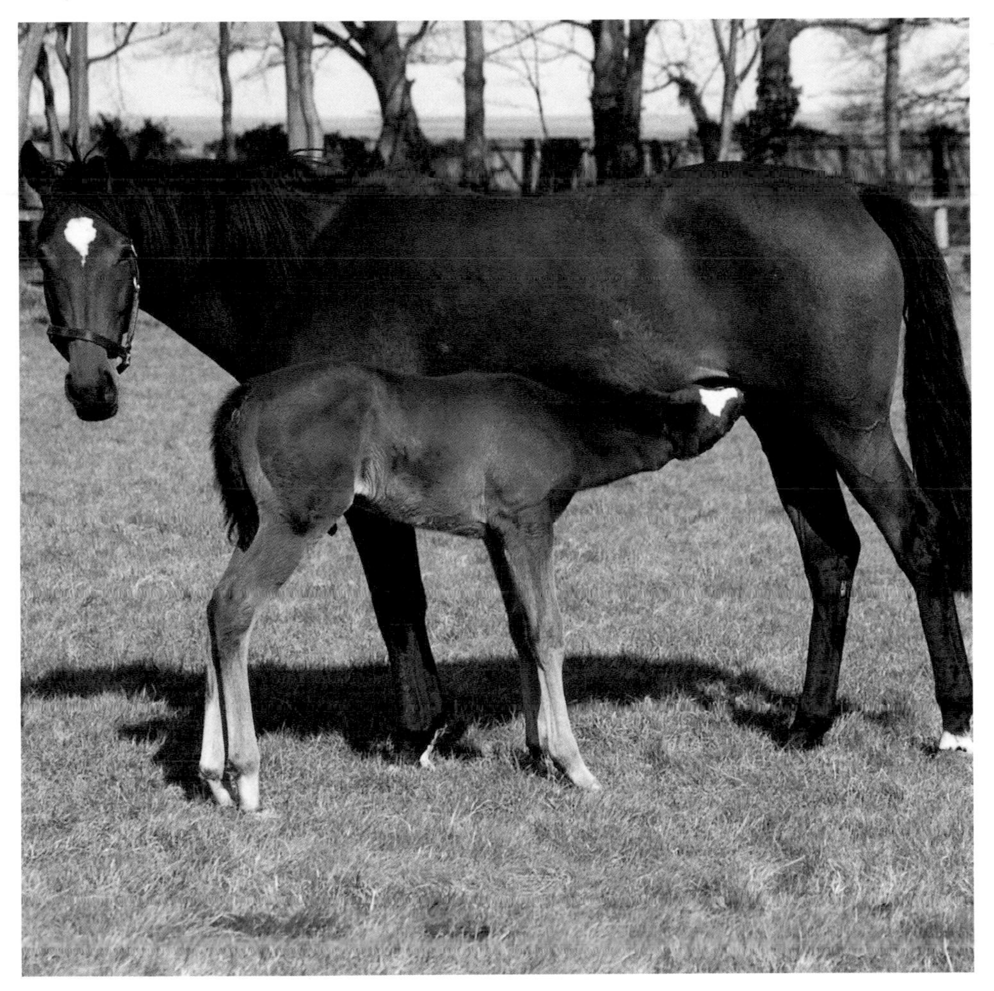

much longer than that maintained in a domesticated environment. Most studfarms provide supplementary concentrates and forage for the growing foals from an early stage and this may be the reason why the foals become independent much sooner than in the wild (Figure 14.3).

Foals at about six months of age may still suck, but the milk percentage of their diet is very small and it is now not essential. Most studfarms wean the foals completely at about six months, especially if the dam is in foal again, to give the mare a chance to regain condition and concentrate on her developing pregnancy. Mineral supplements in the form of paddock blocks and licks are very useful and some research has indicated that the provision of mineral blocks reduces the amount of tail and fence chewing by youngstock.

Handling

Just like children, foals are very impressionable at an early age and usually very cooperative when the dam is close by. This is an ideal time to begin initial

Figure 14.3

Fence mounted creep feeders can be useful in paddocks with small groups of mares and foals. However, any fixed protrusion from the fencing must be considered a hazard to youngstock

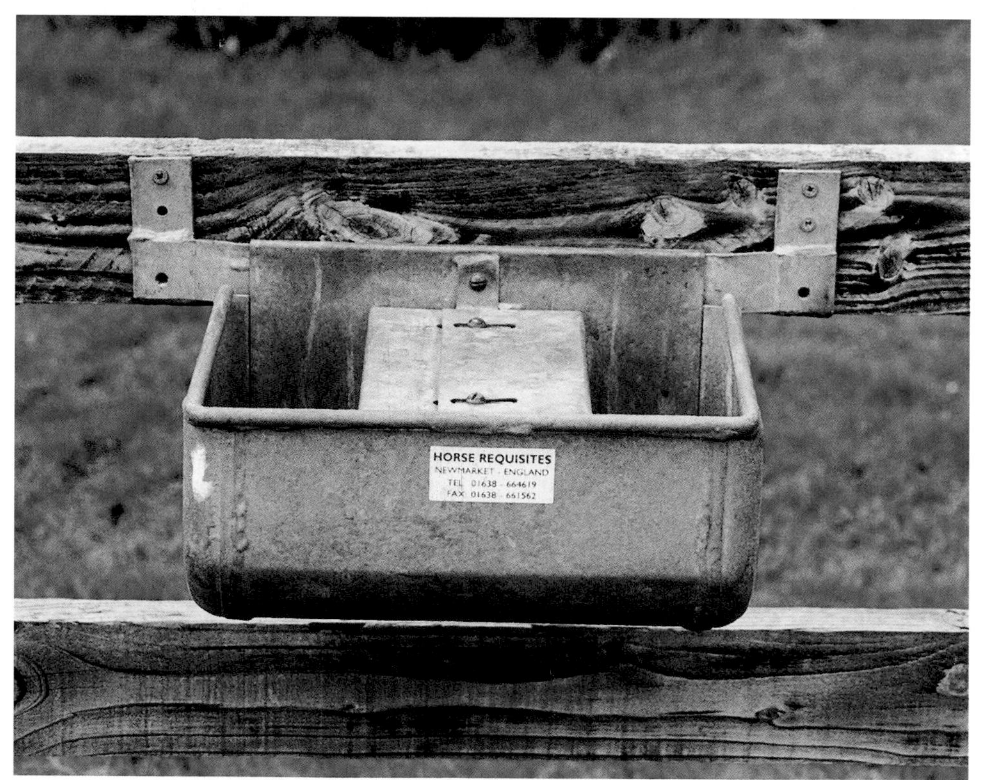

training, such as accustoming the foal to wearing a headcollar and being led. Most handlers also like to teach the foals to be groomed lightly and to have their feet picked up and handled at this early age.

One of the most important aspects of foal management is hoof care, but sadly this is an area that is often overlooked. Regular farrier visits and trimming from about three or four weeks of age will also allow the foal to be assessed for structural development. Foals born with limb deviations may need to be seen by a specialist from very early on to prevent lasting damage (Figures 14.4, 14.5 and 14.6).

In the wild state, horses rely on their quick reactions to run from predators and this instinct remains the primary

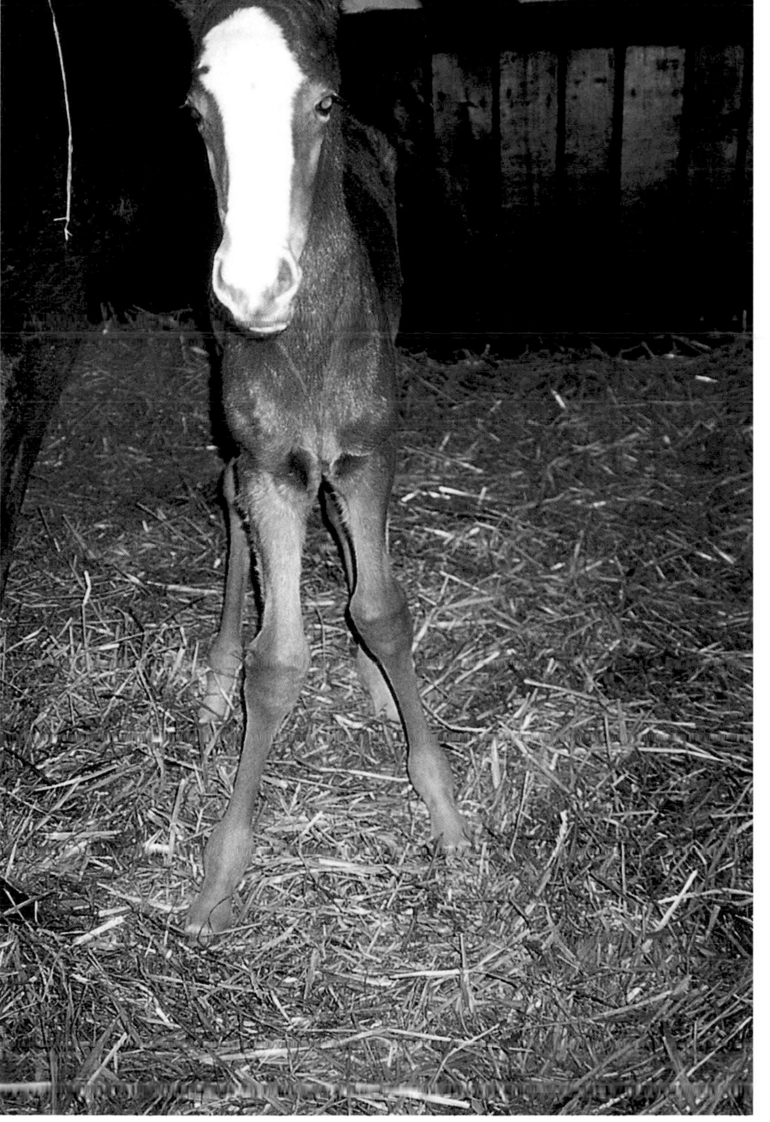

Figure 14.4

Foals with limb weaknesses and deviations require conservative care and restricted exercise

response of any horse to a dangerous or frightening situation. One of the most important aspects of early training is to teach the horse to resist the urge to flee and to accept levels of restraint. The earlier this is started the better, and many studfarms begin to handle the foals regularly from a few days of age. Foals who are particularly nervous or shy will become more difficult to train if they are left unhandled until they are older.

It is important to try to make every effort to reduce the amount of emotional and physical stress on a young horse. A horse that panics is a danger to itself and to its handler; these horses also constantly learn that handling is a bad thing as they get hurt when it happens.

Physical battles with a strong foal should be avoided at all costs – these experiences can affect the horse's attitude towards all future training.

It is common for studfarms to use small leather headcollars for their foals, fitting them as early as three or four days of age. This enables the foals to become accustomed to the feel from an early age and also allows the handlers to easily identify each foal, as name discs can be fitted. Foals are rarely led directly from their headcollars at this stage – generally foals are cradled with the handler's arms around the foal's chest and quarters. After a few days the foal can be taught to lead alongside its mother – generally it will be led from its left side by the handler putting a few fingers through the noseband of the

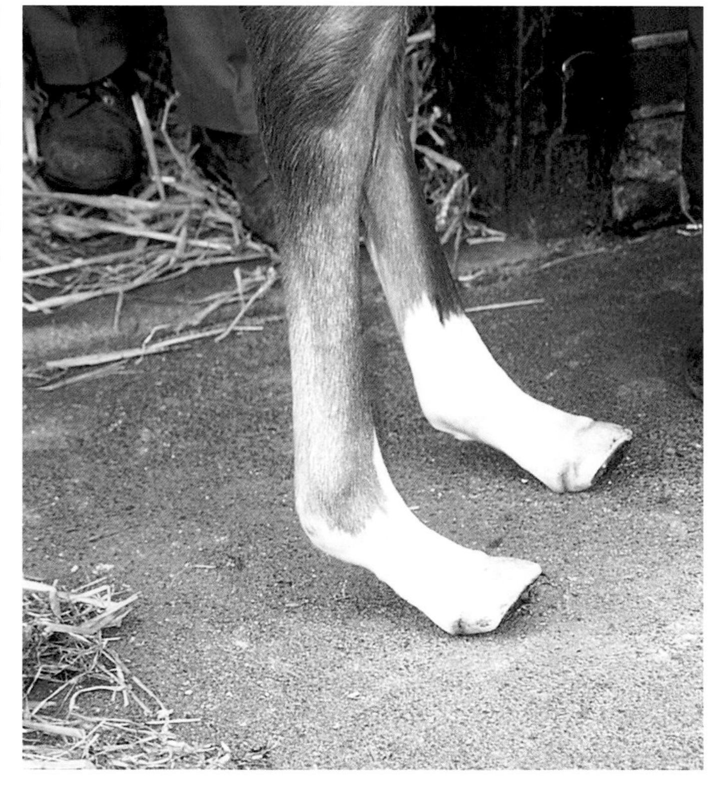

Figure 14.5

Weak or flaccid fetlock joints will require remedial care and conservative management, but generally have a good prognosis

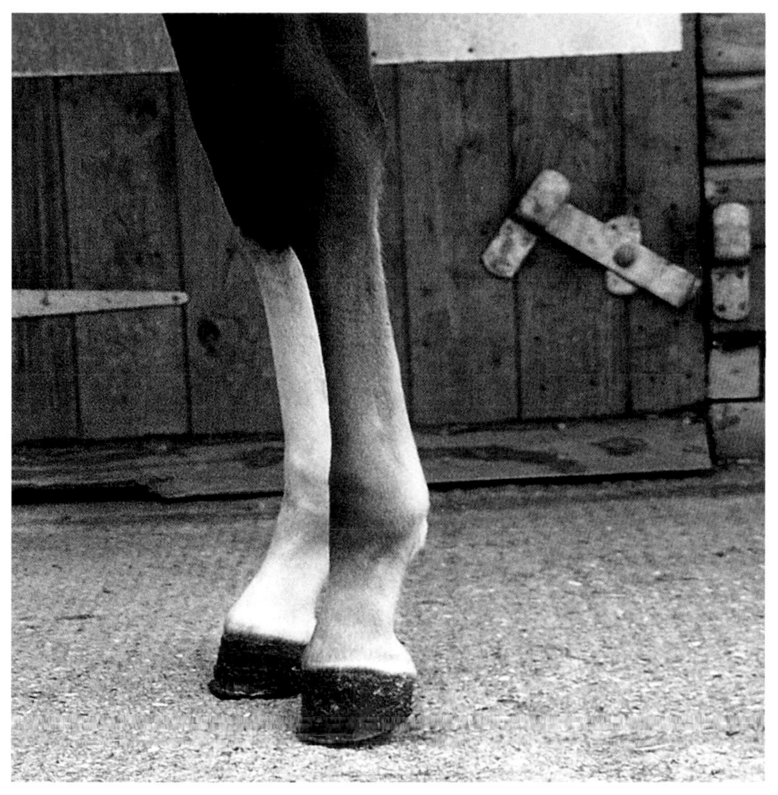

Figure 14.6

Hyperflexion of the front legs in a Thoroughbred foal. This condition can occur almost overnight and requires remedial care. Extreme cases may require surgical correction

headcollar, and its mother led with a rope from her right side.

Foals taught to lead this way will invariably stay up alongside their mothers and progress to being led with a rope very quickly. In the early stages it may be helpful to have another handler to follow beside the foal with a hand on its quarters should it stop or become nervous. Foals do not respond well to being pushed or pulled and many will cause injury to themselves by falling or rearing away from the pressure. As always, it is better to encourage quietly, particularly at this early stage, than force, especially when the foal may simply not understand what is being asked of it. Make use of the mother as the foal will want to follow her at all times – foals learn an enormous amount from following sometimes imperceptible cues given by their mothers and this fact can be fully utilised by the handler during early training.

Exercise

Exercise is very important for a foal's development, both physical and psychological. Most foals benefit from regular free exercise and may suffer developmental problems if this has to be restricted for any reason. Unless there is a problem, most mares will be turned out with their young foals from as early as 12 hours from foaling. In countries where the climate allows, even Thoroughbred mares foal outside and this can be ideal for mares in the

UK if they are foaling during the summer months. Paddocks used for mares with young foals tend to be small with rounded corners and are generally used for only one mare and foal at a time. These nursery paddocks should be sited within easy access of the foaling boxes to avoid the foals having to be walked a long way.

Some farms prefer to use covered schools for turnout of these young foals, especially if it is early in the year. This works well, but consideration should be given to the surface used. Larger paddocks are ideal as the foals get older and able to cope with a higher level and duration of exercise. Foals with weak limbs or other developmental problems should be exercised conservatively to avoid further damage by overtired limbs.

Most farms will reintegrate mares and foals back into an established familiar group from about two weeks of age. Groups restricted to a size of six to eight mares and foals tend to produce a lower rate of injury than larger groups, but this will obviously be affected by the paddock size available.

Foal management programmes tend to follow a similar pattern from stud to stud, but the anticipated aim for the foal should be taken into consideration. It is obvious that some breeds, such as the Thoroughbred, are bred to mature much earlier than, say, a Warmblood, but each have their own specific needs to be met to ensure maximum potential of each individual foal. In general terms, managers are interested in developing a strong musculo-skeletal system and overall soundness in each individual. This is an area where commercial or breed requirements may encourage managers towards extreme measures, although it is possible to have a well-balanced programme that combines good nutrition, disease prevention, sensible exercise and individual attention to achieve optimal results. In a more natural environment, the foal could be allowed to develop steadily instead of being conditioned for maximum early performance – surprisingly, this can sometimes be at a rate that will affect the long-term potential, ability and soundness of that individual as an adult.

Weaning

Weaning from the mother is a stage that all mammals go through – some soon after birth and others several months or even years after their birth. Equines naturally wean their offspring after about a year, or shortly before the birth of the next foal. The bond between a mare and her offspring, if they are kept in a small close-contact group, can remain very strong for many years but the mare will rarely permit the foal to suck once the weaning transition is made.

For commercial studfarms weaning is a necessary procedure performed each year to ensure the optimum condition of both mare and foal. Most mares are bred each year and are normally four or five months pregnant with the next foal by the time the current one is weaned. Weaning at this time gives the mare a chance to regain any condition that she may have lost by nursing and allow her to concentrate on providing for the pregnancy. Additionally, the quality of the milk she is producing will be decreasing as the foal should already be receiving the majority of its nutritional needs from supplemental concentrate feeds and/or grazing.

With all that said, weaning is nearly always a very stressful time for both mare and foal. In the natural course, foals are weaned around the time of the arrival of the next – when the foal is sometimes a year old. The mare gradually dissuades her foal from sucking and her milk dries up. Most farms will try to reduce the emotional stress as much as possible, but it does need careful planning to ensure the risk of any long-term damage is kept to a minimum. There are several methods used for weaning and each has its advantages and disadvantages. The main considerations for choosing a suitable method for an individual farm will be facilities, staff, number of mares, age of the foals and condition of the mares and foals.

When the foal is weaned its life changes immediately and dramatically. It has lost not only its mother but the physical and psychological support a mother provided. Preparation for weaning is therefore vital. There are occasions where a mare may be lost suddenly, or the foal becomes ill and is required to be weaned in order to be cared for properly – it is impossible to plan for every eventuality, but in most normal circumstances preparation for weaning cannot ever be considered unnecessary.

Foals should be given access to some form of supplemental or creep feed several weeks before weaning is planned. They will already have been showing an interest in any concentrate feed that their mothers may have had and will have been making attempts to eat with her from an early age. This behaviour starts as copying and then develops so that the foal's daily intake increases as the milk proportion of its diet decreases. Creep feed can be provided just for the foals in a variety of ways. The individual hand feeding of each foal would be prohibitively time consuming and labour intensive so other methods are much more common. These include providing a separate feed bowl in the stable that both mare and foal are housed in. This feed bowl should have narrow bars to permit only the foal to access the food. For paddock creep feeding, perhaps the ideal way of providing this type of feed for foals, the use of a creep feeding pen is common.

This pen is made of either timber or metal and is constructed so as to allow only the foals access through narrow and/or low entrances. The single most important factor with any structure of this type is that it should be safe. The pen should be large enough to allow all the foals access and space to feed. The feed can be provided in either feed bowls or troughs within the pen – far enough in to stop any mares from being able to reach. It should go without saying that the structure should be sturdy enough to withstand the efforts of any mare who wishes to try and reach the food – it is surprising how determined some greedy mares can be. Normally the pens are set into the ground to provide the necessary strength for the structure, or existing fence lines can be utilised if practical and safe. Even when the foals are only a few months of age they already have a social structure and ranking system, so care should be taken to ensure that there is sufficient space and bowls for each foal to eat without being bullied by another.

Creep feed is normally provided on an ad lib basis as the foals will rarely overeat. However, each group of foals should be observed carefully during the first stage of introducing a creep system to ensure that each foal is taking full advantage. It is rare that foals will have to be shown the food inside the pen as they are naturally so curious; each stage of the pen construction will have been monitored closely!

The foals will normally start to eat well within a week or so of the creep feed being provided and, with this increase in their concentrate diet, they will naturally begin to spend less time nursing.

Foals can be weaned completely from as early as three months of age and some farms report that these foals grow more quickly than those weaned at six months. However, the emotional stress on such a young and immature foal is greater than that suffered by an older, more independent individual. Research has also suggested that by the time foals are yearlings the growth rate difference has reduced sufficiently so as to be negligible, so early weaning may not be as productive for routine use as once thought.

Large studfarms normally establish groups of mares and foals according to foal age. This assists with reducing some of the stress of separation for both groups. The foals will already be familiar with each other and there should be less risk of bullying as tends to happen with a group of mixed-age weanlings. The mares will also be established as a herd group and normally will settle more quickly than if put together with an unfamiliar group. However, on smaller farms this may not be practical and all the foals may need to weaned together regardless of age. If this is the method to be used, the weanlings should be carefully monitored for a long period to ensure that they are all eating well and not being intimidated by older foals.

Planning the weaning process should be well thought out. Several methods are used and each method should be evaluated as to its use and practicality for each studfarm situation. Traditionally, the mares and foals were separated completely with the mares being moved to a far part of the farm and the foals generally left alone in a stable for a few days – some farms still prefer to keep weaned foals in a darkened stable by closing the top door and windows. This is about the most traumatic way of separating the pair. It takes anything from three to six days of complete separation for the mare and foal to settle. Although it is a very successful method, it can be an anxious time for the handlers as the mares can become very distressed, sometimes causing injury to themselves by attempting to return to their foals. The foals are also at risk of injuring themselves and can become quite frantic. They may also cease to eat during this period and can lose considerable condition, making them more susceptible to infection and, in some cases, causing considerable setbacks in their development to date. If this method is to be used it is best to separate the pair at the end of the day, when the foal has had the benefit of paddock exercise all day. A tired foal is less likely to injure itself than one that has been confined. Bearing this in mind, foals that have been confined following weaning should be released in a safe, small enclosed environment when first turned out to allow them to 'let off steam' before being moved to a larger turn-out area. For these reasons, other methods are now more commonly used.

Familiarity will help to reduce the stress to the foal – maintaining some of the elements of the foal's normal environment will also tend to help. For this reason, gradual weaning is the most common method currently used on studfarms. This process takes much longer than the traditional methods but is closer to the ideal for all concerned. One or two mares will be removed from an established group at a time. Their remaining foals may call and show some levels of anxiety for a short while but generally settle down with the remaining mares and foals quickly. The fact that the other horses in the group are all familiar and that they are not all distressed greatly helps the weaned foals to return to normal routines. The mares are generally taken to another part of the farm and may also show some levels of anxiety and distress for a short while but this is generally short lived, and some seem almost relieved no longer to have the responsibility of their foals. Additional mares are removed at intervals of a few days to a week until the group is completely separated. Some breeders believe that this method only prolongs the anxiety but research has shown that this is not the case when compared to traditional methods.

Another method used more commonly on smaller farms, is that of gradual separation where the foals are put into stables or paddocks close to the mares. This enables the contact between both groups to be maintained but prohibits nursing. The foals are reassured by the close presence of their dams and this method is extremely useful if there is no way that the two can be kept out of sight and sound of each other. However, the fencing does need to be particularly carefully maintained to ensure that it is of a suitable type and strength for this purpose.

Mares generally settle more quickly than the foals but this will vary with individuals and also be dependent on the number of foals she has had before. The most important aspect of weaning for the mare is encouraging her milk supply to cease. Care of her udder is therefore paramount to avoid the risks of mastitis and secondary infections. Decreased nutritional quality of her diet for the initial period is helpful – some farms use relatively sparse and bare paddocks for the weaned mares. Plenty of free exercise will also help to reduce the size and discomfort of a full udder – hand milking should be kept to an absolute minimum, as the more she is milked the more milk she will produce – the pressure of a full udder will actually decrease and eventually stop milk production completely. Once the mare has completely 'dried up' then the quality of her feeds and/or grazing is usually increased.

CHAPTER FIFTEEN

The Worm Menace

The control of internal parasites in the horse is one of the most important routine management practices. A proper programme of control is as important to the person with one pony as it is to the most prestigious commercial stud-farm. Regardless of how much meticulous care is taken with the feeding and preparation of young horses, they will never be able to reach their full potential if they are compromised by parasites.

Sadly, all too often the adage of 'what you can't see can't hurt' means that many horses are carrying a totally avoidable parasite burden to a greater or lesser degree from just a few days after they are born. Young horses (less than three years) are particularly vulnerable to infestation, as some degree of immunity is developed as the horse matures. These horses are still developing and maturing physically so any infestation at this time will probably cause permanent damage. Just because the horse does not look 'wormy' does not mean that it does not have a parasite infection – the majority of infections produce only sub-clinical signs.

The main clinical signs of infection are poor condition, weight loss, intermittent colic, depression and diarrhoea. Younger horses may display a general unthriftiness and, due to intestinal ulcerations, may be prone to constant low-grade digestive upsets with diarrhoea that contains little more than blood. Severe infections are commonly linked with acute colic. Colic of this type is commonly fatal.

Internal parasites are extraordinarily successful at making the most of every opportunity. It is shocking to realise that an adult egg-laying parasite can produce as many as 10 million eggs every 24 hours. This enormous quantity of eggs is passed out in the droppings of the horse, infecting the pasture that it is grazing. With most equine parasites, each egg will hatch into larvae, which are then ingested again by the horse and so the whole cycle continues.

The term parasite is defined as 'an organism which benefits by nourishing itself at the expense of another, termed as the host, but normally without destroying it'.

The main problem with parasites is the damage they do internally to the horse (Figure 15.1). In simple terms, each of the main equine parasite types has a similar life cycle but, significantly, they may cause damage to different areas of the horse's body throughout their life stages. Understanding the life

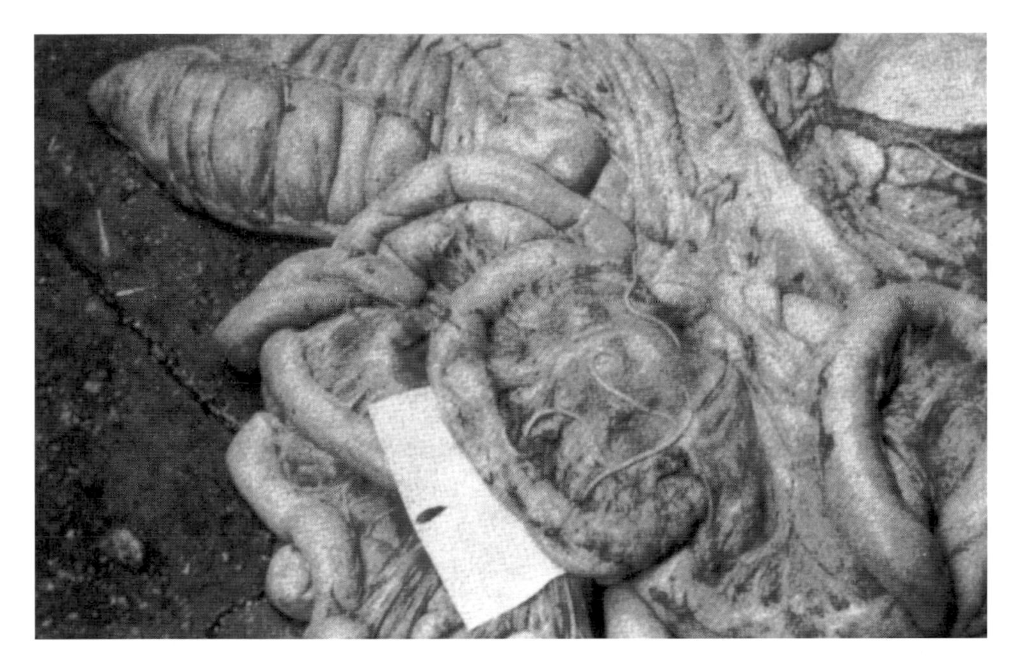

Figure 15.1

White worms may cause rupture of the gut and death of foals between the ages of two and six months

cycles of each of the main parasites that affect our horses is important so that an effective control programme can be maintained.

Over thousands of years, horses in wild herds have roamed free grazing enormous areas of grassland. On this timescale, it is only comparatively recently that horses have been intensively domesticated and kept in restricted areas. Until domestication, internal parasites were a relatively mild threat but now they have learned to make the most of the new conditions and become a constant threat to the health of every domesticated horse.

There are five main groups of parasites that commonly affect horses; these are the strongyles (redworms), ascarids (roundworms), pinworms, bots and tapeworms.

Typically, the life cycle of each is completed within six months, but perhaps most significantly, the small strongyle can remain in an encysted form in the gut wall of the horse for up to three years until environmental conditions are at an optimum.

Strongyles

This group includes both large and small forms. They are actually colour less but become red because they suck blood from the gut wall. The small

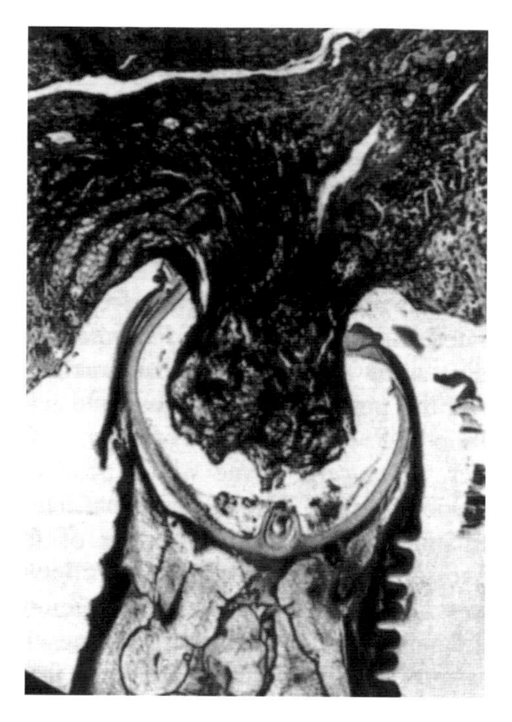

Figure 15.2

A highly-magnified view of a redworm (below, centre) attached to the lining of the gut from which it sucks blood

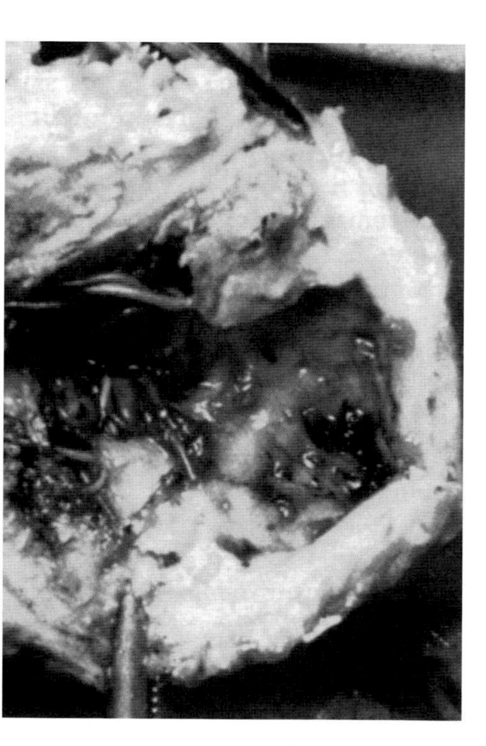

Figure 15.3

Redworm larvae (*S. vulgaris*) seen in the artery leading to the gut

strongyle is about 1–1.5 cm in length and the large strongyle about 1.5–4.5 cm in length. This group probably represents the most sinister threat to the horse's health (Figure 15.2).

The cycle starts with eggs laid onto the pasture from an infected horse. In warm and moist conditions, these eggs develop into three stages of larvae whilst still in the faeces. The third stage larvae migrate from the manure to blades of grass so that they can be eaten. Typically, this migration occurs during warm, wet weather; if the weather conditions are unsuitable, they can remain in the manure for some time. The development of the larvae through the three stages relies on optimum temperatures of between 8–10°C. It can be slowed during low temperatures so that it takes many weeks for the infective stage to be reached or, conversely, speeded up by higher temperatures. This great adaptability means that the larvae optimise their chances of survival. Strongyle larvae can be killed by prolonged freezing, heating or dryness. In the UK, the optimum time for infection with strongyles is during late spring and summer.

Figure 15.4

A (highly magnified) view of the intestinal wall, showing encysted redworm lava which has been sectioned at four (arrowed) places

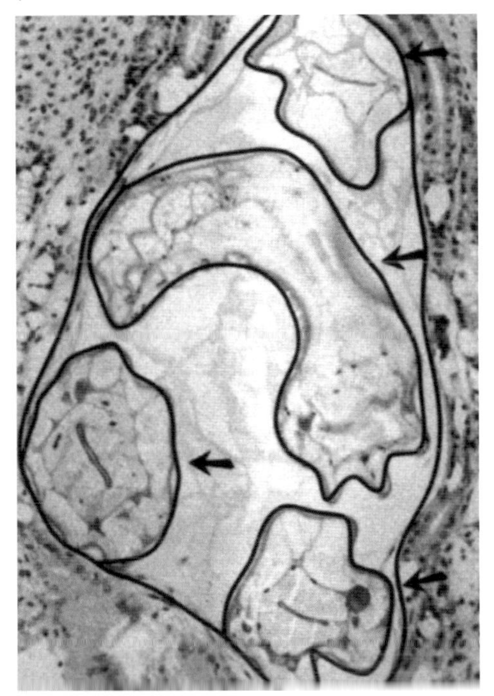

Once the larvae are eaten, they migrate extensively through the body. One type, *Strongyle vulgaris*, migrates through the gut wall into the main mesenteric artery, which supplies blood to the intestine (Figure 15.3). They will follow the path of this artery until they reach the point where it meets the aorta, which is the main artery of the body. The larvae can remain here for several weeks or months until they return to the intestinal wall, emerging back into the intestine as adults. Typically, with *S. vulgaris*, the adults will start egg-laying about six months after the horse was first infected. Other less common strongyle types migrate to other organs such as the liver and/or pancreas before returning to the intestine and they commonly form nodules in the peritoneal lining of the abdomen that bleed. *S. vulgaris* is the most dangerous of the large strongyles because it enters the circulatory system and can cause serious arterial aneurysms as it migrates (Figure 15.4).

The small strongyles (cyathostomes) have a more straightforward life cycle, but infection is no less serious. The main differences with the cycle of the small compared to large strongyle is that it does not migrate further than the intestinal wall and it has the ability to become encysted in its larval stage in the wall of the intestine for up to three years, allowing it to survive sub-optimal conditions, for example during the winter months. Under optimum conditions, the larvae of the small strongyle will emerge from the intestinal wall into the lumen and begin egg-laying about three months after infection. The encysted larvae pose little threat to the health of the horse while they remain dormant. However, the larvae typically emerge simultaneously in large numbers and in doing so they release their own metabolic waste products that cause significant damage to the gut wall. The emergence of such a large number of the larvae also causes the formation of ulcerated lesions on the lining of the gut, causing disruption of the digestive processes. Until recently, most routine drug treatments for parasite control were not effective against the encysted stage of the small strongyle. However, a relatively new wormer, containing the drug moxidectin, is reported to be effective against the encysted stage.

Roundworms

Roundworms or ascarids is the common name for *Parascaris equorum*. These parasites can grow up to 50 cm in length and they are found in the small intestine. Roundworms are particularly significant in younger horses. Large populations are commonly found in foals and yearlings, whereas adult horses carry few if any of these worms. Foals develop a rising level of immunity to this parasite, so that by the time they are yearlings any re-infection will result in the larvae being killed before they reach the adult stage.

The adults lay an enormous quantity of eggs, up to as many as 200,000 per day. The eggs are passed out in the droppings where the larvae develop into the infective stage whilst still within the shell of the egg. This process takes about ten days to three weeks, depending on the weather conditions. As with the strongyles, the roundworm is remarkably adaptable to weather conditions and the eggs are almost completely resistant to freezing and drying. On studfarms this factor is of particular importance, as each year's foals will be at risk of infection. The infective larvae have a sticky outer shell which will adhere to many surfaces, multiplying the risk of infection being passed not just whilst grazing, but also in the stables. When young horses eat the infective eggs, the larvae hatch and migrate through the intestinal wall to the lungs and the liver. It is in the lungs that the larvae can cause havoc. They emerge through the bronchioles (the air sacs) and travel up the trachea to be swallowed. Once back in the small intestine, the larvae develop into egg-laying adults. Once the infective larvae are eaten, the cycle to egg-laying adulthood takes about three months.

Infected foals display clinical signs such as dull coats, nasal discharge, coughing, poor condition, typically with a pot-bellied appearance; as well as intermittent colic and diarrhoea. Severe infections may result in pneumonia and acute colic. The sheer size of the roundworm means that complete intestinal blockages are common with heavy infections.

Strongyloides westeri

The parasite *S. westeri* has the common name of threadworm due to its appearance. *S. westeri* has a complicated life cycle and, remarkably, can be transferred to the foal directly through the mare's milk as early as a few days after birth. Infection can also be transmitted through infected bedding. For this reason, this parasite is of particular importance on studfarms. If adult horses are infected the larvae migrate to body tissues and, with the exception of infected lactating mares, do not develop any further. In an infected mare, the larvae are triggered to re-emerge and travel to the udder only when lactation starts.

Contrary to the other parasites discussed so far, *S. westeri* does not have to depend on an intermediate development stage outside of the horse's body. The worms develop very quickly in the newborn foal and within ten days have reached egg-laying adulthood. Eggs passed out through the faeces will re-infect foals if eaten directly and the parasite also has the unusual ability to develop to adulthood outside of the host if required.

Not only does this optimise every possible chance of infecting as many hosts as possible, it greatly increases the survival chances of each individual parasite, regardless of environmental conditions. The parasite migrates via the circulatory system to the liver and lungs. Similar to roundworms, they are then coughed up and swallowed to develop into adults in the intestine.

S. westeri infections used to be very common in foals, causing severe diarrhoea and intestinal ulceration. Today, with the increased awareness of the need for routine preventative treatment of broodmares during pregnancy, severe infestations of this parasite have reduced in number. The ability of this parasite to survive and develop outside its host further emphasises the need for a high level of stable hygiene, particularly in foaling boxes and nursery paddocks.

Pinworm

Oxyuris equi or pinworm affects all age groups of horses. It lives in the large intestine and grows to about 15 cm in length.

The female pinworm will remain in the intestine until she is fertilised by the male worm. She then moves down through the gut until she reaches the anus, where she lays her eggs in large numbers under the horse's tail. The eggs will drop off the horse, falling into bedding, grazing and feeding bowls, within a few days. The eggs are not resistant to environmental stresses and die quickly if shed on pasture. Stables are where pinworms have optimum conditions to re-infect.

Infected horses are irritated by the presence of the eggs and will rub their tails, producing a characteristic broken-haired appearance. The eggs can irritate so much that the horse actually rubs its tail to the point of causing sores.

Tapeworm

Tapeworm is the common name for *Anoplocephala perfoliata* and *Anoplocephala magna*.

This is a flat-segmented parasite that lives in the small and large intestines of the horse. *A. perfoliata* is the most common. The adults are tapered, finely segmented and develop to about 4 cm wide and 8 cm long. *A. magna* can grow to 80 cm long and is termed as ribbon-like in appearance.

Tapeworms continually grow eggs in segments which are then passed out in the droppings. The eggs are then eaten by a mite that lives in grassland. The tapeworm develops as a cyst in the body of the mite and the horse becomes re-infected by eating the mite when grazing. The adult can develop only when the mite is ingested by a suitable host.

For many years, tapeworm infection was not thought to be significant in horses and it may be true that heavy infestations are uncommon. However, tapeworms do regularly affect the health of the horse by causing damage to the intestinal wall where their heads have attached, leaving lesions and ulcerations, together with a marked degree of inflammation. Their very presence in any number will invariably mean that the horse will look poor in condition and fail to thrive; some horses also suffer from chronic diarrhoea. Recent research has suggested that as many as 20 per cent of spasmodic colics may be tapeworm-related.

Tapeworm are resistant to most routine worm doses and require double dosage rates of specific drugs to be affected.

Bots

Bots, or *Gastrophilus intestinalis* and *Gastrophilus nasalis*, infect the horse during their larval stage. Almost all age groups of horses are infected. The adult bot fly is similar to a bee in that it has yellow and dark banding on its body. The female bot fly has an ovipositor that is often mistaken for a sting; she uses this to place her eggs on the horse's coat. The larval bots are commonly found in the stomach of the horse. They are normally red brown in colour and about 2 cm long. They have hooks at one end of their body with which they attach to the stomach lining.

G. intestinalis attaches its eggs to the forelegs, neck and shoulders of the horse. The eggs are stimulated by moisture and warmth and by the friction of the horse's tongue as it licks itself. The larvae emerge from the eggs and once eaten penetrate the mucous lining of the mouth. They remain here for some time before they are actually swallowed. The second and third stage infective larvae attach themselves to feed from the stomach lining. *G. nasalis* has a similar cycle, except that the eggs are usually laid around the horse's head and hatch spontaneously, migrating to the horse's mouth without stimulation. The bot larvae leave ulcerations and inflammation throughout the stomach lining and they remain in place for up to ten months. Occasionally a heavy infection can cause the stomach to be perforated, with fatal results. The valve called the pyloric syphincter which is located between the stomach and the small intestine can also become blocked by bot larvae – this can cause acute colic as it will directly interfere with the passage of food through the gut. At the end of this stage, the larvae release their hooks and are passed out in the droppings. Once in the soil they develop into the adult fly within about a month.

Preventative Management

Most adult horses seem able to cope with remarkably high levels of parasitic infection before they show any clinical signs. Most owners are horrified to learn that their horse has a high worm count, particularly if it looks healthy in every other way. Discussing the life cycles of each of the main horse parasites reveals the very serious threat to our horses on a daily basis. The good news is that parasitic infection is controllable and today, with the availability of well-researched and effective drugs, most well-managed horses have low levels of infection that pose little long-term risk to their health. But it is not just a case of giving the horse a regular dose of a worm drug – there are several key management practices that can dramatically reduce the number of parasites present on the land and, therefore, the risk to all the horses kept there.

A routine policy of administering appropriate worming drugs to every horse on the property at the same time should be practised. The interval between treatments is normally recommended to be every six to eight weeks. Wormers such as 'Equest' are reported to be effective for up to 13 weeks ('Equest' is not suitable for foals under four months of age).

Administer the dose according to weight and age. Giving too much of a wormer to a horse is false economy and too little is pointless, as it will rarely be effective.

Administer the correct wormer at the correct time of year. Understanding the life cycles of the main parasites is important when deciding which worm drug to administer. Some parasites require treatment at specific times of the year; others may be resistant and require a specific drug and dosage to be effective (see Figure 15.5).

Controlling the level of infection on grazing land is one of the prime factors in preventative management. This can be labour- and time-consuming but it is essential. Large studfarms that have an ever-changing population of horses are particularly at risk, but no less important is any land used for grazing horses, however small the numbers.

Perhaps the simplest method of control is the regular removal of all droppings. Twice a week is normally recommended and many large farms have mechanical methods of removing droppings quickly and effectively. For small paddocks, or where tractor-driven machinery is not practical, picking up the droppings into a wheelbarrow is the best alternative. As discussed, most parasites develop rapidly during the warm, wet months of spring and summer – this is the time when regular, twice-weekly removal of droppings is essential. In the colder months of autumn and winter, it is just as important, but need not be so regular to be effective.

Avoid over-stocking paddocks. If the competition for available grazing is too great, horses will be forced to graze close to their 'toilet' areas where they would not normally eat and where the risk of larval infection is at its highest.

Maintain high levels of stable hygiene, particularly in areas used for foals. The removal of soiled bedding away from the stable area is also vital. It is surprisingly still common to see muck heaps very close to the stables and these provide another source of infection.

Grazing horses as much as possible in their age groups can also help to reduce the numbers infected with parasites such as roundworm.

Resting grazing to interrupt the life cycle of parasites is also an effective control measure. As discussed earlier in this chapter, many of the parasites have

Chemical Group	Brand Name	Effective Control					Known Resistance	Dosing Interval
		Large and Small Strongyles	*Encysted Strongyles*	*Roundworm*	*Bots*	*Tapeworm*		
Fenbendazole 22%	Panacur Guard	Yes	Yes	Yes			Yes	6 weeks in adults
Fenbendazole 22%	Panacur Granules	Yes					Yes	6 weeks in adults [suitable for foals from six weeks old]
Fenbendazole 22%	Panacur Paste	Yes					Yes	
Mebendazole 22%	Telmin Granules	Yes					Yes	6 weeks in adults [suitable for foals from six weeks old]
Mebendazole 22%	Telmin Paste	Yes					Yes	
Pyrantel 43.90%	Pyratape	Yes				Yes 2 x dose	Yes	6 weeks in adults [suitable for foals from four weeks old]
Pyrantel 76.70%	Strongid P Granules	Yes				Yes 2 x dose	Yes	
Pyrantel 43.90%	Strongid P Paste	Yes				Yes 2 x dose	Yes	
Ivermectin 1.87%	Eqvalan	Yes			Yes		No	8 weeks in adults [suitable for foals from six weeks old]
Ivermectin 1.87%	Furexel	Yes			Yes		No	
Moxidectin 18.92mg/g	Equest	Yes	Yes	Yes	Yes		No	13 weeks in adults [suitable for foals from 16 weeks old]

Figure 15.5

Worming drug types detailing known effectiveness

developed ways to survive sub-optimal conditions for several months, if not years. It may not be possible to allow paddocks to be rested from horses for over a year, but the use of a combination of rest and cross-grazing with sheep or cattle can significantly reduce parasite population levels. Sheep and cattle will eat the infective larvae but most parasites are not able to infect different host species and develop to adults successfully.

Treat any newly-arrived horses immediately with an anthelmintic drug, preferably one that is effective against as broad a range of parasites as possible. Keep the new horse isolated for 48 hours after treatment.

Routinely sample resident horses all year round to assess the level of infection present. Almost all veterinary surgeries can provide a worm egg count from a faecal sample. This will give some idea as to how many adult egg-laying worms are present in the individual horse. It will also give some indication as to the type of worm present. However, this is not a completely conclusive test. Not all the worms present will be at the egg-laying stage when the sample is taken and false negatives are common. Also, the life cycles of the common parasites should again be considered and it should be remembered that the immature larval stage of the worm is carrying out untold damage within the horse's body during its migratory course. A one-off worm egg count will provide no clue as to the quantity of immature larvae that may be present. Blood sampling is an effective assessment method, but is normally considered practical only if the horse is showing clinical signs that may indicate a high level of infection. On a large farm, most veterinary surgeons recommend taking random routine faecal samples for worm egg counts several times throughout the year to assess the levels of infection that may be present.

CHAPTER SIXTEEN

Maturity and What It Means

The content of this book has covered the story of the horse from conception to maturity. We all know about what is meant by conception but maturity is a term that has many interpretations according to the context in which it is used. Children are said to be mature in intellect and behaviour and some adults are described as being immature! The newborn is mature if it has, as we have seen with regard to the foal, a gestation of normal length and development; the horse is sexually mature (that is, capable of breeding) as a yearling, although full

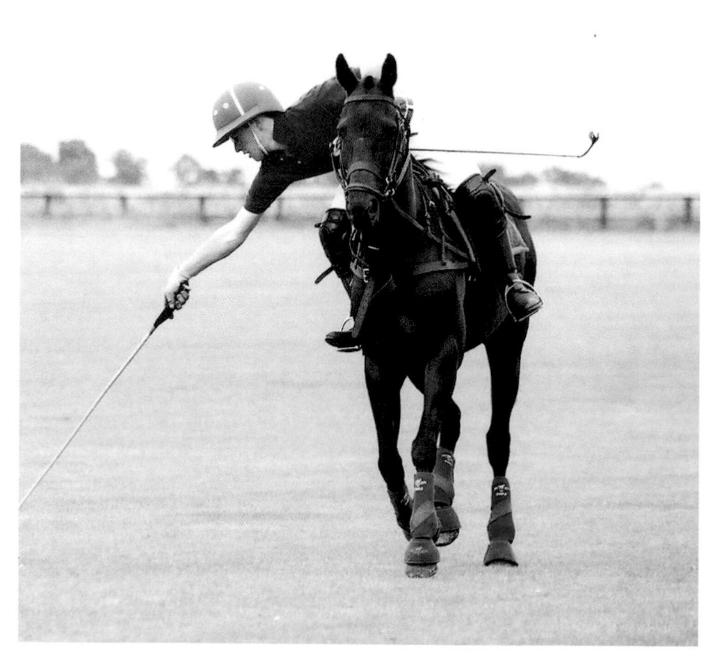

Figure 16.1

Polo ponies commence their training at age four years, aiming for peak performance at between six and seven years

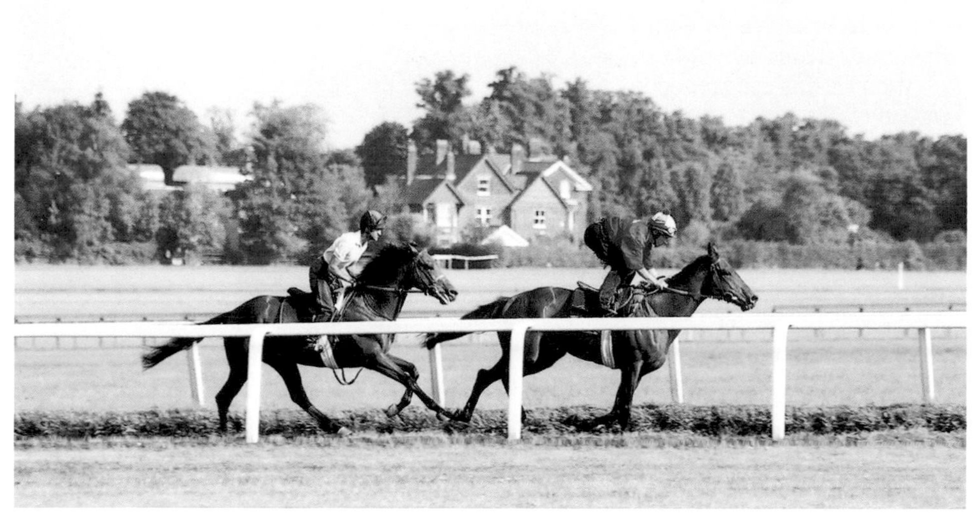

Figure 16.2

Thoroughbred horses are broken and trained to race from age 18 months

Figure 16.3

An event horse is considered mature enough for top-class competition at about age six to eight years

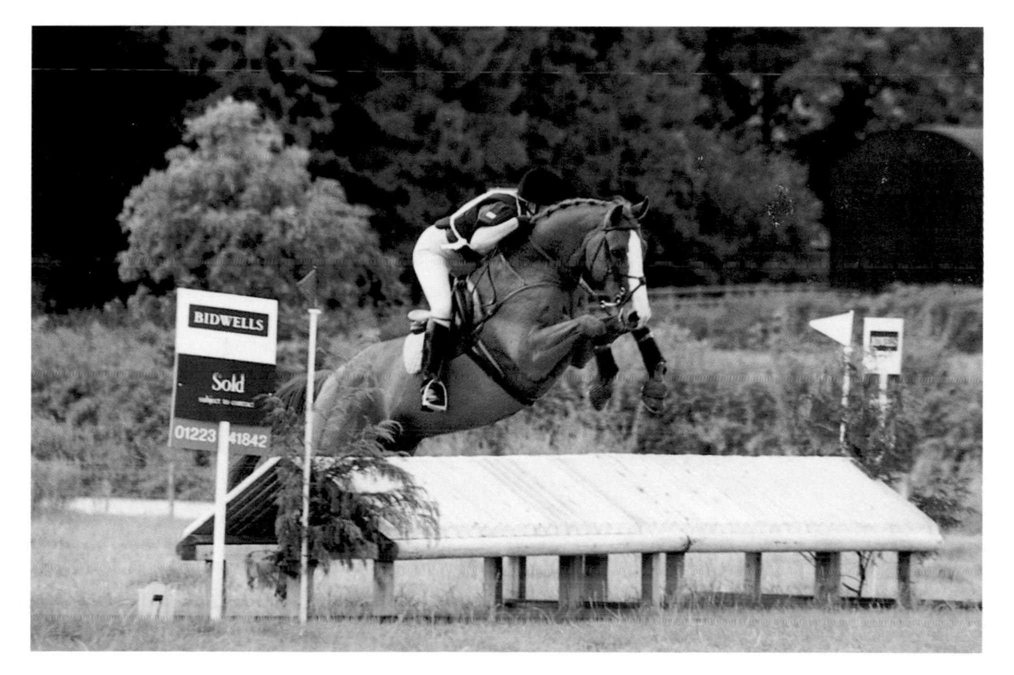

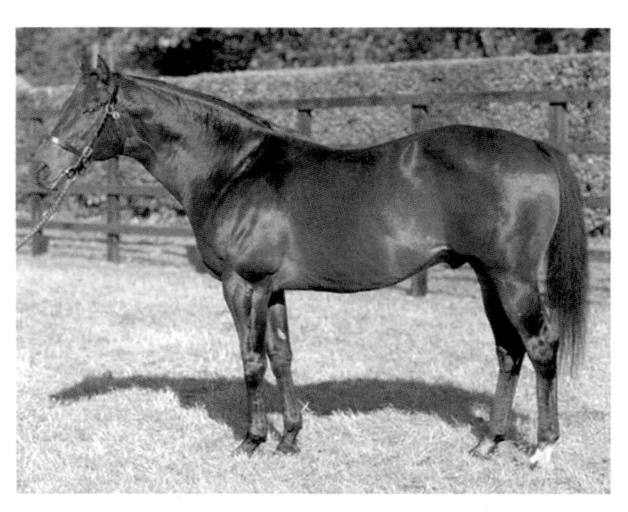

Figure 16.4

Primo Dominie (Cheveley Park Stud) began to cover mares when aged five in 1987. Since then he has succeeded in siring 27 individual stakes winners and in excess of 130 individual two-year-olds, including First Trump and Primo Valentino

maturity of sexual powers is not reached until two or three years of age. The skeleton is the last part of the body to mature in biological terms; that is, for the growth plates of the skeleton to close. In the horse, this process does not reach a conclusion until four and a half to five years of age.

The title of this book, with regard to maturity, implies that the horse has reached a stage of development in which it can be used for our purposes. But these purposes again vary depending on the breed and usage of the individual. Thoroughbreds are used when they are only 18 months of age,

Figure 16.5

Serious training for a dressage horse begins at around age five years

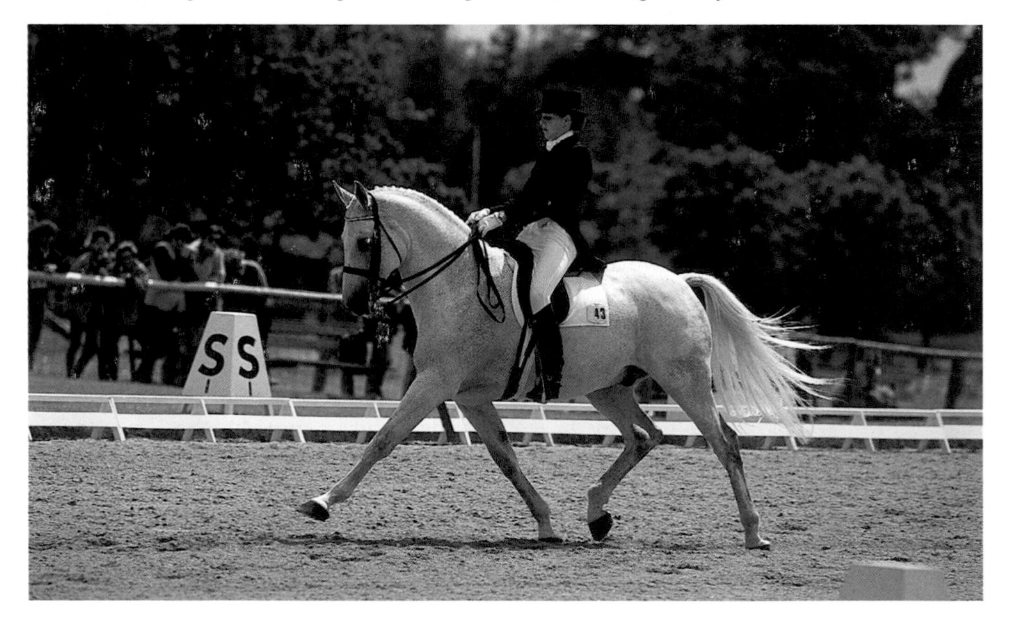

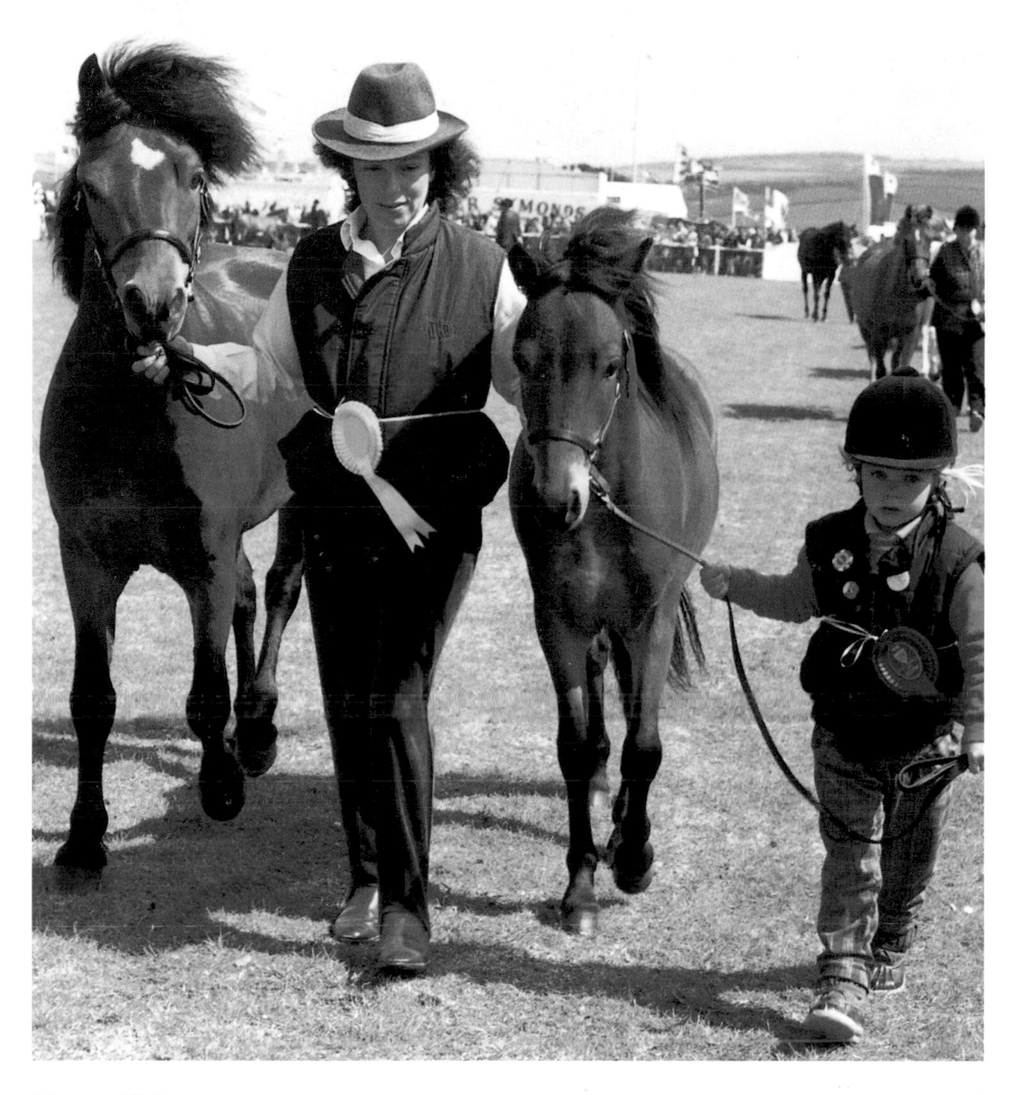

Figure 16.6

Exuberant competitors. Stock are shown in-hand almost from birth

for breaking and training to race eventually as two-year-olds (some are, even, less than 24 months of age when they first race). Horses used for National Hunt racing and Three-Day Eventing or for pleasure riding are generally put to use at an age that corresponds with biological maturity; and they should, therefore, be less prone to injury from precocious use. However, selection in breeding programmes plays an important role in lessening these effects when the horses are used at an age before structural maturity is reached. Structural, and its correlate, functional, maturity are two sides of the coin of

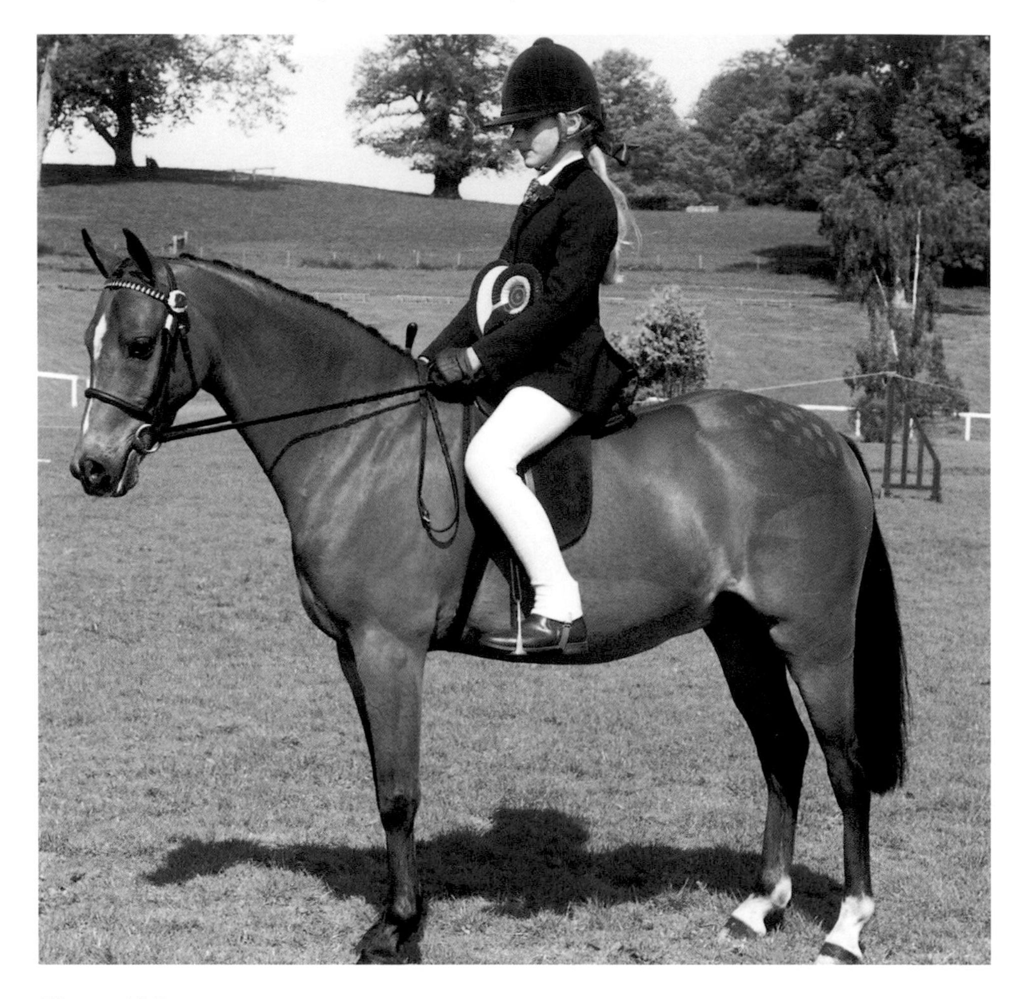

Figure 16.7

A pony cannot be exhibited under saddle until it is age four years

usage. Although not viewed in similar terms, children who make supreme athletic effort in running, tennis, baseball, etc., are faced with the same equation of structural maturity versus the effects of the stressful action on particular bones, joints, muscles, etc., of the body.

Maturity, as far as the horse is concerned, is reached in an individual when function and performance are not limited by the immaturity of the various structures involved. This varies with the individual and, of course, ill effects such as degenerative joint conditions may not necessarily be related to immaturity, but to pathological processes developing at any stage in the journey from conception to maturity.

Glossary

ABORTION
term used to describe expulsion of the fetal foal from the mare in a non-viable state.

ADRENOCORTICOTROPHIC HORMONE (ACTH)
non-reproductive hormone produced by the anterior lobe of the pituitary.

ACUTE
term used to describe a condition that is of sudden and severe nature; for example, endometritis in a young mare due to air contamination after foaling.

ALLANTOIS
the placental membrane which is an outgrowth of the fetal urinary system. The allantois fuses with the chorion (to form the placenta) which is attached to the uterus, and it contains allantoic fluid, formed of placental waste products and fetal urine.

AMNION
the membrane which surrounds the fetal foal and contains amniotic fluid which provides it with protection and nourishment.

ANAEMIA
term used to describe a deficiency of haemoglobin or red blood cells.

BARREN
term used to describe a mare that has been bred but failed to get in foal.

BIOPSY
method used to aid veterinary diagnosis whereby a small portion of living tissue is removed by a special tool so that it can be examined in laboratory; for example, a uterine biopsy to examine the uterine lining.

BLASTOCYST
name given to the fertilised ovum during the first stages of development following its arrival in the uterus from the fallopian tube.

CARRIER
term used to describe an individual who continues to infect other individuals with a disease while displaying no clinical signs of infection.

CERVICAL SWAB
swab taken during oestrus from the cells lining the cervix.

CHRONIC
term used to describe a condition that is long-standing; for example, chronic endometritis in older mares which have bred many foals.

CLITORAL SWAB
swab taken from the clitoral sinuses and fossa of the mare.

COITUS
the act of mating.

COLOSTRUM
first milk produced by the mare, rich in mare's antibodies, which provide passive immunity necessary to protect the foal from infection until its own immune system responds.

DYSMATURE
term used to describe a foal that is born in a premature-like condition but during the full-term range of 320–360 days of pregnancy.

ENDOSCOPE
fibreoptic instrument used to view inside the body.

EQUINE CHRONIC GONADOTROPHIN
hormone produced by special placental cells, which invade the uterine lining at about 35 days of pregnancy. This hormone helps the ovaries produce numerous follicles that ovulate and supplement the corpus luteum of pregnancy formed at the time of fertilisation.

FLUSHING (LAVAGE)
irrigation of the uterus (or other hollow organ) performed by the veterinary surgeon with saline and/or an antibiotic solution.

FOAL PROUD
term used to describe a mare that is particularly protective of her newborn foal, often to the point of displaying extreme aggression towards her handlers. This behaviour generally becomes less intense within a few days of foaling.

FOLLICLE STIMULATING HORMONE
produced by the anterior lobe of the pituitary gland. In the mare, this hormone acts on the ovaries and stimulates the production of follicles. In the stallion, it stimulates the growth and formation of spermatozoa in the testes.

GESTATION
term used to describe the length of pregnancy in a female. In the mare, this is a period of 320–360 days (approximately 11 months) from the time of fertilisation to the actual birth.

GONADOTROPHIN-RELEASING HORMONE (GNRH)
produced by the hypothalamus of the brain. Acts on the pituitary, causing it to release follicle stimulating and luteinsing hormones (FSH, LH).

HIGH RISK
term used in the Codes of Practice (see Chapter 10) or in other circumstances to describe an individual infected in recent years and therefore a possible carrier of disease.

HUMAN CHORIONIC GONADOTROPHIN
hormone found in the urine of pregnant women. It is widely used in equine reproductive practice as a therapy to cause ovulation.

INTERSTITIAL CELL-STIMULATING HORMONE (ISCH)
a male hormone produced by the anterior lobe of the pituitary gland. The hormone stimulates interstitial cells to produce testosterone.

IMMUNOGLOBULINS (IgG)
antibody protein produced in response to stimulation by antigens.

INFLAMMATION
reaction of the body to injury or infection. The main clinical signs are pain, heat and swelling of the affected site.

INVOLUTION
term used to describe the return of an organ to its normal state, such as the uterus after foaling.

LUTEINISING HORMONE
produced by the anterior lobe of the pituitary gland. In the mare, this hormone causes maturation (ripening) of the follicle and ovulation, as well as the formation of the corpus luteum (yellow body). In the stallion, it causes the interstitial cells to liberate testosterone into the bloodstream.

MAIDEN
term used to describe a mare who is being mated for the first time. A maiden foaler is the term used to describe a mare carrying her first pregnancy.

OEDEMA
term used to describe swelling where fluid has collected in the limbs or elsewhere in the body.

OESTROGEN
hormone produced by the follicles in the ovaries. It is the hormone of oestrus. Oestrogen causes the genital tract to be prepared for mating, as well as the psychological changes in the mare's behaviour towards the stallion. Oestrogens are also produced by the fetal gonads during pregnancy.

OXYTOCIN
hormone produced by the posterior lobe of the pituitary gland which causes contraction of muscle. It is instrumental in stimulating the contraction of the uterus during birth.

PARTURITION
term used to describe the actual act of birth or foaling.

PATHOLOGY
study of causes and symptoms of disease.

PHEROMONE
substance produced by the body to affect the behaviour of another, usually associated with substances produced to attract the opposite sex for mating.

POSTCOITAL
after mating.

PREMATURE
term used to describe a foal born before day 320 of pregnancy.

PROGESTERONE
hormone produced by the ovaries in the mare. The hormone of dioestrus and pregnancy.

PROLACTIN
hormone produced by the pituitary gland which stimulates milk production in the udder.

PROSTAGLANDIN (f2 alpha)
hormone produced specifically by the uterine lining. It acts to dissolve the corpus luteum and stops it producing progesterone.

RECTAL PALPATION
technique used by veterinary surgeons to examine the reproductive organs of the mare. This examination method is also used to assist in diagnosing intestinal disturbances such as colic.

RESISTANCE (chemical)
term used to describe the ability of an organism (for example, bacteria, parasite) to remain unaffected by a chemical that would previously have killed it. For example, the ability of some equine internal parasites to become resistant to certain chemical groups of wormers.

SEROPOSITIVE
term used to describe a rise in blood antibody levels denoting previous or existing infection.

SPERMATOZOON (pl. spermatozoa)
the male sex gamete.

SPERMICIDAL
causes the destruction of sperm.

STILLBIRTH
term used to describe a foal born dead but during the full-term range of gestation.

TESTOSTERONE
male sex hormone. This is produced by the interstitial cells in the testes. Testosterone promotes the male physical characteristics as well as libido.

WALKING IN
term used to describe the practice of transporting a mare to the stallion's studfarm for the purpose of being mated, then returning her to her home studfarm.

Index